The Biology of Ageing and Its Clinical Implication

A PRACTICAL HANDBOOK

Edited by

AZA ABDULLA

Geriatrician and Consultant Physician
Department of Elderly Care
Princess Royal University Hospital
South London Healthcare NHS Trust
Orpington, Kent

and

GURCHARAN S RAI

Consultant Physician in Geriatric Medicine
Care of Older People
Whittington Hospital, Lond

Foreword by

PROFESSOR DAVID BL
Senior Censor and Vice President
Education and Training, Royal College of Physicians

Radcliffe Publishing
London • New York

Radcliffe Publishing Ltd
33–41 Dallington Street
London
EC1V 0BB
United Kingdom

www.radcliffehealth.com

British Library Cataloguing in Publication Data

A catalogue record for this book is available from the British Library.

ISBN-13: 978 184619 556 3

The paper used for the text pages of this book is FSC® certified. FSC (The Forest Stewardship Council®) is an international network to promote responsible management of the world's forests.

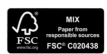

Typeset by Darkriver Design, Auckland, New Zealand
Printed and bound by Hobbs the Printers, Totton, Hants, UK

Contents

Foreword

The future of healthcare is the management of health problems in older adults. In some parts of the world such as the UK this challenge has come on gradually while in other parts of the world, such as China, it will arrive very rapidly. The problem eventually faced by all countries is how to manage the complexity of medical and ethical challenges as well as the financial and human resource challenges of ageing including frailty, ill health and, sadly, dependency.

At the heart of all clinical care is diagnosis. In older people without proper understanding of the biology of ageing and senescence it is impossible to come to a secure and useful diagnosis. It is also important when trying to predict prognosis. Yet both diagnosis and prognosis drive effective care management. The more we understand the interaction of ageing and health as part of the fundamental challenge of geriatric medicine, the more effective we will become as physicians working with older people. Luckily the science of senescence and ageing is growing at the same time as our knowledge of clinical medicine increases.

This book describes itself as a practical handbook. It is exactly that as it helps both trainees and those in independent practice to get a better understanding and remain up-to-date in how biology in ageing is influencing clinical care. Each chapter provides a succinct overview of the current state of biology of ageing and senescence for the relevant clinical system. It then sets that in the context of important and common clinical syndromes and illnesses in old age. Finally, each chapter ends with a short self-testing module to help consolidate the learning within that chapter.

This is a practical, up-to-date and useful book.

Professor David Black
Senior Censor and Vice President for Education and Training
Royal College of Physicians
September 2012

Preface

One of the problems geriatricians are confronted with in everyday clinical practice is differentiating disease from the process of old age. The challenges of ageing, including frailty, co-morbidity, different patterns of disease presentation and slower response to treatment requires a better understanding of the essential biology of ageing in order to separate ageing from disease and, indeed, ageing worsened by disease. This book aims to improve knowledge on the biology of ageing.

Knowledge of biology of ageing has become a requirement for trainee doctors specialising in geriatrics. It is highlighted as a core knowledge objective in the new curriculum for geriatric medicine, in which trainees are required to be able to explain the process of normal human ageing and its effects on the different organ systems, homeostasis and functional ability.

This short textbook is produced primarily for doctors training in geriatric medicine, practising geriatricians and those with an interest in the management of older people. Other people in disciplines working with older people, for example nurses, and professions allied with medicine should also find it useful.

The main aims of the book are:
1 to provide a learning guide on the biology of ageing through an overview of the changes that occur with ageing at both the cellular and system levels
2 to provide knowledge on how biological changes of ageing affect physiology and their clinical relevance in the practice of medicine
3 to relate these changes to certain disease presentations in older people and how these changes may affect disease management in older people.

The book discusses the implications of the biology of ageing on disease management and explores the concept of frailty of ageing in relation to clinical practice.

Although the topic is large and diverse, the intention is to produce for the busy clinician, an easily readable textbook that provides a concise understanding of the changes that occur in the different systems and focuses on the clinical implications of ageing rather than a large comprehensive desk reference. It is for this reason we opted, whenever possible, not to include references but instead ended each chapter with a short list for further reading. The chapters have mostly been written by clinicians and/or scientists who have hands-on experience in their field. Each of the chapters on the ageing systems concludes with a question section.

The idea for the book followed two seminars organised by the editors at the Royal Society of Medicine.

We believe better understanding of the molecular basis and physiological processes of ageing should lead to better patient care.

Aza Abdulla
Gurcharan S Rai
September 2012

About the editors

Aza Abdulla is a consultant physician and geriatrician at the Princess Royal University Hospital in the South London Trust. He has a special interest in medical education and was college tutor and training programme director for core medical training until 2011. He has been secretary for the Membership of the Royal College of Physicians Specialty Question Group in Geriatrics at the Royal College of Physicians since 2004, and is a member of the South East London Training Committee in Geriatrics at the London Deanery and chair of the Clinical Effectiveness Committee at the British Geriatric Society.

Gurcharan S Rai is a consultant physician in geriatric medicine at the Whittington Hospital. Since his appointment as consultant physician, he has been actively involved in the teaching and training of undergraduates and post-graduates, and is presently lead training programme director and the regional advisor for geriatric medicine for North Thames (East).

List of contributors

Aza Abdulla
Geriatrician and Consultant Physician
Department of Elderly Care
Princess Royal University Hospital
South London Healthcare NHS Trust
Orpington, Kent

Munir Ahmed
Consultant Urological Surgeon,
Princess Royal University Hospital
South London Healthcare NHS Trust
Orpington, Kent
Honorary Senior Lecturer,
  Undergraduate Sub Dean
King's College of Medicine, University of
  London
London

Tanvir Ahmed
Specialist Registrar in General Medicine
  and Care of the Elderly
  University Hospital of Wales
  Cardiff

Terry Aspray
Consultant Physician and Honorary
  Senior Lecturer
Musculoskeletal Unit
Freeman Hospital
Newcastle upon Tyne
Institute for Ageing and Health
Newcastle University
Newcastle upon Tyne

Barbara J Bain
Professor in Diagnostic Haematology
St Mary's Hospital Campus of Imperial
  College
London

Daniel Baylis
Doctoral Research Fellow and Registrar
  in Geriatric Medicine
MRC Lifecourse Epidemiology Unit
University of Southampton

Mark Birch
Senior Lecturer
Institute for Cellular Medicine
Newcastle University
Newcastle upon Tyne

Oliver J Corrado
Consultant Physician
Leeds Teaching Hospitals NHS Trust
Leeds

Sultan Darvesh
Professor and Clinician-Scientist
Departments of Medicine (Neurology
  and Geriatric Medicine) and Anatomy
  and Neurobiology
Dalhousie University
Halifax, Nova Scotia, Canada
Department of Chemistry and Physics
Mount Saint Vincent University
Halifax, Nova Scotia, Canada

Deborah Dunn-Walters
Reader in Immunology
Department of Immunobiology
King's College London School of
  Medicine
London

Tamara Griffiths
Consultant Dermatologist & Honorary
  Lecturer
Salford Royal NHS Foundation Trust
Dermatology Research Centre,
Faculty of Medical & Human Sciences,
Manchester Academic Health Science
  Centre
The University of Manchester
Manchester

Hasan Haboubi
Academic Gastroenterology SpR
Swansea University
Swansea

Nadim Haboubi
Consultant Physician in Adult Medicine
  and Gastroenterology
Nevill Hall Hospital
Abergavenny

KO Lee
Professor and Senior Consultant
  – Endocrinology
National University of Singapore
Singapore

Stephen R Lord
Senior Principal Research Fellow
Falls and Balance Research Group
Neuroscience Research Australia
University of New South Wales
Sydney, Australia

Finbarr C Martin
Consultant Geriatrician
Guys and St Thomas' NHS Trust
Professor of Medical Gerontology
King's College London
President – British Geriatrics Society

Victoria Martin
PhD student
Department of Immunobiology
King's College London School of
  Medicine
London

Jasmine Menant
Post Doctoral Fellow
Falls and Balance Research Group
Neuroscience Research Australia
University of New South Wales
Sydney, Australia

Martin R Miller
Professor of Medicine
Institute of Occupational and
  Environmental Medicine
University of Birmingham
Birmingham

Marissa Minns
SpR in Geriatric and General Medicine
Bradford Teaching Hospitals NHS Trust
Bradford

Glyn Nelson
PhD
Institute for Ageing and Health
Newcastle University
Newcastle upon Tyne

William Ogburn
SpR General Medicine and Geriatrics
Princess Royal University Hospital
South London Healthcare NHS Trust
Orpington, Kent

Gurcharan S Rai
Consultant Physician in Geriatric
  Medicine
Care of Older People
Whittington Hospital
London

Chakravarthi Rajkumar
Professor of Geriatrics and Stroke
  Medicine
Brighton and Sussex Medical School
Brighton

Isobel Ramsay
Academic Foundation Trainee
Brighton and Sussex University Hospitals
Brighton

Kenneth Rockwood
Professor of Medicine (Geriatric
  Medicine and Neurology) and
Kathryn Allen Weldon Professor of
  Alzheimer Research
Dalhousie University and Queen
  Elizabeth Health Sciences Centre
Halifax, Nova Scotia, Canada

Avan Aihie Sayer
Professor of Geriatric Medicine
MRC Lifecourse Epidemiology Unit
University of Southampton
Southampton

Roxanne Sterniczuk
Postdoctoral Fellow
Department of Psychiatry
Dalhousie University and Queen
  Elizabeth II Health Sciences Centre
Halifax, Nova Scotia, Canada
Department of Psychology
Dalhousie University
Halifax, Nova Scotia, Canada

Daina L Sturnieks
Post Doctoral Fellow
Falls and Balance Research Group
Neuroscience Research Australia
University of New South Wales
Sydney, Australia

Alice M Taylor
Haematology Specialist Registrar
Imperial College
London

Tharani Thirugnanachandran
Registrar in Geriatric and General
  Medicine
Leeds Teaching Hospitals NHS Trust
Leeds

Thomas von Zglinicki
Professor of Cell Gerontology
Institute for Ageing and Health
Newcastle University
Newcastle upon Tyne

Rachel Watson
Senior Lecturer in Aesthetic Dermatology
Dermatology Research Centre
Faculty of Medical & Human Sciences
Manchester Academic Health Science
  Centre
The University of Manchester, UK.
Manchester

James Wordsworth
PhD Student
Institute for Ageing and Health
Newcastle University
Newcastle upon Tyne

List of abbreviations

$1,25(OH)_2D_3$	1,25-dihydroxyvitamin D_3
3MS	Modified Mini-Mental State
25(OH)D	25-dihydroxyvitamin D
^{32}P	radioactive phosphorus
ACE	angiotensin-converting enzyme
ACTH	adrenocorticotrophic hormone
AD	Alzheimer's disease
ADP	adenosine diphosphate
AF	atrial fibrillation
AGEs	advanced glycation end products
AIH	autoimmune hepatitis
ALL	acute lymphoblastic leukaemia
AML	acute myeloblastic leukaemia
AMPA	2-amino-3-(5-methyl-3-oxo-1,2-oxazol-4-yl)propanoic acid
ANAs	antinuclear antibodies
APC	adenomatous polyposis coli
ATP	adenosine triphosphate
BBB	blood–brain barrier
BCC	basal cell carcinoma
BCR	B-cell receptor
BDNF	brain-derived neurotrophic factor
BFU-E	burst-forming units, erythroid
BHF	British Heart Foundation
BMD	bone mineral density
BMI	body mass index
BMP	bone morphogenetic protein
BOF	best of five
BPH	benign prostatic hyperplasia
CAP	community-acquired pneumonia
CASP-19	Control, Autonomy, Pleasure and Self-realization
CC	closing capacity
CCF	congestive cardiac failure
CCK	cholecystokinin

CFU-E	colony-forming units, erythroid
CFU-GM	colony-forming units granulocyte-macrophage
CG	Cockcroft–Gault
CIHR	Canadian Institutes of Health Research
Cin	inulin clearance
CKD	chronic kidney disease
CLL	chronic lymphocytic leukaemia
CNS	central nervous system
CO_2	carbon dioxide
COPD	chronic obstructive pulmonary disease
CR	calorie restriction
CrCl	creatinine clearance
CRP	C-reactive protein
CSR	class switch recombination
CT	computed tomography
CV	closing volume
CYP_{450}	cytochrome P_{450}
DC	dendritic cell
DCC	deleted in colon cancer
DDR	DNA damage response
DEJ	dermal–epidermal junction
DFLE	disability-free life expectancy
DHEA	dehydroepiandrosterone
DHEAS	dehydroepiandrosterone sulphate
DLBCL	diffuse large B-cell lymphoma
DNA	deoxyribonucleic acid
DPP-IV	dipeptidyl peptidase-4
DEXA	dual-energy X-ray absorptiometry
EBV	Epstein–Barr virus
ECG	electrocardiography
ECM	extracellular matrix
ED	erectile dysfunction
eGFR	estimated value of glomerular filtration rate
ENS	enteric nervous system
EPCs	endothelial progenitor cells
EPO	erythropoietin
EWGSOP	European Working Group on Sarcopenia in Older People
FEV_1	forced expiratory volume in 1 second
FoxO	forkhead box class O
FRC	functional residual capacity
FSH	follicle-stimulating hormone
FVC	forced vital capacity
G-CSF	granulocyte colony-stimulating factor

GABA	gamma-aminobutyric acid
GAGs	glycosaminoglycans
GFR	glomerular filtration rate
GH	growth hormone
GIP	glucose-dependent insulinotropic polypeptide
GLP-1	glucagon-like peptide-1
GM-CSF	granulocyte-macrophage colony-stimulating factor
GORD	gastro-oesophageal reflux disease
HA	hyaluronic acid
Hb	haemoglobin
HbA1c	glycosylated haemoglobin
HLE	healthy life expectancy
HSCs	haematopoietic stem cells
ICC	interstitial cells of Cajal
Ig	immunoglobulin
IGF-1R	insulin-like growth factor-1 receptor
IGF	insulin-like growth factor
IL	interleukin
KDOQI	Kidney Disease Outcomes Quality Initiative
LDL	low-density lipoprotein
LH	luteinising hormone
LPS	lipopolysaccharide
LRP	low-density lipoprotein receptor-related protein
LTP	long-term potentiation
LUTS	lower urinary tract symptoms
mAChR	muscarinic acetylcholine receptor
MCQs	multiple-choice questions
MDRD	Modification of Diet in Renal Disease
MDS	myelodysplastic syndromes
MGUS	monoclonal gammopathy of undetermined significance
MHC	major histocompatibility complex
MI	myocardial infarction
MIBG	metaiodobenzylguanidine
MPN	myeloproliferative neoplasms
mRNA	messenger ribonucleic acid
MS	multiple sclerosis
MSCs	mesenchymal stem cells
mtDNA	mitochondrial DNA
mTOR	mammalian target of rapamycin
NAD^+	nicotinamide adenine dinucleotide
NADPH	nicotinamide adenine dinucleotide phosphate
NES	neuroendocrine system
NGF	nerve growth factor

NHANES III	National Health and Nutrition Examination Survey 1988–94
NK cell	natural killer cell
NMDA	N-methyl-D-aspartate
NOX	nitrous oxide
NPY	neuropeptide Y
NSAIDs	non-steroidal anti-inflammatory drugs
O_2	oxygen
ONS	Office for National Statistics
OPG	osteoprotegerin
OPQOL	Older Peoples' Quality of Life
$PaCO_2$	partial pressure of carbon dioxide in the blood
PCI	percutaneous coronary intervention
PHN	post-herpetic neuralgia
PP	pancreatic polypeptide
PPAR-γ	peroxisome proliferator-activated receptor-gamma
PPIs	proton pump inhibitors
PSA	prostate-specific antigen
PTH	parathyroid hormone
PYY	Peptide YY
QoL	quality of life
RANKL	receptor activator of nuclear factor kappa-B ligand
RAS	renin–angiotensin system
RNA	ribonucleic acid
ROS	reactive oxygen species
RSD	residual standard deviation
RV	residual volume
SASP	senescence-associated secretory phenotype
SCC	squamous cell carcinoma
SCF	stem cell factor
SCN	suprachiasmatic nucleus
SHM	somatic hypermutation
SR	standardised residual
TAVI	transcatheter aortic valve implantation
TCR	T-cell receptor
TGF-beta	transforming growth factor-beta
TLC	total lung capacity
$T_{L,CO}$	lung transfer factor
TLR	toll-like receptor
Tm	tubular maximum
TNF	tumour necrosis factor
TRs	transitional B-cells
TSH	thyroid-stimulating hormone

UK	United Kingdom
US	United States
UV	ultraviolet
VDR	vitamin D receptor
VO$_2$ max	maximum oxygen consumption
VOR	vestibulo-ocular reflex
WCC	white-cell count
WHAS	Women's Health and Aging Study
WHO	World Health Organization
WHOQOL-OLD	World Health Organization Quality of Life Assessment of Older People

Section 1

General

CHAPTER 1

Epidemiology of ageing

GURCHARAN S RAI AND AZA ABDULLA

INTRODUCTION

'Epidemiology' has been defined in many different terms, but generally it refers to the study of disease in populations and attempts to answer questions relating to prevalence, incidence and the association of the disease with a particular risk factor. This definition also includes evaluation of healthcare services. The first person known to have examined relationships between the occurrence of disease and environmental influences was Hippocrates, the Greek physician – some call him the 'father of epidemiology'.

Three common approaches in epidemiology studies are shown in Box 1.1.

BOX 1.1 Common approaches in epidemiology research

Case-control observational studies compare groups of patients with a disease/condition with those without the disease/condition.

Cohort studies compare groups of people exposed to a particular risk factor with those who have not been exposed to this risk factor, with the aim of establishing the cause of disease.

Randomised controlled studies look at a treatment and compare those who have received treatment with those who received a placebo or another treatment to examine the treatment's effectiveness.

Although the epidemiology of old age can involve any area related to geriatrics, there are three main areas of focus: life expectancy and its demographics, disability, and the natural history of diseases common to old age. In studying these aspects, older population epidemiology may therefore employ both qualitative and quantitative methodologies and include cross-sectional/longitudinal studies of age-related distribution and causes of disease, associated disabilities and mortality, and aim to determine why older people are at increased risk of developing specific diseases, disability and death.

There are a few technical problems when conducting epidemiological studies in older people. Problems with selection bias and confounding variables are notably common in older age studies. Narrowing down the selection through tightening exclusion criteria may make it difficult to identify a sample size large enough to render the findings significant. In contrast, widening the selection may result in including older people with many confounding variables that could make interpretation of results unreliable because of background noise and conclusions difficult to draw. Furthermore, the use of techniques such as questionnaires and interviews, commonly used in qualitative research, requires special skills and time, given the high prevalence of visual impairment, memory problems, hearing difficulties and disability from arthritis in this age group.

This chapter will look at ageing in the United Kingdom (UK), considering population projections, life expectancy, common causes of disability and mortality in older people.

AGEING

The population of UK has been changing since the early part of the nineteenth century. Over the last 25 years, the percentage of the population aged 65 years and older has increased from 15% in 1985 to 17% in 2010. This trend is likely to increase (*see* Figure 1.1).

There is expected to be further increase in the percentage of those aged over 65 years during the next 25 years. By 2036, it is estimated that the number of 65–74-year-olds will increase by 50%, while the number of those aged 75 years and older will rise by 70%. The picture is the same across most developed countries. In 1900, only 4% of the United States (US) population was aged 65 years and over, whereas at the end of the twentieth century, this section of the population comprised over 13% of the total. By 2030, this population group is expected to grow to over 20%.

These changes will affect the number of centenarians. In the UK, the number of centenarians has increased from 2600 in 1981 to 11 600 in 2010, and it is estimated that by mid-2034 there will be 87 900. In fact, if the pace of increase in life expectancy in developed countries continues through the twenty-first century, it is predicted that most babies born since the year 2000 will live to reach 100 years of age.

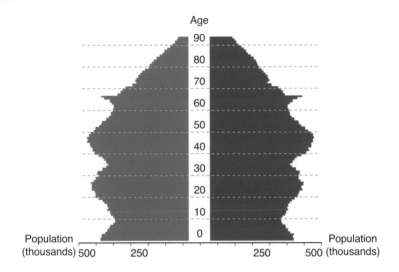

FIGURE 1.1 UK population by sex and age, mid-2010. Age and sex of the population, expressed structurally as a population pyramid, the structure of which is determined by births, deaths and migration. Each bar represents a particular year of age and its length shows the population of that age. Males: blue; females: purple. Reproduced from Office for National Statistics licensed under the Open Government Licence v.1.0. *Annual mid-year population estimates 2010*. Statistical Bulletin. Newport: Office for National Statistics; 30 June 2011. Available at: www.ons.gov.uk/ons/rel/pop-estimate/population-estimates-for-uk--england-and-wales--scotland-and-northern-ireland/mid-2010-population-estimates/annual-mid-year-population-estimates--2010.pdf (accessed 11 August 2012)

Factors influencing ageing patterns and trends include:

- low fertility rates
- the impact of the post-war baby boom on the accelerated growth of the older population in the second and third decades of the twenty-first century
- improving mortality rates
- increasing longevity
- advances in medical treatment
- migration.

LIFE EXPECTANCY

Life expectancy is an estimate of average relating to all persons still alive at a given age, regardless of their state of health. The Office for National Statistics (ONS) defines healthy life expectancy (HLE) as years in good or fairly good perceived general health, and disability-free life expectancy (DFLE) as years free from limiting long-standing illness. The difference between the estimates of life expectancy and HLE/DFLE is the number of years a person can expect to live in poor general health or with a limiting persistent illness or disability.

Life expectancy is usually taken from the interim life tables that are published yearly by the ONS, and HLE is calculated using data from the General Household Survey in Great Britain and the Continuous Household Survey in Northern Ireland. The data in these two surveys are based on responses to following two questions:

1 Do you have any long-standing illness, disability or infirmity – by long-standing illness I mean anything that has troubled you over a period of time or that is likely to affect you over a period of time?

If the answer is 'yes', the respondent is then asked:

2 Does this illness or disability (do any of these illnesses or disabilities) limit your activities in any way?

Life expectancy is increasing with each generation (*see* Figure 1.2).

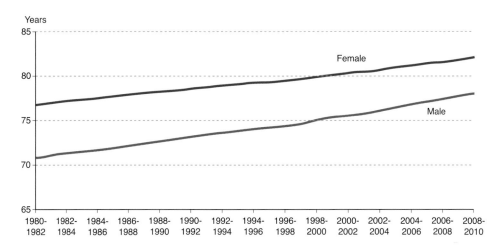

FIGURE 1.2 Life expectancy at birth, UK, 1980–1982 to 2008–2010. Source: Office for National Statistics licensed under the Open Government Licence v.1.0.

In 1983, based on data for years 1980–1982, life expectancy was 70.81 years at birth and 12.96 years at age 65 for males and 76.80 years at birth and 16.91 years at age 65 for females. In 2000, based on data for the years 1997–1999, life expectancy was 74.73 years at birth and 15.19 years at age 65 for males and 79.70 years at birth and 18.47 years at age 65 for females. By 2010, based on data for years 2007–2009, life expectancy had increased to 77.71 years at birth and 17.60 years at age 65 for males and 81.88 years at birth and 20.24 years at age 65 for females (*see* Table 1.1).

TABLE 1.1 Life expectancy by sex in the UK

	Sex	Year		
		1983	2000	2010
At birth	Male	70.8	74.7	77.7
	Female	76.8	79.7	81.9
At age 65	Male	12.9	15.2	17.6
	Female	16.9	18.5	20.4

This data show that between 1983 and 2010, life expectancy increased by an average of 7 years for males and 5 years for females.

The major impetus for increased life expectancy worldwide since the mid-1800s has been a decline in mortality from respiratory diseases, especially tuberculosis and pneumonias, through improved living standards and the discovery of antibiotics.

However, as already suggested, not all these years will be spent in good health. In 2006–2008, males in the UK could expect to live in 'good' or 'very good' health (i.e. disability-free life years) for 62.5 years at birth and 10.1 years at age 65. Figures for females were 64.3 years at birth and 11.3 years at age 65. Subtracting these figures from the life expectancy figures, the years individuals could expect to live in 'poor' or 'very poor' health can be calculated: based on data for 2006–2008, males in the UK could expect to live in poor or very poor health for 14.9 years and females for 17.3 years (i.e. disabled life expectancy).

FACTORS INFLUENCING DISABILITY IN OLDER PEOPLE

Many factors influence the percentage of disabled life expectancy (i.e. in the presence of disability). Some of these can be influenced during life to reduce the period an individual may spend in poor or very poor health. Canadian research has highlighted five types of chronic illness that contribute to disability in older persons aged over 65 years: cognitive impairment, impaired vision, arthritis, foot problems and heart problems. Other studies have highlighted hearing impairment, chronic obstructive airways disease and falls and hip fractures as important factors that increase disability in older persons.

Of course, the normal ageing process itself, which is associated with a 1%–2% decline in functional ability per year, may influence disability. With ageing, there is a decline in performance of generic tasks that require strength in limbs, fine dexterity and balance (which in turn increases the risk of falling); mild cognitive decline; and increased risk of developing diseases that affect cognition directly (e.g. Alzheimer's disease) or indirectly through development of depression.

Other risk factors that can influence functional disability include lack of schooling, diabetes, sedentary lifestyle, limited diversity in social relations, depression, obesity, poor self-perceived health and presence of co-morbidities, such as stroke, coronary heart disease, Alzheimer's disease, depression and hearing and visual impairment.

SUCCESSFUL INTERVENTIONS/APPROACHES THAT CAN REDUCE DISABILITY WITH AGEING

Certain interventions (preventive measures and specific treatments) can reduce disability with ageing. Examples of successful interventions/approaches include:

- exercise – this can improve strength, mobility and balance, thus reduce the risk of falls, and may protect the individual from risk of hip fracture
- social support to reduce isolation and depression
- financial and housing support that aids independence and therefore increases functional ability
- nutritional advice and support
- multi-professional intervention in the community
- treatment of medical conditions such as wax removal to improve hearing; cataract surgery to improve vision; treatment of vitamin D deficiency, hypothyroidism and heart failure.

AGE-RELATED DISTRIBUTION OF DISEASE AND COMMON CAUSES OF AGE-ASSOCIATED MORTALITY

With increasing age, there is not only an increase in the incidence and prevalence of disease and disability but also death. However, it is important to distinguish disease from ageing and to identify the role and contribution of the ageing process (if any) in a particular disease. The possible reasons for the difficulty in differentiating between ageing and disease in older people are reduced immunological surveillance, the influence of environmental and social factors, and genetics.

Several major age-associated causes of death are detailed following.

- *Cardiovascular disease*: for example, ischaemic heart disease, hypertension, peripheral vascular disease, and abdominal aortic aneurysm where the incidence in men with a history of hypertension, coronary artery disease, cerebrovascular disease or peripheral vascular disease is 7%–8% (compared with 1%–2% in women with same conditions).
- *Cancer*: the cancers that have increased incidence and death rates with age include colorectal cancer (incidence rate rises from 4 per 100 000 of the population aged below 50 years to 380 per 100 000 of the population aged over 80 years), breast (over half of all cases of breast cancer

diagnosed are in women aged 70 years or older), lung (50% of cases occur in patients aged over 60 years) and ovarian cancer.

- *Diabetes*: the prevalence of diabetes not only increases with age but also shows marked increase in older people of South Asian origin in the UK. Since 1996, the number of people diagnosed with diabetes has increased from 1.4 million to 2.6 million and it is estimated that by 2025 over 4 million people will have diabetes. Most of these cases will be type 2 diabetes because of the ageing population and the rapidly rising number of overweight and obese people. Obesity also increases the probability of disability, reduces chances of recovery and increases risk of death.

   People with diabetes are two to three times more likely to have a stroke than those without the condition. It is the leading cause of blindness in people of working age in the UK and the rate of lower-limb amputation in people with diabetes is 15 times higher than in people without diabetes.

   Diabetes is responsible for 11.6% of deaths among 20–79-year-olds in England. Around 80% of people with diabetes will die from cardiovascular disease.

- *Chronic obstructive pulmonary disease (COPD)*: there are an estimated 3 million people with COPD in the UK. COPD is the fifth largest killer and third largest cause of respiratory death in the UK. In 2005, 124 160 people in the UK died as a result of COPD.

   The mean age at death of patients with severe COPD is 74.2 years compared with 77.2 years in patients with mild disease and 78.3 years in individuals who do not have COPD.

- *Dementia*: the prevalence of later onset and young onset dementia increases with age, doubling every 5 years. The Expert Delphi Consensus estimates the prevalence with age range as follows:

Age (years)	Females	Males
65–69	1.0%	1.5%
70–74	2.4%	3.1%
75–79	6.5%	5.1%
80–84	13.3%	10.2%
85–89	22.2%	16.7%
90–94	29.6%	30.0%

Dementia shortens lives; the estimated median survival with Alzheimer's disease at 7.1 years (95% confidence interval, 6.7–7.5 years) and for vascular dementia 3.9 years (95% confidence interval, 3.5–4.2 years).

   The proportion of deaths due to dementia also increases with age, from 2% at age 65 years to a peak of 18% at age 85–89 years in men and from 1% at age 65 to 23% in women at age 85–89 years.

FURTHER READING

Ferri CP, Prince M, Brayne C *et al.* Alzheimer's Disease International. Global prevalence of dementia: a Delphi consensus study. *Lancet.* 2005; **366**(9503): 2112–17.

Office for National Statistics. *UK Interim Life Tables, 1980–82 to 2008–10.* Available at: www.ons.gov.uk/ons/rel/lifetables/interim-life-tables/2008-2010/sum-ilt-2008-10.html
——. *Life Expectancies.* Available at: www.ons.gov.uk/ons/taxonomy/index. html?nscl=Life+Expectancies

Stewart A. *Basic Statistics and Epidemiology: a practical guide.* 3rd ed. London: Radcliffe Publishing; 2010.

CHAPTER 2

The concept of ageing: theories and mechanisms

AZA ABDULLA AND GURCHARAN S RAI

INTRODUCTION

Ageing is almost a right, imposed on 'nearly' all living creatures. Beyond the stage of reproductive maturity, time inevitably brings on ageing. No being is immune and all are affected, albeit at a variable rate. Since it is a universal process occurring in virtually all organisms, ageing is not a disease, although it may itself lead to pathology or disease. However, as geriatricians, it is important to appreciate that the greatest risk factor for most diseases that cause mortality is old age. Cases of diseases like cerebrovascular events, myocardial infarction and cancer are highest in old age.

'Ageing' may be defined as progressive wear and tear of body organs and systems, in both structure and function, eventually leading to the detriment and death of the individual. All physiological functions lose efficiency with time and the individual is no longer able to maintain the internal milieu (homeostasis) when exposed to the stress of the external environment. At a cellular level, ageing is characterised by progressive loss of molecular fidelity in which an inability to maintain molecular structure gradually ensues, leading to loss of function. The impact can be local or systemic.

Unlike humans, animals in the wild rarely achieve old age and death is usually due to extrinsic events, mostly predation, infection, extremes of temperature and lack of food. Whether we, as human beings, are programmed to die may be viewed as a philosophical question. However, the concept of ageing as a programmed event has been refuted by most biogerontologists. Similarly, views that maintain that ageing is nature's attempt to limit population and prevent competition, thereby allowing the best utilisation of its limited resources for regeneration of life, lack scientific support and are merely of historic value.

The process of ageing is inherently complex and our poor understanding of how ageing occurs has produced a vast array of theories. In 1990, Medvedev listed more than 300 of such theories. However, recent studies and research developments have narrowed the focus down to only a few.

THEORIES OF AGEING

Evolutionary

The evolutionary theory of ageing is in essence based on the Darwinian law of natural selection and views ageing as the result of declining fitness, which is detrimental. It assumes that natural selection works at a young age but decreases after the onset of reproductive maturity and will have little impact on the effect of genes at ages exceeding the natural life expectancy. Therefore, mutations causing deleterious effects at advanced age are not removed from the population.

Although ageing is essentially a continuous process, most of the phenotypic manifestations appear after the reproductive period of the organism, at an age that is beyond the reach of natural selection. Therefore, ageing is seen as a genetically determined but non-adaptive process.

Mutation accumulation (Medawar, 1952)

This theory postulates that genetic mutation occurs with time, producing late-acting alleles that positively affect longevity over successive generations. Unlike defective genes that appear phenotypically at an early age, these 'bad' mutant genes, expressing themselves only at an older age, will not be picked off by natural selection at an early developmental age. Over successive generations, these deleterious mutations will accumulate, leading to increased mortality in later life.

Antagonistic pleiotropy (Williams, 1957)

Antagonistic pleiotropy proposes the existence of genes with dual antagonistic effects at the opposite ends of the spectrum of age; where they would have increased benefits in early life, they become detrimental at a later age. The genes here are 'pleiotropic' in that they can change their function with age. Ageing according to this theory is the result of the cumulative effect of many late-acting detrimental alleles.

Somatic mutation (1943)

The somatic mutation theory postulates gradual accumulation of somatic mutations arising through genome instability during a single generation. The theory has been the prevailing paradigm in cancer, where a single somatic cell accumulates multiple DNA mutations, producing oncogenes that lead to cell proliferation.

Disposable soma (Kirkwood, 1977)

This theory predicts that ageing results from the progressive accumulation of un-disposed molecular damage within cells and proposes a trade-off between resources dedicated to reproduction and those for somatic repair to maintain function and survival. The more the animal expends on reproduction, the less it can expend on bodily maintenance. The theory suggests a direct correlation between longevity and the resources dedicated to cellular and bodily mainte-nance and proposes that longevity is primarily controlled through genes that regulate the levels of somatic repair and maintenance. Nonetheless, the mech-anisms of cellular and molecular ageing are inherently stochastic (strongly influenced by chance).

The disposable soma theory is considered by many as a variant of the antag-onistic pleiotropy theory that elaborates on how the same gene could at one end of life be beneficial yet have deleterious effects at the other.

MOLECULAR MECHANISMS OF AGEING

The main molecular mechanisms of ageing are:
- Free radical theory
- Telomerase loss theory
- Somatic mutation theory/DNA damage and repair
- Mitochondrial theory
- Altered protein and waste accumulation theory.

Free radical theory (Harmen, 1956)

Noted also as a mechanical theory of ageing, this theory proposes that free radi-cals derived from oxygen are responsible for oxidative damage associated with ageing and that the antioxidant systems in the cells are unable to counteract all the free radicals continuously generated.

A 'free radical' is any chemical particle (atom, ion or molecule) contain-ing an unpaired or odd number of electrons. In biological systems, the most common source of free radicals is molecular oxygen (O_2), which, on utilisa-tion during cellular energy production, produces highly reactive agents that have the potential to cause significant damage to biological tissues. The most abundant source of free radicals is mitochondria (which use some 90% of the O_2 consumed by the human body), in which oxygen is reduced in sequential steps to produce water. This produces a number of short-lived intermediates, including superoxide (O_2^-), hydrogen peroxide (H_2O_2) and the hydroxyl radical ($^.OH$). Free radicals, collectively called 'reactive oxygen species' (ROS), oxidise and cross-link proteins of enzymes and connective tissues, leading to damage.

The effect of oxygen radicals on DNA can be strand breakage or base dissociation, with the potential to produce harmful or lethal error.

The potential damage from ROS production is counteracted by an intricate antioxidant defence system that includes superoxide dismutase, catalase and glutathione, among others.

Although the rate of ageing generally varies with metabolic rate, a good correlation has been demonstrated between the rate of free-radical leakage and the lifespan of many animals. This indicates that free-radical production, rather than metabolic rate, is the primary driver, although the two are generally related. Given that mitochondria utilise the bulk of intracellular oxygen and are therefore responsible for the majority of intracellular free-radical (ROS) production (*see* below, 'Mitochondrial theory'), the theory was expanded in 1972 to include the possibility that lifespan could be determined by the rate of damage to the mitochondria.

Telomerase loss theory

Telomeres are specialised nucleoprotein complexes that serve as protective end caps to linear eukaryotic chromosomes. During cell division, replication of chromosomal DNA may result in loss of terminal DNA. Telomeres can counter this effect by engaging telomerase, a ribonucleoprotein polymerase enzyme that is required to synthesise DNA (telomeric) repeats at the ends of each chromosome. Therefore, telomeres participate in processes of chromosomal repair. In the absence of the telomerase enzyme, telomere loss occurs through the end-replication problem that arises: the inability of conventional DNA polymerases to fully replicate the ends of chromosomes.

Loss of telomere function is associated with loss of cellular viability and renewal potential. The strongest indication that telomeric decline could play a role in cellular ageing comes from studies of primary human fibroblasts grown in culture. These cells lose telomeres with each division and eventually stop dividing. Remarkably, there is a good correlation between the number of divisions the fibroblasts undergo before they senesce and their initial telomere length. It is now clear that in most tissues (skin, fibroblasts, T-cells, kidney cells, mammary epithelium, endothelial cells and cervical cells) chromosomes gradually lose their terminal nucleic acid repeats with each division. It has been proposed that telomeric decay represents a 'mitotic clock' that counts cell divisions and limits the replicative potential of primary cells in most tissues apart from germ-line tissue. Indeed, telomeres of somatic cells appear significantly shorter than germ-line (sperm) telomeres from the same individual. Critical telomere shortening in human tissues may therefore activate senescence responses or lead to cell depletion, either of which could contribute to impaired tissue function with ageing.

Accelerated telomere shortening has been implicated in certain genetic diseases such as dyskeratosis congenita (a multi-system disorder characterised by cutaneous abnormalities, bone marrow failure and an increased predisposition to cancer) and Werner syndrome (characterised by early greying and loss of hair, scleroderma-like skin changes, osteoporosis, atherosclerosis, cataracts, diabetes mellitus, hypogonadism and increased risk of cancer at an early age). These patients have premature onset of many age-related diseases and early death. Other studies have shown that loss of telomere function induces endothelial dysfunctions observed in aged 'atherosclerotic' arteries and an association between telomere length and poor survival from heart disease and infections in older people has also been noted.

DNA damage and repair/Somatic mutation

A great many studies have provided evidence that DNA damage accumulates with age. Such damage may arise by physiological processes, during normal DNA replication or accumulation of ROS (endogenous), but more commonly as result of environmental factors (exogenous) such as ultraviolet light, ionising radiation and chemicals like those in tobacco products and aflatoxins in food. Since cellular function relies heavily on the integrity of its genome, cells have evolved multiple mechanisms to detect and repair DNA lesions, which are collectively termed the 'DNA damage response' (DDR). Important components of the DDR include protein kinases and nuclease, polymerase and ligase enzymes. A specific enzyme, poly (ADP-ribose) polymerase-1, involved in the immediate cellular response to stress-induced DNA damage, is positively correlated with increased lifespan.

The accumulation of DNA damage within cells may result not only from ongoing damage but also from declining capacity for DNA repair over time. Failure to repair DNA damage may lead to cell dysfunction and loss of homeostasis over time, which leads to ageing. DNA damage may occur independently of and without accompanying telomere shortening.

Genetic models that involve enhanced expression of antioxidant enzymes/pathways have been shown to increase lifespan. For example, transgenic mice over-expressing mitochondrial catalase have increased both median and maximum lifespan. Such models demonstrate that increased resistance to oxidative stress and reduced oxidative damage is associated with longevity.

Mitochondrial theory

Mitochondria are organelles present in all cells. They contain their own genetic material, mitochondrial DNA (mtDNA), and are involved in important activities. They are the energy source of the cell, producing the cell's adenosine triphosphate (ATP) requirement through oxidative phosphorylation. However, the process of energy production also produces free oxygen radicals. Under physiological conditions, it is estimated that up to 2% of the total oxygen consumption will result in superoxide radicals.

Many studies, including those in mammals, have shown that mutations, especially deletions, of mtDNA increase with chronological age. The accumulated damage to the mtDNA, as well as to the membranes and proteins of mitochondria, increases with age, leading to impaired function, reduced efficiency in ATP production and slower replication. The modified free-radical theory is based on the hypothesis that with increasing age, mutations of the mitochondrial DNA will accumulate, leading to loss of function with subsequent acceleration of cell death.

Altered protein and waste accumulation theory

Failure to remove defective protein molecules results in accumulation of abnormal proteins over time, leading to impaired function. Common examples of diseases in support of this theory are Alzheimer's disease and senile cataract.

The mechanisms summarised thus far predict that ageing is the result of the lifelong impact of molecular damage that accumulates in cells and eventually results in frailty and death.

Network theory of ageing

Based on the premise that no single mechanism can fully explain the ageing phenomenon, the effects of mitochondrial defects, aberrant proteins, DNA repair defects and free-radical accumulation have all been brought together under one umbrella theory termed 'network theory of ageing'. This theory acknowledges the contributions of the various mechanisms mentioned here (*see* Figure 2.1) and suggests that they should be considered together to explain the process of ageing.

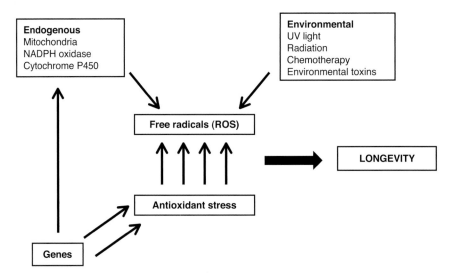

FIGURE 2.1 Mechanisms of ageing depicting interplay between genes and environmental causes

AGEING VERSUS LONGEVITY

Longevity is different from ageing. According to Hayflick, ageing is a catabolic process driven by chance whereas longevity is an anabolic process designed to maintain body integrity that is to a certain extent genome driven.

Limiting food intake or caloric restriction has been shown to extend lifespan in a wide range of species. Rodents who have their diet restricted to only 60% of their normal consumption live 40% longer than controls on a free diet. Not only is lifespan increased but many of the consequences of ageing are also delayed. The intervention is most effective when initiated at an early age (before puberty). Such experiments have been conducted since the 1930s and have been repeated in several species with similar results. The mechanism by which caloric restriction (the reduction of food intake without loss of essential nutrients and minerals) increases lifespan is not known, but it has been proposed that this may be achieved through decreasing oxidative stress and increasing metabolic efficiency.

THE GENETICS OF AGEING

Most of the advances in our understanding of the genetics of ageing and longevity have come from research studies on the nematode worm *Caenorhabditis elegans*, the *Drosophila* fly and rodents. These studies have shown that mutations in single genes can extend lifespan.

The worm *C. elegans* is comparatively easy to study, given its short natural lifespan of about 20 days, and a mapped genome on six chromosomes only.

In *C. elegans*, mutations of certain genes like *age-1*, *daf-2* and *daf-16* have produced surprising results. In their native form, the two genes *age-1* and *daf-2* suppress the function of a third gene, *daf-16*, which encodes proteins involved in regulating energy use and protects cells from oxidative and other forms of stress. Mutations of the *age-1* gene with loss of function produced a mean increase in lifespan of about 65% and maximum lifespan by 110%. These worms also demonstrated increased resistance to oxidative stress, suggesting that the allele is a negative regulator of the gene encoding for superoxide dismutase, which promotes antioxidant protection. Similarly, mutations of the *daf-2* gene produced worms exhibiting prolonged lifespan by an average of two- to threefold. Conversely, loss of function mutations of *daf-16* not only abolished longevity conferred by *age-1*, *daf-2* mutations, but also eliminated resistance to stress. Interestingly, the long lifespan *age-1* mutant *C. elegans* is correlated with a slower rate of accumulation of mtDNA deletions, which provides a link between genes, mitochondrial loss and the free radical theory.

Similar studies in the *Drosophila* fly, have demonstrated that the mutation of certain genes, which leads to enhanced antioxidant activity, results in extension of lifespan by 30%–50%.

Another gene involved in longevity and enhanced response to stress in

C. elegans is *clk-1*, the clock gene. Mutations of this gene have been shown to extend lifespan by up to 50% and appear to do so by slowing down the rate of worm development. In contrast, over-expression of *clk-1* leads to reduction in lifespan. Both *age-1* and *clk-1* genes are also found in humans, though their role remains to be defined.

In *C. elegans*, *age-1* and *daf-2* genes are associated with an insulin-like signalling pathway (insulin-like growth factor [IGF]-1). Disruption of this signalling cascade can significantly extend lifespan and allow the worm to survive periods of food scarcity. Similar results are seen in rodents, in which gene mutations leading to reduced production of IGF-1 result in prolongation of lifespan.

In vertebrates, the somatotrophic axis, consisting of pituitary-derived growth hormone, IGF-1 and its receptor IGF-1R, is the key determinant of somatic growth. IGF-1R is activated by its ligand IGF-1, which is secreted in response to growth hormone.

Suppression of the pathway as well as the lactotroph and thyrotroph process has been shown to accelerate ageing in mutant mice. Mice in which IGF-1R has been inactivated displayed greater resistance to oxidative stress and lived on average between 26% and 33% longer than wild-type controls. Similarly, mutated dwarf mice with a pituitary defect impairing production of growth hormone, prolactin and thyrotropin have an increased lifespan of more than 40% compared with controls with the normal allele responsible for normal pituitary development on the same locus. Further studies in these mice have identified delay in the development of senescence in many organs including the kidneys and joints in these mutants. These studies indicate that IGF-1R may be a central regulator of mammalian lifespan.

The role of IGF-1 in humans is interesting. Insulin sensitivity normally declines with age and humans become more insulin resistant. Insulin resistance is an important risk factor notably in metabolic syndrome and is associated with a variety of diseases such as hypertension and atherosclerosis. In contrast, centenarians have been found to have greatly enhanced sensitivity to insulin compared with less aged subjects, and to have a reduced incidence of diabetes. The data suggest that an efficient insulin response has a positive impact on longevity. Therefore, IGF-1, a potent anabolic hormone during developmental years, appears to be deleterious in later life. This finding provides impetus to the antagonistic pleiotropy theory of ageing, which proposes that the expression of particular genes is beneficial early in life but becomes detrimental with age.

It has been suggested that genes probably account for only around 20%–30% of the variance in human lifespan. However, the genetics of ageing is complex and, in the last two decades, the discovery of the associations between ageing and genetics has brought the role of genes back to the fore. Such studies argue that genetic changes do in fact modulate the ageing process, indicating that the ageing process is subject to regulation rather than being purely random and stochastic. However, the extent to which genes such as those identified by mutant screening and transgenic studies account for 'natural' lifespan is unclear. Furthermore, whether these genetic influences in lower animals transcend to affect higher mammals remain to be seen. The current view is that genes do not drive the ageing process but instead determine longevity.

RELATIONSHIP BETWEEN LONGEVITY AND STRESS RESISTANCE

Based on the current theories of ageing, an important requirement for longevity is the need to combat stress. This, at least in part, is genetically determined and a positive relationship has been demonstrated in lower organisms. As already discussed, most of the mutations that prolong life do so through strengthening stress resistance. Caloric restriction and decreases in the response to oxidative stress and in IGF signalling all efficiently extend lifespan in mice. However, it is unclear how these mechanisms cooperate and the extent to which they are independent.

CONCLUSION

Ageing is a complex, multifactorial process. Although different theories propose various mechanisms and processes, none provides a comprehensive explanation. Furthermore, many of the claims are not supported by hard evidence. The recent discovery of single genes affecting ageing has widened the debate on the role genetics plays in the process.

Our understanding of the interplay between these factors and the degree of interaction is important for geriatricians. Managing the mechanisms involved is likely to have an effect on the well-being of older people.

FURTHER READING

Bartke A. Minireview: role of the growth hormone/insulin-like growth factor system in mammalian ageing. *Endocrinology*. 2005; **146**(9): 3718–23.

Garinis GA, van der Horst GT, Vijg J *et al.* DNA damage and ageing: new-age ideas for an age-old problem. *Nat Cell Biol*. 2008; **10**(11): 1241–7.

Kirkwood TB. Understanding the odd science of aging. *Cell*. 2005; **120**(4): 437–47.

Miller RA. Biology of ageing and longevity. In: Halter JB, Ouslander JG, Tinetti ME *et al.*, editors. *Hazzard's Geriatric Medicine and Gerontology*. 6th ed. New York: McGraw-Hill; 2009. pp. 3–14.

Viña J, Borrás C, Miquel J. Theories of ageing. *IUBMB Life*. 2007; **59**(4–5): 249–54.

CHAPTER 3

The ageing cell

JAMES WORDSWORTH, GLYN NELSON AND
THOMAS VON ZGLINICKI

INTRODUCTION

Before 1961, it was widely accepted that cells in culture could go on dividing indefinitely. When cells ceased to divide, it was thought to have resulted from poor culture conditions or technique. However, by culturing old and young cells together, Hayflick and Moorhead showed that the old cells arrested first, followed by the young cells, demonstrating that it was not an effect of the culturing but rather an intrinsic limitation to cellular division. Both the young and old cells arrested with a similar number of total divisions, which was termed the 'Hayflick limit'. The state of permanent arrest was termed 'cellular senescence' (hereafter referred to as 'senescence').

The Hayflick limit differs between cell types, and even within a homogeneous population, according to the levels of endogenous and exogenous stress. The science of cellular ageing has yielded some intriguing discoveries relevant to the ageing of organs and organisms as a whole, and indeed any understanding of the decline of these more complicated structures would be incomplete without knowledge of the ageing process of their cellular makeup. This chapter will describe the mechanisms of cellular deterioration and their relevance to organ and organismal function, along with implications for healthy ageing and successful treatment.

Before describing the processes of cellular ageing, it is important to distinguish between old cells and cells from old individuals, as these can be easily confused. An 'old cell' is one that has reached or is close to reaching the end of its replicative cycle – that is, is nearly or fully senescent. Even in the oldest individuals, most of the cells will not have reached this state and should still be considered young cells.

THE DNA DAMAGE RESPONSE

Cells do not simply have an internal clock counting down the number of divisions before they senesce; their arrest is a response to stress forcing them to exit the cell cycle. In culture, increasing the exogenous stress causes the cells to reach their Hayflick limit after fewer divisions or immediately if the stress is severe. Various stresses have been shown to activate senescence, including hyperoxia, hypoxia, reactive oxygen species (ROS), ionising radiation, ultraviolet radiation and oncogenic activation.

Such a range of stresses could be thought to instigate senescence via multiple pathways; however, there is a single dominating one: the DNA damage response. Through direct damage or via stimulating replication, stressors induce DNA damage, including its most severe form, DNA double-strand breaks. Such breaks activate a specific kinase cascade that marks the break and initiates its repair: the DNA damage response. Activation of the tumour-suppressor p53 is one outcome of the DNA damage response, halting the cell cycle until repair is completed.

If the damage cannot be repaired by the cell, or if damage is continuously generated so that signalling through the DNA damage response pathway persists, the cell will progress towards an irreversible growth arrest: cellular senescence. High doses of X-rays or γ-rays can cause sufficient DNA damage to induce senescence; however, stress rarely reaches these levels in the body. The reason our cells still senesce under physiological conditions is mainly due to telomeric attrition. The ends of all linear chromosomes are defined and actually protected by stretches of heterochromatin known as 'telomeres', consisting of repetitive DNA sequences organised into a tight and stable structure. Telomeres shorten with each cell division for two reasons: (1) the DNA replication machinery cannot work well at the very end of a DNA molecule and (2) the compactness of the telomere inhibits DNA repair, so that DNA breaks can accumulate with time and induce loss of distal DNA during replication. Eventually, short telomeres can no longer form the protective chromosome caps and are recognised as double-strand breaks in the same way as those induced by ionising radiation. In human somatic cells, telomere shortening cannot be rectified, providing a persistent signal through the DNA damage response to p53.

A close association between DNA damage and ageing is evident in human progerias. These rare genetic diseases, which cause striking acceleration of the appearance of many – but normally not all – markers of ageing and early death, are all caused by mutations in genes that seriously influence the maintenance of DNA integrity. Werner syndrome, the most common progeria, results from the mutation of a helicase involved in DNA maintenance, causing symptoms to begin manifesting at around 10 years of age, with skin wrinkling and hair loss by 40 years of age that can make patients appear decades older. Patients develop a variety of endocrine problems and severe cataracts, and death usually occurs between 40 and 60 years of age due to myocardial infarction or cancer.

Hutchinson–Gilford's progeria results from a defect in the lamin proteins that make up the nuclear envelope, inducing severe and widespread DNA damage. Sufferers are symptomatic within months of birth and normally develop atherosclerosis, kidney and cardiovascular problems, hair loss, scleroderma and wrinkling prior to death in their teens or early 20s. Other segmental progerias, including Bloom's disease, Fanconi's anaemia, Cockayne syndrome and tri-chothiodystrophy are all caused by mutations in genes relevant to DNA damage repair and transcription control. Where it has been examined, senescence was accelerated in cells from these patients. Whether accelerated senescence con-tributes significantly to these diseases is not known.

THE SENESCENT PHENOTYPE

While cell senescence starts with a p53-mediated persistent proliferation block by an ongoing DNA damage response, it does not stop there. On the contrary, cells change almost beyond recognition during the establishment of irreversible growth arrest (*see* Figure 3.1). In consequence, senescent cells look different, function differently and interact differently with their neighbours and with the extracellular matrix.

Mitochondria are among the first cell compartments to change. About 2 days of a persistent DNA damage response are sufficient to trigger, via activation of the p38 mitogen-activated protein kinase and other signals, mitochondrial dysfunction – that is, loss of membrane potential together with increased production of ROS. This reduces mitochondrial energy output, changes the dynamics of the mitochondrial network (*see* Figure 3.2) and increases oxida-tive damage both within mitochondria and throughout the cell, including the nuclear DNA. In turn, this stabilises the DNA damage response; thus, mito-chondrial dysfunction is part of a positive feedback loop, or vicious cycle, that maintains cell senescence.

There are major changes in gene-expression patterns in senescent cells invol-ving thousands of different genes. Some of these are induced in response to mitochondrial dysfunction; many are associated with changes in chromatin structure and condensation state. Thus, heterochromatinisation is often used as a marker of the senescent cell state. Pro-inflammatory transcription factors – specifically, nuclear factor-kappa B – bind more tightly to senescent chro-matin. Accordingly, senescent cells express and secrete more pro-inflammatory cytokines and other bioactive peptides including growth factors and matrix-remodelling enzymes. It is because of this so-called senescence-associated secretory phenotype (SASP), together with ROS release, that senescent cells impact differently on their tissue environment (*see* below, 'The bystander effect').

Mitochondrial dysfunction and the pro-oxidant milieu put a heavy strain on the turnover mechanisms in senescent cells. Dysfunctional mitochondria are targeted for clearance in the lysosome/autophagosome system, while oxidised proteins are mainly degraded in the proteasome. While these systems are both highly evolved for the disposal of cellular debris, during senescence they are overwhelmed. The products of oxidative damage such as protein carbonyls can make proteins resistant to degradation through non-specific hydrophobic interaction with other proteins. As a result, the proteins act as nucleating sites for further aggregation. Growing in size, these aggregates may incorporate a diverse range of macromolecules, forming bonds that become increasingly resistant to cleavage. Thus, a chemically polymorphous brownish-yellow highly autofluorescent pigment known as 'lipofuscin', or 'age pigment', accumulates in non-dividing cells. As it builds up in the cell, it interferes with cellular trafficking and, importantly, acts as a competitive inhibitor of lysosomal and proteasomal function, which may foster the build-up of other cytotoxic protein aggregates. In the extreme, it can lead to lysosomal bursting, which releases the catalytic enzymes and acid into the cytoplasm. Conversely, activation of the cellular protein turnover machinery via, for example, caloric restriction or inhibition of mammalian target of rapamycin (mTOR) signalling can reduce frequencies of cells with a senescent phenotype and extend lifespan.

SENESCENCE AND STEM CELL DYSFUNCTION

Senescent cells accumulate with age in multiple organs and may therefore lead to deterioration through the autonomous depletion of functional cells. Stem cells are responsible for maintaining homeostasis of organ cellularity by differentiating into the lineages responsible for making up tissues and organs. When organs suffer damage or cellular depletion, stem cells divide to replace the lost or badly functioning cells with fresh ones, while at the same time maintaining their own number. The senescence of stem cell compartments has long been considered as a possible cause of ageing, especially of highly proliferative tissues. However, even less proliferative organs such as the heart and brain have stem cell reservoirs.

Evidence now suggests that many of the factors associated with cellular senescence are responsible for depleting stem cell populations. One study elevated ROS in murine haematopoietic stem cells (HSCs), which activated pathways and led to stem cell depletion. Another study discriminated between HSCs with high and low levels of ROS, finding that this could be used to determine proliferation potential. Cells with low ROS levels were multi-potent with long-term repopulation potential, exhibiting stem cell properties including quiescence and interaction with niche osteoblasts, while cells with high ROS were lineage restricted and unable to sustain serial transplantation. Studies implicating ROS as instigators of stem cell differentiation are not unanimous; recently, one study showed that ROS were integral to the maintenance of neuronal stem cells (NSCs). However, ROS-induced stem cell decline has been demonstrated in a diverse range of stem cells, from cardiac to embryonic.

Other senescent phenotypes such as mitochondrial dysfunction have also been linked with stem cell compromise. Most directly, mice lacking p16, a potent inducer of senescence, show enhanced HSC and NSC function with age. Combined, these data suggest that the vicious cycle controlling the maintenance of senescence is causally involved in the deregulation and depletion of stem cells. However, the exact mechanisms involved are still unknown. Although the term 'stem cell senescence' is widely used, its meaning is contentious. As stem cells age, for the most part they do not appear to enter a state of permanent cell-cycle arrest characteristic of differentiated cells, but instead appear to lose their potency and to some extent their potential for proliferation. Contrarily, a recent study has shown that when HSCs are exposed to ROS many of the cells enter apoptotic cell death, but the survivors are long-lived with a continually activated DNA damage response and a senescent-like phenotype. While an in-depth discussion of whether stem cells actually permanently arrest like differentiated cells is beyond the scope of this chapter, the important factor is that, as a result of cellular ageing, they exhibit many of the same markers of deterioration as senescent differentiated cells.

THE BYSTANDER EFFECT

Multiple studies have demonstrated that the exposure of cells to ionising radiation, in the form of α particles, γ or X-rays, does not have purely autonomous effects. While the target cells exhibit a strong DNA damage response, they also instigate a DNA damage response in surrounding cells that were not hit by the radiation. The spread of DNA damage from stressed to unstressed cells has been termed 'the bystander effect'.

Senescent cells also induce bystander effects. Given the multitude of biologically active substances secreted from senescent cells, it is unsurprising that the net biological response depends largely on the type of bystander cells targeted. Senescent cells stimulate growth and invasion of adjacent tumour cells, presumably via release of growth factors and matrix-degrading enzymes as part of the SASP. They activate macrophages and other immune cells by the release of chemoattractant cytokines. They also instigate DNA damage in bystander cells. This has no practical consequences if the bystander cells are tumour cells with compromised DNA damage checkpoints. However, normal bystander cells have intact checkpoint mechanisms, and bystander signals from senescent founder cells can induce them to senescence themselves. Thus, senescence may spread from cell to cell in a tissue, possibly faster than senescent cells can be cleared away by the immune system. *In vitro*, the induction of DNA damage in bystander cells can be abrogated by the addition of antioxidant enzymes to the medium, revealing that ROS were potent inducers of this bystander effect.

Even when considering stem cell senescence, it is clear that this is not a purely autonomous process. Under some conditions, stem cell ageing appears to be completely non-autonomous – such as with murine muscle satellite cells, in which function can be fully restored to old cells by exposure to the extracellular milieu of young mice. The niche is the micro-environment surrounding the stem cells, made up both of other cells and, just as important, the extracellular matrix in which they reside. Together, these factors provide stem cells with the necessary stimuli to maintain their potency. It has also been well documented that the stem cell niche changes as organisms age and that this could play a causal role in stem cell decline. At present, the net effect of senescent niche cells upon residing stem cells is completely unclear. However, the interplay of matrix remodelling, paracrine growth factor stimulation and activation of a DNA damage response might well account for some of the complex changes in tissue-resident stem cells with age.

Finally, there are systemic effects driven by senescent tissue-resident cells to consider. Fractions of apparently senescent cells as high as 20%–30% have been measured in some tissues of old mammals. This indicates that senescent cells may be a significant source of systemic pro-inflammatory signals in old organisms. Persistent low-level inflammation has long been shown to be associated with ageing and often been speculated to be a driver of age-related functional decline.

SENESCENCE, AGEING AND CANCER

If cellular senescence counteracts the health of individuals and contributes to ageing, why has it evolved at all? Or, assuming that it is a very ancient phenotype (a senescence-like permanent arrest can be found in unicellular organisms), why has it been retained through evolution? Telomeres shorten by necessity with every cell division; however, a specific enzyme, telomerase, can compensate for this. Telomerase is able to re-elongate telomeres by using its own template RNA. It is active in human germ-line and stem cells, enabling genomic stability through generations, but it is switched off in most human somatic cells. Artificially expressing telomerase in such cells overcomes their telomere-dependent senescence and can efficiently immortalise human cell clones. So, why are we not made only of telomerase-positive cells that are potentially immortal? Would that not increase lifespan and slow down ageing?

The first answer to this question is of course that evolution does not care about ageing – genes that ensure healthy ageing are only very weakly or not selected for because progeny is generally produced from young parents. Mechanistically, this question has been addressed using mouse models. Mice have long telomeres and active telomerase in most of their cells. Knocking out telomerase shortens not only telomeres but also, ultimately, the lifespan of these mice. Recent research suggests that both cell senescence and apoptosis contribute about equally to this life-shortening effect of telomere loss. In accordance with the knockout data, carefully controlled activation of telomerase can somewhat enhance the life expectancy of transgenic mice. The important term here is 'carefully controlled'. Ubiquitous over-expression of telomerase increases tumour risk significantly, thus shortens lifespan. Cellular senescence is an important tumour-suppressor mechanism in long-living animals including humans, and telomerase, by removing one limit to proliferation, enhances tumour risk. About 90% of all human tumours are positive for telomerase. This might be because they emanate from telomerase-positive stem cells or that they have reactivated the enzyme at some step during tumour progression. In addition, the vast majority of human tumours are negative (by mutation and/or epigenetic silencing) for at least one of the main checkpoint proteins that control the main pathway for induction of senescence, namely, p53, pRb, p21^{CIP1,WAF1} and p16^{ARF}.

Human naevi are a very instructive case for the power of cell senescence as a tumour suppressor: they typically consist of cells in which an oncogene has been activated. However, if this happens in a cell with intact senescence mechanisms, oncogene activation induces cell senescence after few cell divisions and these potentially tumorigenic cells become arrested. Only in very rare cases have further cooperating mutations occurred that disable senescence induction, and then malign melanoma might be formed. The frequent occurrence of moles compared with the low frequency of melanoma illustrates the efficiency of senescence as a tumour suppressor.

Thus, senescence is a cell-autonomous tumour suppressor. However, as already indicated, this is not the whole story. The reprogramming of senescent cells towards production and release of a great variety of bioactive factors, including ROS, cytokines, chemokines, growth factors and matrix-remodelling enzymes, means that senescent cells have profound bystander effects on premalignant and malignant cells in their vicinity. By inflicting DNA damage, they can further enhance genomic instability in bystander cells in which growth is not checked by intact checkpoints and senescence and apoptosis systems. Furthermore, by degrading local extracellular matrix components, they can facilitate invasion.

This dual effect of cell senescence to both inhibit and promote cancer exemplifies the concept of antagonistic pleiotropy (*see* Chapter 2, 'Theories of ageing'). Genes can be pleiotropic; that is, they can control more than one phenotypic trait in an organism. George Williams hypothesised in 1957 that genes would be selected for during evolution if they were beneficial for the organism's fitness at young age (when reproduction occurs), even if the same gene or the same trait was detrimental in later life. He reasoned this because, in the wild, most organisms die young due to starvation, cold or predation, irrespective of the ageing process. Therefore, the late disadvantage of such mutations would be heavily outweighed by the early life advantage, causing such individuals to be selected for. Cell senescence is clearly such a trait: it is beneficial as it prevents cells from becoming neoplastic; however, as senescent cells increase with age, the bystander effects become increasingly important in stimulating the malignancy of other cells, as well as contributing to organismal decline.

SENESCENCE AND THE DISEASES OF AGEING

Thus far, this chapter has described what cell senescence is and why it occurs, detailing the mechanisms that lead to cell, organ and organismal decline in ageing. However, ageing does not normally result in universal organismal decline; rather, it results in the onset of diseases associated with ageing, which affect the function of specific organs or organ systems. These may differ between individuals, making it more difficult in the clinic to spot the cellular dysfunction that is the underlying cause. These last sections examine how cell senescence may contribute to the diseases of ageing, and its implications for treatment.

Neurodegenerative diseases

Neurodegenerative diseases such as Alzheimer's and Parkinson's involve the accumulation of aggregates that inhibit neuronal function. As discussed previously above ('The senescent phenotype'), senescent cells have defects in the proteasome and autophagosome/lysosome systems responsible for 'rubbish' clearance. Thus, it is tempting to speculate that similar mechanisms might cause deficiencies of turnover systems in senescent cells and in neurons from dementia patients. Indeed, specific mutations have been identified that deregulate the labelling of proteins for destruction at the proteasome, which cause Alzheimer's disease. Many Alzheimer's brains have been found to have defects in the proteasome pathways. Dementia is also a common manifestation of lysosomal storage diseases such as Hurler syndrome, in which the lysosomal clearance mechanisms are disrupted. However, it is unclear at present whether signalling pathways related to the development of the senescent phenotype in proliferation-competent cells are activated in old post-mitotic neurons.

Atherosclerosis

This is also linked with senescence-associated factors. The primary instigator of atherosclerotic plaques is considered to be oxidised low-density lipoprotein (LDL) binding to damaged sites in artery walls, where it attracts macrophages, resulting in inflammation and further damage. It has been shown that the oxidation of LDL from artery wall cells increases according to their secretion of ROS. Fittingly, atherogenic sites have been associated with shortened telomeres and, more recently, a high concentration of senescent cells, indicating that they are responsible for the heightened ROS. Additionally, *in vitro* studies have shown that senescence induces several gene-expression changes in human aortic endothelial cells that have been implicated in atherogenesis.

The senescence of endothelial progenitor cells (EPCs), which are circulating cells involved in the regeneration of damaged endothelium, has also been suggested as allowing plaque formation through the decreased healing of the vessel walls. Therefore, senescence is likely to play a role in atherogenesis through both autonomous cellular depletion and non-autonomous damage to artery walls.

Diabetes mellitus

This disease is heavily linked with the decreasing efficacy of the insulin/IGF pathways, which are intricately connected with the ageing process. However, there is growing evidence that senescence also plays a causal role. Pancreatic β-cell senescence has been demonstrated in early type 2 diabetes progression, which can be predicted by the rate of telomere shortening. Additionally, analysis of mitochondrial DNA (mtDNA) mutation revealed that β-cells were particularly sensitive to mitochondrial dysfunction, as much lower levels lead to pathology than in other cell types. Concordantly, mitochondrial dysfunction has long been known to cause diabetes, with mtDNA mutation associated with Kearns–Sayre syndrome and mitochondrial encephalopathy lactic acidosis and stroke-like episodes, the symptoms of which include diabetes.

Notably, diabetes mellitus is known to contribute to EPC senescence via raising blood glucose levels. As diabetes increases risk of atherosclerosis, hypertension and neurodegenerative disease, senescence could be considered a causal mechanism in these diseases via the induction of diabetes. Equally, the ROS and aggregates associated with these plaques can cause cellular senescence.

Key to understanding senescence and the ageing process is that they are not looked at as a chain of events, but rather as a cycle of increasing degradation made up of multiple agents, all of which feed into each other. As such, removing specific components will not necessarily slow the ageing process, making treatment more difficult.

CELL SENESCENCE AND IMPLICATIONS FOR TREATMENT

Has treating cell senescence the potential to postpone ageing? The fact that cellular senescence is a pleiotropic trait warrants caution. In mouse models, suppressing cell senescence by over-activating telomerase or disabling senescence-inducing checkpoint proteins generally led to early life cancers and sometimes dramatically reduced lifespan. Therefore, inhibition of the mechanisms that induce cells to senesce is not a therapeutic option.

However, it might be possible to leave the senescent growth arrest intact while suppressing the aspects of the senescent phenotype that induce non-autonomous bystander effects, thus preventing stressed cells from damaging normal cells and from promoting cancer development. However, general antioxidant or anti-inflammatory treatments have had little proven success for various reasons. Many antioxidants, such as vitamin C, actually have pro-oxidant properties at high doses, while others lower the activity or expression of the natural antioxidant enzymes. Antioxidants that effectively lower ROS might induce major side effects, as ROS are not just damaging agents but crucially involved in many signalling processes. Therefore, in some cases, vitamin supplementation, such as with β-carotene, has actually been found to be detrimental to health, forcing studies to end prematurely.

The evidence for the beneficial effects of anti-inflammatories on age-related disease is more convincing but still equivocal. Non-steroidal anti-inflammatory drugs have been shown either to reduce the incidence of Alzheimer's disease or to have no effect, depending on the study. While meta-analyses have revealed some effect, the appropriate dosage and duration required to achieve a good benefit to risk ratio were unclear.

In contrast, calorie restriction (CR) is a well-established intervention to slow ageing. It exerts this effect via many targets, improving protein turnover, improving mitochondrial function and reducing expression of various inflammatory cytokines in multiple organs such as the brain, heart and liver. Interestingly, these are all interventions that suppress components of the senescent phenotype; in fact, it has been shown that CR decreases the frequencies of senescent cells *in vivo*. It is thought that many effects of CR are mediated though inhibition of the mTOR-dependent nutrient signalling pathway. In agreement with this, pharmacologic blocking of mTOR has been shown to increase the lifespan of mice. Effects of mTOR activity modulation on cell senescence are now a topic of intense research.

Exercise is another systemic stimulator that has been long associated with improved health and even increased lifespan. While physical activity increases muscle cell secretion of pro-inflammatory interleukin-6, it also stimulates the release of several anti-inflammatory cytokines, and inhibits macrophage accumulation in fat depots. Like CR, exercise has multiple effects on metabolism and metabolic signals that can act to suppress the senescent phenotype and may also play roles in its beneficial effects.

While these systemic interventions suggest potential for anti-senescence treatments, there are no specific interventions yet known that will suppress the senescent phenotype and delay ageing *in vivo*. However, an alternative approach might be just to kill senescent cells specifically. After all, if their only 'positive' purpose is to avoid the establishment of tumorigenic mutations in a cell, they have served this purpose once they are there. A seminal study by Baker and colleagues recently used a targeted inducer of apoptosis to specifically ablate p16-positive senescent cells in mice. The authors demonstrated that starting this treatment in the young delayed the onset of some age-related pathology, specifically in the eyes, adipose and skeletal muscle tissues, while beginning the treatment late in life attenuated the progression of these disorders. As this study was performed in mice that were genetically engineered to develop a very specific pattern of senescent cells extremely dependent on p16 activation, its adaptation to normal ageing mice or humans might still be a long way off.

However, it shows that even a very radical anti-senescent treatment might help to cure diseases of ageing.

CONCLUSION

To suggest that the permanent growth arrest of damaged cells, known as cellular senescence, is the single and most proximal cause of ageing, would be presumptuous, as there is still much we do not understand about the ageing process. Initially, cellular senescence theories of ageing were criticised because many tissues such as the brain and heart were considered post-mitotic and therefore not subject to the effects on cell division. However, these criticisms have since been shown to be incorrect. While both the brain and heart have stem cells, which affect organ function when damaged, more importantly, senescent cells can have widespread damaging effects through their secretions of ROS and inflammatory cytokines. The evidence clearly suggests that cellular senescence is a major contributor to organismal ageing and the development of age-related disease.

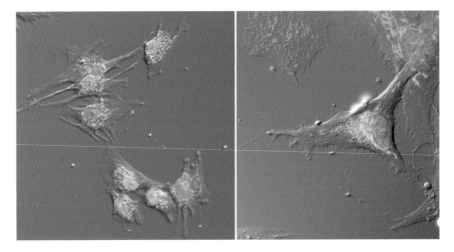

FIGURE 3.1 Combined differential interference contrast and epifluorescent images of young (left) and senescent (right) human fibroblast cells. Cell nuclei are stained with Hoechst (blue) and mitochondria are stained with MitoTracker® (green) and the membrane potential-sensitive dye tetramethylrhodamine, methyl ester (red). Comparison between young and senescent cells shows multiple aspects of the senescent phenotype: enlarged cell size, flattened cell morphology, changed state of chromatin condensation (increased heterogeneity of blue nuclear stain) and increased mitochondrial mass (green), together with decreased membrane potential (less red mitochondrial stain) indicating mitochondrial dysfunction, increased abundance of cytoplasmic granules (lysosomes and autophagosomes), indicating accumulation of waste products due to diminished autophagocytosis in senescent cells

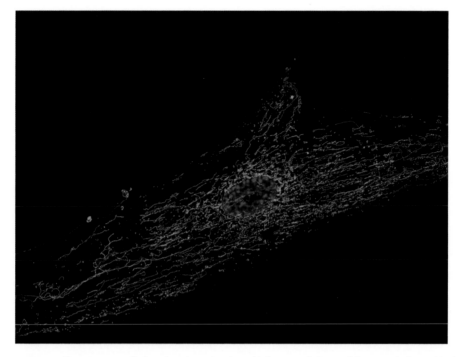

FIGURE 3.2 Senescent cell showing the mitochondrial network (green) in association with the lysosomes (red) around the nucleus (blue)

FURTHER READING

Baker DJ, Wijshake T, Tchkonia T *et al.* Clearance of p16[Ink4a]-positive senescent cells delays ageing-associated disorders. *Nature*. 2011; **479**(7372): 232–6.

Hayflick L. *How and Why We Age*. New York: Ballantine Books; 1996.

Tchkonia T, Morbeck DE, von Zglinicki T *et al.* Fat tissue, aging, and cellular senescence. *Aging Cell*. 2010; **9**(5): 667–84.

von Zglinicki T, editor. *Aging at the Molecular Level*. Dordrecht: Kluwer Academic; 2003.

Section 2

The ageing systems and clinical implications

CHAPTER 4

The immune system

DEBORAH DUNN-WALTERS, VICTORIA MARTIN
AND AZA ABDULLA

INTRODUCTION

Immunity is accomplished by a complex system comprising different types of cells acting in concert to provide effective regulation and clearance of pathogens. Cellular interaction is achieved either by direct cell-to-cell signalling using surface receptors or through chemical messengers such as cytokines and chemokines. The immune system can be broadly divided into two functionally distinguished parts: innate immunity, which provides a broad immediate response to pathogenic challenge, and adaptive immunity, which generates a specific immune response that is highly efficient at recognising and targeting a response towards almost any possible pathogen.

The innate immune system detects pathogens using non-specific receptors designed specifically to identify the presence of any foreign antigen by recognising pathogen-associated molecular patterns. This non-specific reaction is very rapid (within seconds or minutes) and provides a uniform response to different pathogens with no development of immunological memory. Macrophages, neutrophils and dendritic cells (DCs) all play an important role in innate immunity, not only by directly responding to the pathogen with effector molecules, but also by signalling the presence of an invading pathogen to the adaptive immune system, thus facilitating the generation of a more targeted and specific response.

Adaptive immunity evolves later, taking a few days to reach full efficacy but providing a level of specificity that enables precise targeting of the pathogen in order to achieve sterilising immunity. The adaptive response is more complex, involving a wide variety of cellular interaction, and results in long-term immunological memory to protect against future challenge. Upon repeat exposure to the same pathogen, immunological memory enables faster detection of the pathogen, more rigorous and specific responses and therefore enhanced immune efficiency. The cells of the adaptive immune response are B- and T-cells, which express specific antigen-detecting receptors (B-cell receptor [BCR] and T-cell receptor [TCR], respectively).

Within healthy young individuals, the immune system is highly efficient at detecting and eliminating foreign antigens due to the body's ability to tightly regulate each of the cells involved in the immune response, thereby keeping them functioning correctly and efficiently. During the ageing process, the body's ability to tightly control the immune system diminishes, ultimately leading to a decline in the effectiveness of the immune system as a whole. The consequence of this is apparent in the greater rates of morbidity and mortality seen in older people as a result of inflammatory diseases and infections such as pneumonia.

Multiple components within the cellular network are affected as a result of the ageing process, making immune senescence a complex process to understand. The immune environment, the innate immune system and the adaptive immune system are all altered in immune senescence. In this chapter, we outline what is currently known regarding the molecular and cellular changes that occur within each different component of the immune system and discuss how this affects infection, autoimmunity and cancer in older people.

MOLECULAR AND CELLULAR CHANGES

Cellular environment

Pro-inflammatory and anti-inflammatory signals are produced from a range of cells and aid in mediating cell-to-cell communications. Since many different cells can be affected by the presence or absence of a particular signal or cytokine, relatively small changes in the overall level of a cytokine in blood or tissue may have quite a large overall effect. Ageing is accompanied by an increased level of pro-inflammatory cytokines, in particular interleukin (IL)-6 and tumour necrosis factor α, and has led to the use of the term 'inflammaging'. The hypothesis is that a general increase in pro-inflammatory signals can make it difficult for the immune system to detect and respond to specific signals when an infection occurs. At the same time, it will contribute towards the inflammatory milieu that may exacerbate the autoimmune diseases of old age and other age-related diseases in which inflammation has been implicated in their aetiology, such as cardiovascular disease or Alzheimer's disease. The exact cause of the increased levels of pro-inflammatory cytokines is not known, and there is much controversy in the literature around the subject. Controversial results appear to be the consequence of looking at different age groups and different populations and it is not always easy to exclude the possibility of underlying inflammatory diseases in the older populations, which may mean that some results are distorted by subclinical disease states rather than an effect of ageing per se. To complicate matters, it has also been reported that the important anti-inflammatory cytokine IL-10, as well as IL-6, is increased, although not all groups agree. However, there is currently a general agreement that ageing is associated with a chronic pro-inflammatory rather than anti-inflammatory status.

Innate immune system
Neutrophils

Neutrophils are highly important cells, not only in helping to eradicate pathogens but also in both bridging the innate and adaptive immune systems and helping to resolve the response. They are the first cells to arrive at the site of infection, where they phagocytose and degrade bacteria and fungi by releasing reactive oxygen species (ROS) and antimicrobial and proteolytic granule proteins. The secondary role of neutrophils is to recruit macrophages and T-cells to the site of infection and to regulate the activity of these cells, along with their own activity. This recruitment is achieved by releasing signals, called chemokines and cytokines, which act to attract and guide cells to the site of infection. A third role of neutrophils is to produce anti-inflammatory signals that help to resolve and end the immune response once the pathogens are destroyed. It is vital that this occurs, as a continuing immune response would result in inflammatory diseases and autoimmunity. Neutrophils have a natural apoptotic pathway, meaning that they are short-lived cells, dying within 12–24 hours of release from the bone marrow. Although they do not live past the point at which they phagocytose pathogens, these cells need a prolonged lifespan during an immune response. This requires their exposure to survival signals. Without these signals, the apoptotic pathway and anti-inflammatory signals would result in the rapid death of neutrophils.

The overall number of neutrophils does not appear to change considerably with age, although some reports have suggested that the number may actually increase. Despite this, there are several ways in which neutrophils are affected by ageing. Aged neutrophils are less efficiently recruited to the site of infection, due to a decrease in particular adhesion molecules that help guide and roll the cells along the epithelium towards the target area. During the process of errant navigation through tissue, neutrophils can cause bystander damage to healthy tissue. In resting cells, the ability of neutrophils to survive is the same between young and old, but, upon stimulation, the old neutrophils have a decreased ability to respond to survival signals. This is thought to be due to a lack of activation within intracellular signalling pathways, highlighting that the age-related dysregulation in neutrophils occurs at both the molecular and cellular levels.

Aged neutrophils also show functional inefficiencies caused by a decreased phagocytic capacity (the ability to engulf pathogens) and decreased antibody-dependent phagocytosis followed by decreased intracellular killing. Subsequent to phagocytosis, fusion with the lysosome is required to generate ROS, superoxide, hydrogen peroxide and hypochloric acid, all of which are toxic to microbes. There is an antigen-dependent reduction in the production of ROS in aged cells, especially in response to *Staphylococcus aureus*, a Gram-positive bacterium. It is thought that these differences are due to age-specific changes occurring in some but not all signalling pathways, altering the ability of neutrophils to generate ROS in response to only certain types of antigen stimulation. The difference between young and old neutrophil intracellular killing can be dramatic, showing a 44% reduction in the killing of *Escherichia coli* and a 10%–50% reduction in the killing of *Candida albicans*.

The combination of reduced recruitment to the target site of infection, decreased ability to be rescued from apoptosis alongside decreased phagocytic capacity and decreased intracellular killing severely impairs the cells' functional ability to target and eliminate invading pathogens.

Natural killer cells (NK cells)

NK cells are cytotoxic cells that can detect and kill infected cells and some tumour cells. They also have an impaired function with age, when their cytotoxic abilities are decreased and they have decreased cytokine secretion in response to activation. Studies have shown that in those over the age of 85 years, low NK cell count is associated with an increase in all-cause mortality.

Antigen-presenting cells

Cells of the innate immune system that can capture and hold antigen in a form that is recognisable by B- and T-cells are vital bridges between the innate and adaptive immune systems. While B-cells can recognise antigen in unprocessed form, T-cells require antigen to be processed into peptides and presented to them in the context of major histocompatibility complex (MHC) class II molecules. Additional co-stimulatory molecules will be expressed to help activate the recipient cell. Antigen-presenting cells will also secrete pro-inflammatory cytokines, therefore may be partially responsible for the inflammatory phenotype of ageing. Antigen-presenting cells of the innate immune system are monocyte-macrophages and DCs. B-cells of the adaptive immune system are also very effective antigen-presenting cells.

Monocyte-macrophages

Monocytes develop in the bone marrow and are released into the bloodstream where they can migrate into tissues to mature as macrophages. They can differentiate into a variety of tissue-specific macrophages, for example, osteoclasts (bone), Kupffer cells (liver) and microglia (brain). Within tissues, these cells can survive for months or years but without activation most cells die by apoptosis.

Macrophages are involved in both the innate and adaptive immune systems, in both the initiation and the resolution of a response, and function via many different mechanisms: (1) they can interact directly to destroy and remove parasites, viruses, bacteria, tumour cells or damaged/stressed cells; (2) they act indirectly to release cytokines that regulate other immune cells; (3) they act as antigen-presenting cells, breaking down pathogens and presenting pathogen-related antigens to cells of the adaptive immune system; and (4) they can secrete cytokines that promote tissue regeneration. This wide variety of activities means that they have the ability to perform opposing functions, such as secreting both pro- and anti-inflammatory cytokines or secreting both metalloproteinases and metalloproteinase inhibitors; therefore, their functions must be highly regulated towards the activity that is required at a particular stage of the immune process. Classically activated M1 macrophages kill microorganisms, remove debris and secrete pro-inflammatory cytokines. Later, in the resolution phase, alternatively activated M2 macrophages have antigen-presentation properties, immunoregulatory functions and are involved in tissue remodelling.

TABLE 4.1 Age-related changes in monocyte-macrophages

Function	Change with age
Recruitment to the site of injury	↓
Activation	
Production of pro-inflammatory signals – LPS stimulation	↓
Production of chemokine signals – LPS stimulation	↓
Response to LPS signals – LPS stimulation	↓
Downstream signalling signals – LPS stimulation	↓
TLR activation – LPS stimulation	↓
Antigen-presenting capacity – MHC class II molecule expression	↓
Phagocytosis	↓
Wound repair	↓

Adapted from Sebastián *et al.*, 2009.

↓ = decrease

Given their central role and multiple functions, it is clear that any change in macrophage function will have far-reaching effects across the immune system. Many age-related changes have been reported (*see* Table 4.1). Their ability to respond to recruitment signals at a site of injury is decreased, resulting in the delayed attendance of macrophages. Once at the site of infection, aged macrophages are not able to respond as well. Phagocytosis of pathogens by macrophages is an important first line of defence, but aged macrophages have a reduced phagocytic capacity. They are also less able to respond to pathogen-associated molecular patterns such as the bacterial product lipopolysaccharide

(LPS), they express fewer pattern-recognition receptors, such as toll-like receptors (TLRs), on their surface, secrete less cytokines in response to stimuli and have intracellular signalling deficiencies downstream of antigen-recognition receptors. Their antigen-presentation capacity is diminished, with a reduced level of MHC class II molecules on their surface, and their ability to secrete angiogenic and fibrogenic growth factors is also reduced, so they cannot contribute as well towards wound healing during the resolution of the response.

Dendritic cells (DCs)

DCs are potent antigen-presenting cells that also provide a vital link between the innate and adaptive immune systems, both in regulating and enhancing immune protection and also in balancing immune tolerance to protect against autoimmunity. They function efficiently due to their ability to: (1) detect, capture and present antigens to other immune cells (*see* Figure 4.1); (2) migrate to defined sites within tissues in which they are able to present antigen and initiate the adaptive immune system (*see* Figure 4.1); and (3) rapidly differentiate and mature upon activation by a wide variety of stimuli such as pathogens, intracellular pro-inflammatory signals and dying cells.

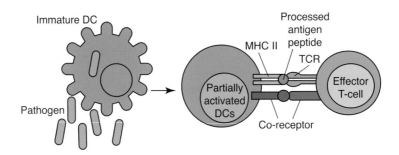

FIGURE 4.1 DC interactions upon contact with antigen

As DCs are found at entry portals into the body – for example, skin and airways – they form protective networks of cells that can quickly detect and respond to pathogens, allowing a rapid immune response and effective protection against pathogens. Another crucial function of DCs is to maintain T-cell tolerance, which protects the immune system from becoming autoreactive by preventing the activation of T-cells against self-antigens. DCs continually sample self-antigens from dying cells, ensuring that T-cells that respond to self-antigens are eradicated or turned off. Upon contact with an antigen, DCs down-regulate their capacity to sense and capture antigens in conjunction with up-regulating molecules that are required for enhancing their antigen-presenting abilities. In addition to direct activation of other immune cells, DCs also secrete inflammatory mediators, giving them a broad influence on the rest of the immune system.

Given the crucial importance of these cells in both enhancing an immune response and protecting against autoimmunity, any age-related changes that affect DCs could have a vast impact on the body's defence mechanisms. Overall, there appears to be no major age-related change in the total number of DCs, although some studies have observed changes in different types of DCs in different locations. For example, Langerhans cells are DCs that are found within the epidermis. There is a decreased density of Langerhans cells within the skin, mucosal tissues and tonsil epithelium, which reduces the protective network of cells at entry sites into the body. Their morphology changes such that they have fewer and shorter dendritic branches and a rounder shape, which decreases their antigen-presentation abilities and causes a degree of functional loss. There is a clear trend towards an increased mature DC phenotype with age – that is, more cells express co-stimulatory molecules on their surface. This might be linked with the age-related decrease in the antigen-capturing capacity that has been observed in DCs for both pathogens and apoptotic cells, since the functions of capture and presentation are not usually present at the same time in one cell. The process of apoptosis, and subsequent phagocytosis of apoptotic cells, is highly important, as necrotic cells would accumulate and release autoantigens otherwise. The age-related decrease in phagocytosis means necrotic cells activate DCs to secrete many pro-inflammatory signals that enhance the immune response and result in a greater uptake of the autoantigens, thereby increasing the chances of chronic inflammation. Defects in the activation of DCs have also been observed in older cells; compared with younger cells, antigen binding results in increased production and secretion of pro-inflammatory signals, which may contribute to inflammaging. There are also possible signs of age-related defects in DC migration towards the site of infection in tissue.

The mechanisms for these age-related changes are much less understood than the defects themselves, but initial research shows that, at least in part, these functional changes occur as a result of changes in signalling pathways downstream of the initial antigen-recognition receptor. Overall, considering the pivotal role that they play in the immune response, the functional changes in DCs with age are highly significant.

Adaptive immune system

The adaptive immune system takes longer to develop but is highly specific, extremely effective and provides immune memory to facilitate a quicker targeted response upon secondary challenge. The adaptive immune system is comprised of B-cells and T-cells, which have specific antigen-recognition receptors (BCRs and TCRs, respectively) on their surfaces. The diversity of these receptors is enormous, with millions of different recognition capabilities, giving the system as a whole the potential to detect almost any antigen. Upon pathogen challenge, the cells carrying receptors that can recognise the challenge expand, thus adapting the repertoire towards recognition of the threat.

T-cells

T-cells play a central role in the adaptive immune system and can be broadly categorised into two types based on their functions: CD4+ helper T-cells and CD8+ cytotoxic T-cells.

CD8+ T-cells recognise antigen from intracellular pathogens that are presented on the surface of an infected cell in the context of MHC class I molecules. The function of CD4+ cells is not to kill infected cells but to provide help to other cells. They are absolutely required by B-cells for an effective humoral immune response against protein antigens (Th2-type T-cells) and can help activate other cells such as macrophages, NK cells and cytotoxic T-cells (Th1-type T-cells). Each T-cell has a unique TCR, formed by rearrangement of genes and heterodimerisation of gene products, such that the repertoire of different TCRs is huge. T-cells differentiate from an initial lymphoid progenitor within the bone marrow and continue their development in the thymus, where positive (for functional T-cells) and negative (against self-reactivity) selection events shape the pre-immune repertoire. Naive T-cells become active upon contact with antigen presented to them by antigen-presenting cells and will expand, thus altering the repertoire so that more cells with the specificity for the activating antigen are present.

The age-related changes occurring in T-cells are well documented. There is no age-related change in the total number of cells, but the thymus shrinks with age, resulting in a decreased output of naive CD8+ and CD4+ T-cells. The smaller number of new cells entering the repertoire ultimately results in a distortion of the T-cell repertoire towards antigen-experienced cells (*see* Figure 4.2). Since naive cells are required for the detection of novel antigens, the reduction of diversity in the T-cell repertoire makes it more difficult for an aged individual to respond to new challenges.

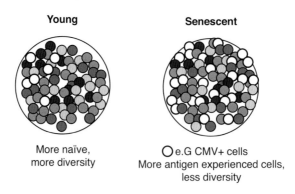

Young   Senescent

More naïve, more diversity   ○ e.G CMV+ cells
More antigen experienced cells, less diversity

FIGURE 4.2 Illustration of the difference in TCR diversity between young and senescent repertoires

In addition to the distortion of the repertoire, there are many reported intrinsic deficiencies in old T-cells. Within the CD4+ T-cells, some reports have suggested there may be a shift towards the Th2 phenotype with age, thus altering the cytokine environment. Aged T-cells are less responsive to stimulation, have defects in their signalling pathways, secrete less cytokine, proliferate less, express lower levels of co-stimulatory receptors on their surfaces and are more resistant to apoptosis. Given that many other cells in the immune system rely on T-cells for help, then these failures have much more serious consequences for effective immunity than just the loss of protection against intracellular pathogens. Humoral immunity, in particular, is severely compromised without T-cell help.

B-cells

B-cells are a vital component of the adaptive immune system as they not only generate large quantities of antibodies against various pathogens and toxins, but they can also act as antigen-presenting cells to activate T-cells. They develop solely in the bone marrow, where they, too, acquire a diverse pre-immune antigen-receptor (BCR) repertoire by gene rearrangement and heterodimerism that is tested to remove self-reactive cells. Upon activation in the periphery, antigen-specific cells expand, skewing the repertoire as a whole towards one with more recognition of the challenging pathogen. Unlike T-cells, B-cells undergo further maturation to improve the affinity of the BCR for antigen by somatic hypermutation (SHM). The cells can switch the functional part of their BCR (e.g. from immunoglobulin [Ig] M to IgG or IgA) by class switch recombination (CSR) before differentiating into memory cells or to plasma cells that secrete the BCR in the form of an antibody (*see* Figure 4.3). B-cells require T-cell help for CSR and affinity maturation, particularly via CD40 co-stimulation.

Less is known about the age-related changes that occur within B-cells than within T-cells, with most research focusing on changes in the cellular populations. During the early stages of development, haematopoietic cells must either commit to a myeloid (monocytes, neutrophils, basophils, etc.) or lymphoid (lymphocytes) lineage. In aged humans, there is a shift in the commitment towards the myeloid lineage, with cells showing less lymphoid potential. This is thought to be due to changes in gene expression, increasing genes that are required in myeloid cells and decreasing those required in lymphoid progenitor cells. Despite a reduction in B-cell precursors, there is no significant change in the overall number of B-cells in aged donors. However, changes have been seen in the proportions of different cells; there is a decrease in naive B-cells and an increase in memory B-cells so there are fewer antigen-inexperienced naive B-cells available to respond to novel antigens. The skewing of the B-cell repertoire in old age can correlate with ill health.

There is no change in the overall concentration of immunoglobulins, but there is a shift towards a different composition of the antibody repertoire with age. Older people can still make high-quality specific antibodies but not in the same quantity as younger people, so there may not be a sufficient quantity of

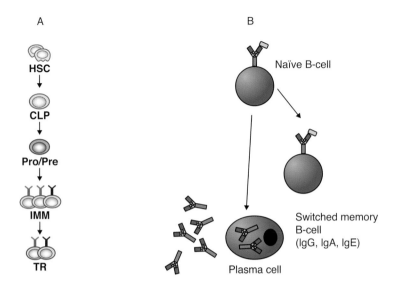

FIGURE 4.3 (A) The stages of B-cell development. Haematopoietic stem cells (HSCs) differentiate into common lymphoid progenitors before the generation of pro-/pre-B-cells (Pro/Pre). These then continue to differentiate into immature (IMM) B-cells through to transitional B-cells (TRs) and, finally, into naive B-cells. (B) The differentiation of naive B-cells upon activation by antigen

good-quality antibodies available when needed. There have also been reports of differences in the relative proportions of different isotypes, although this may not always be the case. Additionally, there may also be defects in the developmental processes that control self-reactivity, since the number of autoantibodies in old people is significantly increased. This may be important in some autoimmune diseases, such as rheumatoid arthritis, that are increased with age.

Very little has been published on B-cell-intrinsic changes with age, although there are reports that the enzyme activation-induced cytidine deaminase, which is a critical catalyst of the SHM and CSR processes, is reduced in older B-cells.

CLINICAL IMPLICATIONS

Infections

There is now increasing evidence that immune senescence contributes to increased incidence, morbidity and mortality associated with infection in older people. In a study evaluating the epidemiology of sepsis in 192 980 patients, the incidence was 3 cases per 1000 members of the general population, increasing to 26 per 1000 members of the population in those aged over 85 years. The changes in immune function in older people may well contribute to greater susceptibility to infection, and the abnormal presentation of infections in older people often delays diagnosis. The adverse serious consequences of infections in older people have prompted the view among many geriatricians that, when a decision is made to treat a significant infection, antibiotics should be: given early, empirical and broad spectrum, and delivered parenterally.

Increasing age is an independent risk factor for community-acquired pneumonia (CAP). The incidence of CAP in older people is up to four times greater than in those aged under 65 years, and it is estimated that around 1 in 20 people aged over 85 years of age will develop a new episode of CAP every year. Mortality rates are also notably high, ranging from 30% in community dwellers to 57% in nursing home residents.

The changes in the older immune system outlined in this chapter, combined with the anatomical and physiological changes in the lungs and airways, are likely to be responsible for the increased incidence of CAP and its complications in older people. Other common bacterial infections in old age occur in the urinary tract, can cause significant morbidity and frailty and are particularly difficult to detect in a timely fashion.

Ageing is also a risk factor for both herpes zoster and post-herpetic neuralgia (PHN). Herpes zoster has a 10-fold higher incidence in people over the age of 85 years than in those aged under 20 years old. In those aged over 70 years, 73% develop PHN, two- to threefold more than those aged under 55 years (27%). Age is also a significant predictor of severity and duration of pain. Herpes zoster is caused by reactivation of dormant virus in sensory dorsal root ganglia from an earlier bout of primary varicella. It is thought that in normal conditions, cellular immunity prevents the clinical re-expression of varicella zoster virus disease. The waning of cellular immunity to the virus with advancing age is at least partly responsible for the clinical reactivation.

Some viral infections may actually contribute to immune senescence, by constant activation of the lymphocytes responsible for protecting against them. *Cytomegalovirus* is a prime example of this, causing a reduction in diversity of the T-cell repertoire. This is also a growing population of individuals with human immunodeficiency virus who may have more severe T-cell repertoire dysregulation than normal and, therefore, accelerated senescence of the T-cell compartment.

Vaccination: influenza and pneumococcal vaccine

Influenza causes high morbidity and mortality in older people; 90% of deaths due to the disease occur in people aged 65 years and older. The response to vaccination in older people is attenuated by immune senescence. Not only is antibody response to vaccination reduced, but vaccination also provides a lower level of protection. Even when the antigen match between vaccine and infecting strain is close, infection is prevented in only 30%–40% of people in this age group compared with 80% of those aged under 65 years. Despite the poor response, older people are most likely to benefit from vaccination given the high incidence of infection and mortality. Vaccination is associated with a significant reduction in morbidity and mortality, including a decrease in secondary pneumonia. It has also been shown to reduce hospitalisation. Similarly, there is a decreased antibody response to pneumococcal vaccine. Nonetheless, the antibody response predicts, at least partly, the clinically observed protection that the vaccine prevents invasive (bacteraemic) pneumococcal disease. However, the overall efficacy of pneumococcal vaccination in older people is moderate at best and only reaches cost-effectiveness due to the low cost of administration as part of the influenza vaccination programme.

Autoantibodies and autoimmune disease

The incidence of autoimmune disorders appears to be higher in older people, but the underlying mechanism(s) is/are unclear. The mild immune dysfunction that denotes immune senescence along with the pro-inflammatory state (inflammaging) associated with ageing may cause dysregulation of cell homeostasis, with a tendency to over-respond to endogenous antigens. Furthermore, the reduction in naive T-cell population and a shift from Th1 to Th2 cytokine production with stimulation may result in augmentation of B-cell-mediated autoimmune disorders and the production of autoreactive antibodies. Rheumatoid factor is one of the most frequent autoantibodies described in older people, with a frequency ranging between 9% and 48%. Similarly, the prevalence of antinuclear antibodies (ANAs), generally at low titres of 1/40–1/80, is higher in healthy individuals over 70 years of age than in younger adults. Several studies have also noted a higher prevalence of anticardiolipin antibodies in older people, approaching 30%. In the majority of cases, these autoantibodies are of low titres and have no clinical relevance. Therefore, they may only be markers of immune senescence. However, it is clear that age is a risk factor for diseases such as rheumatoid arthritis, thus immune senescence may well be an important part of disease aetiology.

Cancer

The incidence of most malignant tumours increases progressively with age. In developed countries, the median age for diagnosis of cancer is 70 years of age. Although this is the result of interplay between different mechanisms, it is thought that immune senescence may be at least partly responsible. The importance of the immune system in preventing tumour formation, termed 'immunosurveillance', has been shown repeatedly in animal models and is supported by epidemiological evidence, such as increased frequency of certain cancer types in immunosuppressed individuals.

The concept of cancer immunosurveillance predicts that the immune system can recognise precursors of cancer and, in most cases, destroy these precursors before they become clinically apparent. However, the diminished function of T-cells with age may be responsible for increased incidence of cancer with age.

Some studies have suggested that decreased cytotoxic activity in older people may favour the development of neoplasia due to a defective recognition of tumour antigens. Immune senescence, therefore, may allow tumours to escape immunosurveillance and subsequent destruction.

CONCLUSION

The immune system is composed of a highly regulated network of cells that interact and function together to quickly and effectively identify, target and destroy invading pathogens. The changes that occur with age are varied and differ between cells; an overview is shown in Figure 4.4. These changes are not always a loss of function; in some cases it can be an increase in function, such as an increase in secretion of pro-inflammatory cytokines. The combined effect of the changes is interference with the tight regulation and balance that keep the immune system working effectively to protect the body against infections and malignancies and which may contribute towards inflammatory diseases.

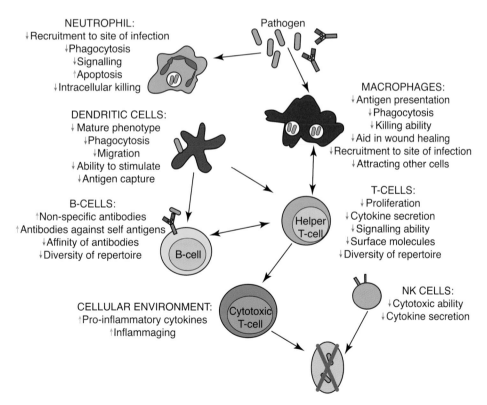

FIGURE 4.4 An overview of the key age-related changes that have been observed in the immune system

FURTHER READING

Bellmann-Weiler R, Weiss G. Pitfalls in the diagnosis and therapy of infections in elderly patients: a mini-review. *Gerontology.* 2009; **55**(3): 241–9.

Fulop T, Franceschi C, Hirokawa K *et al.*, editors. *Handbook on Immunosenescence: basic understanding and clinical applications.* Berlin and Heidelberg: Springer; 2009.

Sebastián C, Lloberas J, Celada A. Molecular and cellular aspects of macrophage aging. In: Fulop T, Franceschi C, Hirokawa K *et al.*, editors. *Handbook on Immunosensecence.* Berlin and Heidelberg: Springer. pp. 919–45.

Wordsworth DTHJ, Dunn-Walters DK. The ageing immune system and its clinical implications. *Rev Clin Gerontol.* 2011; **21**(2): 110–24.

QUESTIONS: IMMUNE SENESCENCE

1 Loss of B-cell or T-cell repertoire diversity in old age is important because:
   A antibody concentrations fall
   B memory for previously encountered pathogens is lost
   C the Th1 and Th2 cytokine balance is changed
   D the cells cannot be activated
   E there is less chance of a lymphocyte recognising new pathogens.

   Answer: E

2 The aged immune system is characterised by:
   A a higher number of B-cells
   B a higher number of T-cells
   C a lower number of DCs
   D a lower number of neutrophils
   E higher levels of inflammatory cytokines.

   Answer: A

3 The most important link between the innate and adaptive immune systems is:
   A antigen-presenting cell
   B chemokines
   C cytokines
   D the pattern-recognition receptor
   E the TCR.

   Answer: A

4 The importance of immune senescence is best demonstrated by:
   A a good response to vaccination against influenza
   B a higher incidence of myocardial infarction with age
   C a higher incidence of viral but not bacterial infections
   D increased mortality following infection
   E reduced response to antibiotics.

   Answer: D

5 Which one of the following statements actually reflects influenza vaccination in older people?
   A compared with in younger individuals, it results in higher side-effect risk
   B compared with younger individuals, vaccination produces a higher antibody response
   C it prevents infection in only a 50% of individuals
   D it provides a lower level of protection
   E it results in reduced mortality but not morbidity.

   Answer: D

CHAPTER 5

The haematopoietic system

ALICE M TAYLOR AND BARBARA J BAIN

INTRODUCTION

Ageing is partly a physiological process and partly the effect of life's events on various organs and tissues. It is possible that crucial stem cells, which could include haematopoietic stem cells, are themselves subject to ageing. Recognising the effect of age per se on haematopoietic function is difficult because of the interplay of haematopoiesis with endocrine and renal function and the effects of systemic disease (sometimes occult) on haematopoiesis. Further confounding factors include nutritional deficiency, which is partly related to social isolation and poverty in older people. It is possible that haematopoietic stem cells and progenitor cells decline in number or function with age, although data are conflicting. Two explanations for such stem cell decline are possible. Undoubtedly there is cumulative DNA damage, partly the result of random events and partly due to exposure to extrinsic influences such as genotoxic drugs, chemicals or irradiation during the course of life. There may also be an intrinsic senescence of stem cells, attributable to telomere shortening, which occurs more rapidly in proliferating tissues.

This chapter explores the changes that may occur in the haematopoietic cells with ageing and discusses their clinical implications as well as some of the more common blood diseases occurring in older people.

EFFECT OF AGEING ON THE HAEMATOPOIETIC SYSTEM

Changes in bone marrow cellularity

With ageing, haematopoietic marrow in distal bones is replaced by fatty marrow, with active haematopoiesis being largely confined to the proximal axial skeleton. Bone marrow cellularity is assessed as the amount of the bone marrow cavity occupied by haematopoietic cells in a biopsy or autopsy speci-men. Cellularity, as assessed in this manner, significantly declines with age, as bone marrow trephine biopsies and other tissue sections reveal. The reduced cellularity that is observed is the result both of a decline in the amount of hae-matopoietic tissue and a loss of trabecular bone, which enlarges the marrow cavity, leading to a larger proportion of fat cells. Early histological studies on the anterior iliac crest, performed at autopsy following sudden death, showed a decline in bone marrow cellularity on average from 70% in childhood to 30% in those over 70 years of age. Similar observations were subsequently made on the iliac crest and on the sternum (*see* Figures 5.1 and 5.2). The decline may be particularly marked beyond the age of 80 years.

The decline in cellularity observed in tissue sections is paralleled by a decline in the cellularity of bone marrow aspirates. The number of nucleated cells in a given volume of marrow declines by about 50% between adolescence and old age. Similarly, the number of granulocytic precursors in the marrow of healthy non-anaemic older people is significantly less than in young subjects; similarly, ferrokinetic measurements show that erythroblast numbers are significantly fewer in non-anaemic older people than in the young.

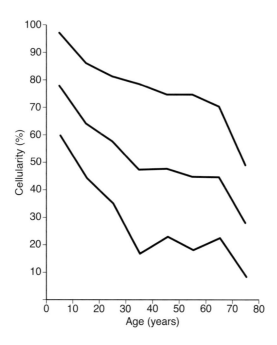

FIGURE 5.1 Means and 95% range of cellularity at various ages in anterior iliac crest bone marrow that has been decalcified and paraffin-embedded. Cellularity is expressed as a percent-age of the bone marrow cavity. Data are derived from Hartsock RJ, Smith EB, Petty CS. *Am J Clin Pathol.* 1965; **43**: 326–31. Reproduced with permission from Bain BJ, Clark DM, Wilkins BS. *Bone Marrow Pathology.* 4th ed. Oxford: Wiley-Blackwell; 2010

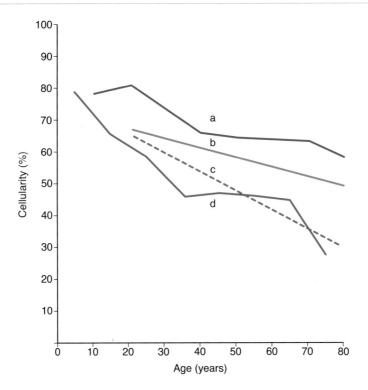

FIGURE 5.2 Mean value of bone marrow cellularity at various ages re-expressed as a percentage of the bone marrow cavity: (a) iliac crest, autopsy, not decalcified (recalculated from Frisch B, Lewis SM, Burkhardt R *et al. Biopsy Pathology of Bone and Marrow*. London: Chapman & Hall; 1985.); (b) iliac crest, autopsy, not decalcified, data from Courpron P, Meunier P, Edouard C *et al. Rev Rheum*. **40**: 469–82; (c) sternum, biopsy, not decalcified, data from Bryon PA, Gentilhomme O and Fiere D (1979) *Pathol Biol*. 1973; **27**: 209–13; (d) ilium, autopsy, decalcified, data from Hartsock RJ, Smith EB, Petty CS. *Am J Clin Pathol*. 1965; **43**: 326–31. Reproduced with permission from Bain BJ, Clark DM, Wilkins BS. *Bone Marrow Pathology*. 4th ed. Oxford: Wiley-Blackwell; 2010

Changes in stem cell and progenitor cell numbers

Studies investigating any effect of age on the number and function of haematopoietic stem cells and progenitor cells have not provided any clear answers. In one study, burst-forming units, erythroid (BFU-E) and colony-forming units, erythroid (CFU-E) in healthy non-anaemic older subjects showed no statistically significant difference from younger controls, although older subjects with unexplained anaemia did show a lower number of CFU-E, suggesting that BFU-E function was abnormal in them. In this study, the number of colony-forming units granulocyte-macrophage (CFU-GM) similarly did not differ between older non-anaemic subjects and younger controls, although CFU-GM numbers were significantly lower in older subjects with unexplained anaemia. However, another study reported conflicting results, in which the number of

BFU-E was significantly lower in older subjects (either anaemic or non-anaemic) than in younger controls ($P < 0.01$ and < 0.05, respectively). Similarly, this same study found a lower number of CFU-GM in older anaemic subjects than in younger controls ($P < 0.05$), but in the non-anaemic older subjects there was no significant difference. Results for CFU-E were inconsistent. In a third study, the proportion of CD34+ cells did not differ between healthy volunteers aged 70–80 years and younger controls. There was likewise no difference between the proportions of the somewhat more mature CD34+CD33+ cells. However, functional differences were found in that, although the maximum number of colonies produced by exposure to granulocyte colony-stimulating factor (G-CSF), granulocyte-macrophage colony-stimulating factor (GM-CSF) and interleukin (IL)-3 was similar, the progenitor cells of older people were considerably less sensitive to lower cytokine doses ($P < 0.01$). In a fourth study, 24 apparently healthy 88-year-olds were compared with controls aged 21–57 years. No difference was found in BFU-E or CFU-E, although the number of CFU-GM was significantly lower in the older probands. In a fifth study, the number of CD34+ cells in eight centenarians did not differ from the number in nine older subjects (aged 66–73 years) or from that in nine younger control subjects (aged 30–45 years). In this study, similarly, the number of BFU-E and CFU-GM did not differ between the three groups.

Although colony-forming ability in response to exogenous stimulants has generally been found to be normal in older people, the situation *in vivo* could differ. This is supported by a study that showed peripheral blood mononuclear cells produced less GM-CSF in older people, including centenarians, than in the young. Production of IL-3 was also significantly lower in centenarians. Unexpectedly, the concentration of serum stem cell factor (SCF), produced mainly by bone marrow stromal cells, increased significantly with age. Thus, it is difficult to determine whether altered cytokine production in older people has any overall impact on the normal functioning of HSCs. The ability of CD34+ stem cells to respond to SCF was retained by older people, including centenarians.

TABLE 5.1 Significant differences in older people in comparison with younger control subjects

BFU-E	CFU-E	CFU-GM	CD34+ cells	Study
No difference	No difference*	No difference*		Lipschitz 1984
Lower	Inconsistent results between groups	No difference*		Hirota 1988
		No difference†	No difference	Chatta 1993
No difference	No difference	Lower		Nilsson-Ehle 1995
No difference		No difference	No difference	Bagnara 2000

*However, lower in anaemic older subjects.
†However, progenitor cells of the older subjects were less sensitive to lower cytokine doses.

The results of the discussed studies are summarised in Table 5.1. Overall, it can be concluded that there is no unequivocal evidence for a decline in stem cell/progenitor cell number or function with age or for a decline in cytokine production that is likely to be biologically significant.

Changes in the peripheral blood count

Haemoglobin concentration (Hb)

As bone marrow cellularity and, possibly, stem cell numbers or function decrease with age, it is logical to think that Hb will similarly decline. However, it can be difficult to identify a physiological decline because of the confounding influence of increased pathology in the ageing population. It is therefore difficult to derive valid reference ranges for a 'normal' Hb in older people with an increased propensity to possibly occult disease. As the population of persons aged 85 years or older is now the fastest growing segment of the US and other populations, trying to establish an appropriate reference range becomes increasingly important. The standardised World Health Organization (WHO) criteria for anaemia, Hb <120 g/L in females and <130 g/L in males, may not be applicable to the older population.

The changes in Hb with age may differ between men and women. In a community study of 3946 unselected US residents over the age of 70 years, Hb was found to show an inverse correlation with age, particularly in men ($P < 0.001$ for both sexes). Another study found a decrease in healthy older white US men, with the 2.5 percentile being 134 g/L for men aged 20–59 years (n = 6709) and 128 g/L for men aged 60 years or older (n = 5615) in one data set; in a second data set, the figures were 134 g/L (n = 1456) and 122 g/L (n = 934). No difference in values for white women who were younger or older than 50 years old was observed. Black men showed a similar decline whereas black women did not. In another US study, reported results for men were similar, but a decline in Hb in women was seen from the age of 50 years old. Conflicting results for women were found in an Italian study, in which Hb was found to be significantly higher in post-menopausal women than in premenopausal, whereas men over the age of 60 years old had a significantly lower mean Hb than younger men. An Italian population study showed that mean Hb was lower in people of both sexes aged over 80 years, but little change was seen in those younger than that; the influence of occult ill health as an explanation could not be excluded. In a longitudinal population study in Sweden, healthy men showed a mean decline in Hb from 152 to 141 g/L between the ages of 70 and 88 years ($P < 0.05$), whereas in healthy women there was no significant change (mean values 140 g/L and 138 g/L, $P > 0.05$).

One can conclude from the published data that with age there is a narrowing of the gap between the sexes in Hb, with a decrease in the Hb of apparently healthy individuals occurring particularly in men and particularly over the age of 70–80 years. If the explanation for any age-related decline in Hb does not lie in the number of stem cells, alternative explanations are needed. Red cell survival does not differ between the young and the old. A declining testosterone concentration in men could provide an explanation of the narrowing difference between the sexes but data are conflicting. Similarly, declining erythropoietin secretion could provide an explanation but data are again conflicting. Some longitudinal studies have seen a mild increase in erythropoietin with age, in individuals with preserved renal function, possibly indicating an increased need for erythropoietin drive. The decline in Hb may relate to a reduced need for oxygen transport, as a result of reduced body mass; the correlation observed in older people between Hb and body mass index in at least two studies supports this hypothesis.

The decline of Hb in older people, particularly in older men, may represent a true age-related decline – an anaemia of senescence; however, on this is superimposed a higher prevalence of anaemia than is seen in younger subjects, this relating to impaired renal function, chronic inflammation and nutritional deficiency.

White-cell and platelet counts

The white-cell and neutrophil count in women decline after the menopause, although not to an extent that is of any clinical significance. However, changes in the function of white cells have been described in both men and women (*see* Chapter 4, 'The immune system'). There is no known age-related change in the platelet count.

Karyotypic changes with age

Older men show an increasing prevalence of Y chromosome loss in bone marrow cells. In one study, this was observed in 10 of 14 men, with the loss being seen in 6%–100% of metaphases. Loss of an X chromosome in some metaphases in women is observed much less often. The loss of Y is a non-clonal abnormality.

Haemostasis and thrombosis

Physiological ageing is associated with increased plasma levels of many blood coagulation proteins together with impairment of fibrinolysis. Plasma concentrations of fibrinogen, factor VII, factor VIII, von Willebrand factor, factor IX, factor XII, high molecular-weight kininogen and prekallikrein increase with progressing age in healthy subjects. Factor VII triggers the coagulation cascade on interaction with tissue factor, the latter exposed with disruption of the vascular wall. Fibrinogen, involved with acute-phase inflammation, is strongly correlated with ageing. With an increase in such pro-coagulant proteins with age, this could have important ramifications for the vasculopathy also known to be inherent in old age.

CLINICAL IMPLICATIONS

The significance of anaemia in older people

There is an increasing suggestion that even mild anaemia is associated with a poorer health outcome, although determining what is cause and what is effect is more contentious. Anaemia has been related to worsened exercise tolerance; reduced bone density, mobility and cognition; and an increased chance of falls and depression. A prospective study of 3607 Dutch people over 71 years of age traced hospitalisation rates over a 4-year period. Anaemic individuals – according to WHO criteria – at baseline were found to spend almost twice as many days in hospital as non-anaemic (25.0 versus 13.7, $P < 0.01$), with more frequent hospitalisation (65.9% versus 54.6%, $P < 0.001$). Mortality was also higher. Similar observations were made in a second Dutch study of 1016 adults over 85 years of age who were well enough to live in the community. Even in those without known medical problems, there was a strong association between anaemia and all-cause mortality. Anaemia (Hb in the lowest quintile) was also independently predictive of mortality in a US study of 1205 individuals aged 65 years or older. Low Hb was an independent predictor of mortality in these patients (relative risk 1.131, 95% confidence interval 1.045–1.224 for each decrease of 10 g/L). Anaemia has been found to be associated with a higher mortality in older patients with heart failure. Studies have been consistent in showing improvement in cardiac and cognitive function as anaemia is corrected.

Although increasing the Hb will improve the maximum potential for oxygen delivery and have an impact on exercise capacity, this is at the expense of increased blood viscosity. Thus, there is an optimal Hb that provides a balance between reduced oxygen-carrying capacity and significant problems related to increased viscosity. Of interest, an Hb in the highest quintile as well as the lowest quintile was predictive of higher mortality in the US study mentioned. In heart failure, the ideal Hb is probably above 125 g/L in most patients, since a meta-analysis has suggested that correcting mild anaemia (Hb >100 g/L), in symptomatic patients with congestive failure can improve exercise tolerance, reduce symptoms and have benefits on clinical outcomes.

Anaemia in older post-operative patients who have had orthopaedic intervention correlates with functional impairment. However, a liberal rather than restrictive transfusion policy does not appear to be of benefit.

Causes of anaemia in older people

Regardless of whether there is an element of physiological alteration explaining a lower Hb in old age, the consensus is that pathological causes of anaemia must be ruled out in the first instance. Chronic inflammation, renal failure and dietary insufficiency are likely causes of anaemia in old age. Myelodysplastic syndromes (MDS), which will be discussed in more detail further on, may account for more cases. However, it has been estimated that at least one-quarter of anaemia cases in older adults are unexplained.

Nutritional deficiency

The National Health and Nutrition Examination Survey 1988–94 (NHANES III) in the US found some type of nutrient deficiency to be related to approximately one-third of cases of anaemia in the older population. Iron deficiency is a common cause of anaemia across this age range. In addition to inadequate iron intake, gastrointestinal loss is a clinically significant cause of iron deficiency in an ageing population.

Megaloblastic anaemias in older people commonly result from cobalamin (vitamin B_{12}) deficiency, with folic acid deficiency being less common. Deficiencies are particularly important to exclude, since they can be corrected with such ease. Folate deficiency due to nutritional insufficiency is now uncommon in the Western world, particularly with the routine fortification of foodstuffs such as bread and cereal now occurring in some countries (e.g. US and Australia but not currently the UK). In the absence of food fortification, the older population may be more vulnerable to folate deficiency, particularly if they are institutionalised, on a lower income or alcoholic. Vitamin B_{12} deficiency in old age is typically due to impaired absorption, either pernicious anaemia or defective absorption of B_{12} from food with retention of the ability to absorb purified B_{12}. More than 10% of the older population in the US has low or borderline B_{12} levels, although it should be noted that low levels do not necessarily correlate with significant tissue deficiency.

Anaemia of chronic disease or chronic inflammation

In the older population, anaemia of chronic disease is important in the differential diagnosis of anaemia. Typical causes are inflammatory disorders, malignancy and infection.

Anaemia due to renal insufficiency

Anaemia was found to be related to renal insufficiency in 8% of anaemic older adults in the NHANES III study.

Other causes of anaemia in older people

The influence of alcohol and medication-related toxicity is difficult to fully elucidate. Alcohol is not likely to be of particular relevance in older people in comparison with younger people, whereas the common requirement for multiple medications is likely to be relevant. The MDS, chronic lymphocytic leukaemia and chronic cold agglutinin disease show a steady rise in incidence with age, thus contribute to anaemia in older people.

The causes of leucopenia and neutropenia in older people

Although there is no age-related change in the total white-cell count or the neutrophil count, there are important causes of neutropenia in older people.

The increasing incidence of MDS and the effects of polypharmacy must be considered.

Alterations in ability to withstand chemotherapy with age

Older patients have been found to be more sensitive to chemotherapy, which has been attributed to decreased haematopoietic reserve. There is a resultant higher incidence of febrile neutropenia following chemotherapy. For example, studies focusing on women receiving chemotherapy for breast cancer have found that patients aged over 65 years are at higher risk of febrile neutropenia, therefore, G-CSF prophylaxis with higher risk regimens has been advised. Similarly, in older non-Hodgkin lymphoma patients, G-CSF has been found to significantly reduce profound neutropenia and febrile neutropenia and to increase the proportion of people able to receive the planned dose of chemotherapeutic agents. Despite the postulated decreased haematopoietic reserve, the response to G-CSF has been found to be preserved in the older patient.

Clonal myeloid disorders in older people

There is undoubtedly an increased prevalence of myeloid clonal disorders with increasing age, of which acute myeloblastic leukaemia and myelodysplastic syndromes are particularly associated with increasing age.

Myelodysplastic syndromes (MDS)

MDS represent an acquired clonal, neoplastic disorder of haematopoiesis, which may occur *de novo* or following chemotherapy or irradiation. They are far more common in those aged 65 years or older and can lead to death from marrow failure or by evolution to AML.

In the early stages, MDS can be very subtle, manifest perhaps only by a macrocytosis, without cytopenias or morphological change. Other laboratory features may include cytopenias, monocytosis, dysplasia of one or more lineages and, eventually, the appearance of blast cells in blood films and in increasing numbers in the bone marrow. The diagnosis of MDS, even in their earliest forms, may increase with more sophisticated genetic markers and may well lead to this diagnosis being made in older patients with previously unexplained anaemia. Therapeutic modalities include erythropoietin with or without G-CSF, blood transfusion and chemotherapy, including, in certain circumstances, the use of lenalidomide or azacytidine. As with other diseases in older people, more intensive treatment may be precluded by toxicity.

Acute myeloblastic leukaemia (AML)

There is certainly an increasing prevalence of AML in the older age group, with over half of all patients being over 60 years of age at presentation. At the age of 40 years, there is 1 case of AML per 100 000 per year, with the annual incidence increasing to 15 per 100 000 in those older than 75 years. AML in older patients is more likely, than in the young, to follow an antecedent haematological disorder such as a myelodysplastic syndrome or to be secondary to chemotherapy or radiotherapy for another malignancy.

In many cases of AML in older people, the disease differs intrinsically from that of AML in younger subjects. There is no age-related increase in the incidence of certain relatively good prognosis types of AML – specifically those associated with balanced chromosomal rearrangements such as t(8;21), t(15;17) and inv(16). The steady increase in AML with advancing age is due to an increase in poor-prognosis AML associated with unfavourable unbalanced cytogenetic abnormalities and multi-drug resistance. There is a higher incidence of expression of the multidrug resistance protein (MDR1) p-glycoprotein, (p-gp), which is associated with a poor outcome. Adverse karyotypic abnormalities often observed include del(5q) or -5, del(7q) or -7, translocations with an 11q23 breakpoint, inv(3), t(6;9), t(9;22) and complex chromosomal rearrangements. As a result of the adverse cytogenetic and molecular characteristics, older patients often have poor disease-free and overall survival, even if they are able to withstand chemotherapy and enter complete remission. Patients younger than 55 years have shown improved survival over the past three decades, but there has been no change for those over the age of 55 years. The adverse outcome of AML in older people can be attributed to inherently adverse disease, worse performance status, frequent co-morbidity and reduced haematopoietic reserve. Older people are more likely to have limited hepatic, renal, pulmonary and cardiac reserves, as well as a lower tolerance of systemic bacterial and fungal infection. Even those with disease that has a relatively good prognosis have a worse outcome; for example, in patients with acute promyelocytic leukaemia who are 60 years of age or older, there are more early deaths and more deaths in remission than in younger patients. Improving the outcome of AML in older people with age-adapted or disease-adapted therapy is yet to be achieved to any major extent, although encouraging results have been obtained in the treatment of acute promyelocytic leukaemia in older people with chemotherapy-free regimens based on all-*trans*-retinoic acid. However, in patients with poor-risk AML, the perceived benefits of achieving remission must be offset against the greater risks of morbidity and mortality from chemotherapy and in some patients it is better not to attempt to induce remission.

Myeloproliferative neoplasms (MPN)

MPN are a group of clonal neoplastic disorders in which there is effective haematopoiesis leading to overproduction of end cells of one or more haematopoietic lineages, at least in the early stages of the disease. They comprise mainly polycythaemia vera, essential thrombocythaemia and primary myelofibrosis. They increase in prevalence with age, although the increase is not as striking as in AML and MDS. The clinical features are similar to those in younger patients except that there is an increased likelihood of vascular events because of the interaction of the MPN with vascular disease. Polycythaemia vera requires venesection to lower the haematocrit and reduce viscosity and, in the long term, possibly hydroxycarbamide as a cytoreductive agent. Essential thrombocythaemia may be managed with aspirin alone or with aspirin plus hydroxycarbamide. Treatment in older people is mainly as in younger patients with two exceptions relating to the indications for cytoreductive treatment and the role of radioactive phosphorus (^{32}P). There is a stronger indication for active treatment in older people than in the young because of coexisting vascular disease; in the British Committee for Standards in Haematology guidelines (2010), one criterion for assigning a patient with essential thrombocythaemia to the high-risk group warranting aspirin plus hydroxycarbamide is an age over 60 years. ^{32}P is well tolerated and effective but is usually avoided in younger patients because of its potential to induce acute leukaemia in a minority of patients. Its usefulness should not be forgotten in older patients when ease of management is very important. It is particularly valuable in older patients whose memory is poor, who may suffer adverse effects as a result of errors in self-medication with hydroxycarbamide. The use of ^{32}P also means that the patient does not have to make frequent visits to outpatient clinics for blood count checks.

Acute lymphoblastic leukaemia, lymphomas and plasma cell neoplasms

Acute lymphoblastic leukaemia (ALL)

ALL is rightly seen as mainly a disease of childhood. However, there is a second peak of incidence later in life, which is the result of increasing incidence of Ph-positive *BCR-ABL1*-positive disease. It is important that adults with ALL, particularly older adults, be investigated for the presence of the t(9;22) translocation and a *BCR-ABL1* fusion gene. This cytogenetic/molecular subset has an adverse prognostic significance and requires use of tyrosine kinase inhibitors and consideration of the need for stem cell transplantation.

Hodgkin lymphoma

There is a second peak of incidence of Hodgkin lymphoma in the older population aged above 60 years, this peak being related to an increase in cases with neoplastic cells carrying the Epstein–Barr virus (EBV). Therapy is similar in principle to that in younger patients, but toxicity related to treatment is a recurring problem.

Non-Hodgkin lymphoma

Aggressive non-Hodgkin lymphoma in the older patient is treated with multiagent intensive systemic chemotherapy, but the dose may need to be modified at the expense of the therapeutic aim because of age and co-morbidity. For example, doxorubicin, which is often used in first-line therapy, may not be possible to use in a patient with impaired cardiac function.

Low-grade lymphomas can be more indolent, thus it is often more prudent to adopt watchful waiting as a policy, particularly in an older person at higher risk of treatment-related morbidity. Waldenström macroglobulinaemia is a syndrome resulting from a low-grade lymphoplasmacytic lymphoma. The effects of immunoglobulin M paraprotein can include hyperviscosity, cryoglobulinaemia, cold agglutinin disease, bleeding diathesis and peripheral neuropathy. Such effects may be particularly burdensome in the older patient.

A newly recognised age-related lymphoma is EBV-positive diffuse large B-cell lymphoma (DLBCL) of older people. In those over 90 years of age, this subtype can comprise as many as 25% of DLBCL. This lymphoma is attributed to declining immune function with senescence.

Monoclonal gammopathy of undetermined significance (MGUS)

This is a term used to define the presence of a monoclonal protein in the serum or urine of a patient with no evidence of multiple myeloma, amyloidosis or any related disorder.

MGUS undeniably increases with advancing age. In a study of a Minnesotan population, MGUS was seen in 1%–2% of people in their sixth decade, 3% in their seventh decade and 4%–5% in their eighth decade. Based on this study, the overall risk of progression of MGUS to myeloma is deemed to be 1% per year. Risk of progression may be influenced by the type and level of M-protein, level of bone marrow plasmacytosis and the presence of an abnormal serum-free kappa to lambda light chain ratio. However, the high proportion of cases occurring in older people means that many patients never progress to myeloma. Guidelines are available indicating which patients with MGUS should be referred to a haematologist and which patients should be further investigated (Bird *et al.*, 2009).

Multiple myeloma (plasma cell myeloma)

Multiple myeloma is yet another disease that preferentially afflicts older people. In addition to a paraprotein (in the great majority of cases), there is evidence of myeloma-related organ or tissue impairment, which may include hypercalcaemia, renal failure, lytic bone lesions or symptomatic hyperviscosity. It is important to be alert to the possibility of myeloma in older patients presenting with backache, anaemia or renal failure.

Chronic lymphocytic leukaemia (CLL)

CLL occurs mainly in older people. The diagnosis is often an incidental one, made as a result of findings from a blood count done for another reason. The need for active treatment is indicated by the stage of disease and its rate of progression. Many patients do not need active treatment, although vaccination against pneumococcal infection and the influenza virus is usually advised. It is also important to be alert to herpes zoster infection, which requires early antiviral treatment to avoid morbidity. A combination of chemotherapy and immunotherapy with rituximab (a monoclonal antibody to the CD20 antigen) is now considered optimal therapy.

Haemostasis and thrombosis

Venous stasis and arterial disease both increase with advancing age, leading to an increased prevalence of thrombosis. However, age-related changes in coagulation proteins may also contribute. The great majority of coagulation changes are adverse. A rare exception is von Willebrand disease, which may be ameliorated by an age-related increase in the concentration of factor VIII and von Willebrand factor. In addition, studies of centenarians have found an apparent state of hypercoagulability: high levels of atherosclerotic risk markers (such as von Willebrand factor) and high-risk thrombophilic alleles (such as the prothrombin gene mutation G20210A). If such markers do correlate with longevity, there may be a different biological relevance in older age.

With an increased tendency to autoimmune phenomena in old age, acquired coagulation factor inhibitors may develop. Acquired haemophilia, resulting from the presence of a factor VIII inhibitor, is associated with pregnancy but is otherwise more common in men and shows an increasing incidence with age. The median age of presentation is around 69 years. Differing from inherited haemophilia, factor replacement has no major role; these patients must be managed with immunosuppression or recombinant factor VII in cases of severe bleeding. The lupus anticoagulant may also occur, but it predisposes to thrombosis rather than haemorrhage.

Thrombocytopenia

Although there are no age-related changes in the platelet count, there are many possible causes of thrombocytopenia at an older age. Autoimmunity, drug toxicity and MDS should be considered.

Anticoagulant therapy

Anticoagulation needs to be carefully monitored in older people. There is an increased rate of bleeding complications, which are more worrisome in a frail patient, and more scope for interference by polypharmacy deranging the stability of anticoagulation.

CONCLUSION

Physiological changes occur in haematological variables with ageing, most of them disadvantageous. Among these, unexplained anaemia and thrombotic disorders are the most prevalent. Many haematological disorders are particularly prevalent in older people and their management is complicated by reduced bone marrow reserve, frequent co-morbidity and reduced ability to tolerate treatment-related infections and other adverse effects of treatment.

FURTHER READING

Beutler E, Waalen J. The definition of anemia: what *is* the lower limit of normal of the blood hemoglobin concentration? *Blood.* 2006; **107**(5): 1747–50.

Bird J, Behrens J, Westin J *et al.* UK Myeloma Forum and Nordic Myeloma Study Groups: guidelines for the investigation of newly detected M-proteins and the management of monoclonal gammopathy of undetermined significance (MGUS). BCSH guidelines, *BJ Haem.* 2009; **147**: 22–42.

Carmel R. Anaemia and aging: an overview of clinical, diagnostic and biological issues. *Blood Rev.* 2001; **15**(1): 9–18.

Lipschitz DA, Udupa KB, Milton KY *et al.* Effect of age on haematopoiesis in man. *Blood.* 1984; **63**(3): 502–9.

Penninx BW, Pahor M, Woodman RC *et al.* Anaemia in old age is associated with increased mortality and hospitalization. *J Gerontol A Biol Sci Med Sci.* 2006; **61**(5): 474–9.

Steensma DP, Tefferi A. Anaemia in the elderly: how should we define it, when does it matter, and what can be done? *Mayo Clin Proc.* 2007; **82**(8): 938–66.

QUESTIONS: HAEMATOLOGY

1 Anaemia associated with ageing is in part due to:
A increased haemopoietic reserve
B increasing prevalence of inflammatory and malignant disease
C increased need for vitamin B_{12} and folate
D increased splenic activity
E shortened red cell lifespan.

Answer: B

2 An 80-year-old woman complains of fatigue and is found to have a Hb of 80 g/L and a mean corpuscular volume of 110 fL. Her neutrophils are hypogranular and many are bilobed. The most likely diagnosis is:
A acute myeloid leukemia
B folate deficiency
C iron deficiency
D myelodyplastic syndrome
E vitamin B_{12} deficiency.

Answer: D

3 There is a decreasing prevalence with age of:
A acute myeloid leukemia
B chronic lymphocytic leukemia
C EBV-positive DLBCL (diffuse large B-cell lymphoma)
D Ph-negative acute lymphoblastic leukemia
E myelodyplastic syndrome.

Answer: D

4 Vitamin B_{12} deficiency in a 70-year-old Indian man is unlikely to be due to:
A decreased thyroid function
B malabsorption of dietary B_{12}
C pernicious anaemia
D previous surgery for Crohn's disease
E use of proton pump inhibitors.

Answer: A

5 There is improvement with age in the severity of:
A factor VII deficiency
B factor IX deficiency
C hypofibrinogenaemia
D thrombophilia due to factor V Leiden
E von Willebrand disease.

Answer: E

CHAPTER 6

The cardiovascular system

ISOBEL RAMSAY AND CHAKRAVARTHI RAJKUMAR

INTRODUCTION

With an ever-expanding older population, the burden of cardiovascular disease is set to increase. Age provides a background of anatomical, metabolic and physiological changes that makes the ageing heart and vasculature more vulnerable to the effects of a multitude of factors that contribute to the development of disease. In the older cardiovascular system, it is often difficult to disentangle the effects of age per se from the effects of prolonged exposure to other cardiovascular risk factors (smoking, diet, etc.). Thus, an understanding of age-related changes in the cardiovascular system and their effects on the management of cardiovascular disease becomes increasingly essential to the practice of geriatric medicine.

This chapter will discuss the molecular and cellular changes in the cardiovascular system, the changes in metabolic processes and cellular signalling and the anatomical and physiological changes in the myocardium and vasculature that occur with age. The effects of age-related changes on common cardiovascular diseases and their management will also be addressed.

THE HEART

Molecular, anatomical and physiological changes in the myocardium

The cells of the myocardium are designed to undergo synchronous contraction in response to electrical excitation to eject blood from the heart. In the older heart, the cardiac myocytes decrease in number (through both apoptosis and necrosis). The human heart loses around a third of its myocytes between the ages of 17 and 90 years, independently of cardiovascular disease. Therefore, the burden of providing enough mechanical force to maintain cardiac function falls upon the surviving myocytes, which undergo hypertrophy.

Ageing is also associated with increased deposition of amyloid, lipofuscin (seen in many senescent cells) and collagen in myocardial tissue. This collagen undergoes increased cross-linking, leading to myocardial fibrosis. The heart valves are similarly affected, becoming calcified and fibrosed.

Fibrosis occurs in the conduction system as well as in the cardiac myocytes. There is a decrease in the number of sino-atrial node pacemaker cells and the neurons supplying the atria undergo axonal degeneration, which leads to attenuated atrial sympathetic innervation.

As with other eukaryotic cells, cardiac myocytes and vascular endothelial cells contain chromosomal DNA. At the ends of these chromosomes are telomeres, which are thought to protect the chromosome. Telomeric length is a possible marker of cell age, as telomeres progressively shorten with each mitotic cycle (*see* Chapter 3, 'The ageing cell'). At a critical point, cells enter replicative senescence (i.e. they lose the ability to divide), become increasingly susceptible to DNA damage and, finally, undergo apoptosis. Studies on telomeres have shown a number of associations with cardiac disease. Shorter telomere length is associated with type 1 and 2 diabetes, hypertension, insulin resistance, heart failure, risk of myocardial infarction (MI) and appears to be linked to the endothelial dysfunction seen with age.

In addition to structural cellular changes, metabolic processes and cellular signalling in the cardiac myocyte also alter with age. Myocytes have a limited capacity to regenerate and the balance between cell-cycle inhibitors and anti-apoptotic factors shifts to favour cell death. Errors occur more frequently in the mitochondrial respiratory chain, creating more reactive oxygen species, and cells become more susceptible to oxidative damage and have a decreased ability to respond to stress. This is evidenced by a change in the array of stress response factors (e.g. heat shock proteins and antioxidant enzymes).

The expression of proteins involved in calcium signalling pathways alters with age, resulting in prolongation of the cardiac action potential and cardiac contraction through a decrease in the sensitivity of myofilaments to calcium.

Studies in rodent models suggest that these effects are in part due to modification of the expression of components of the sarcoplasmic reticulum, including the Ca^{2+}/Na^+ ATPase pump and Na^+/Ca^{2+} exchanger, resulting in protracted rise in cytosolic calcium. This prolonged intracellular calcium transience is thought to contribute to lengthened contraction and impaired relaxation of the myocardium in early diastole.

The myocytes become less sensitive to β-adrenergic signalling as they age, with β-adrenergic stimulation resulting in an attenuated cyclic adenosine monophosphate response and a decreased influx of calcium into the cell.

In rat models, cardiac myocytes contain the α isoform of the contractile protein myosin; however, with age, this is replaced by the β isoform. The β isoform is a slower type of myosin and produces a more efficient contraction than the faster α form. This shift appears to be more marked with hypertension. This, combined with the calcium signalling changes already detailed, results in a more prolonged contraction. Although it is unclear whether these isoform switches occur during normal human ageing, similar isoform shifts have been noted in human hearts in cardiac failure.

Studies in rat models suggest that there is a switch in the ageing cardiac myocyte from fatty acid metabolism to carbohydrate metabolism, with a decrease in the expression glycolysis-related genes. Caloric restriction appears to decrease this effect as well as increase cardiac tolerance to ischaemic insults. This may be due to its effects on mitochondrial function, as it is associated with a decrease in oxidative stress.

At a macroscopic level, the changes in the cardiac myocytes are seen as left-ventricular hypertrophy, fibrosis and dilatation. Data from the Framingham Heart Study (2010) suggest that left-ventricular wall thickness increases with age and left-ventricular dimensions decrease. Age-associated wall thickening appears to be more marked in women and those with diabetes, whereas the decrease in left-ventricular dimensions is attenuated in these groups. As with the rest of the vasculature, the coronary arteries dilate and calcify, becoming more tortuous.

The molecular, metabolic and anatomical changes result in alterations in the different parameters of cardiac and vascular function with age.

Heart rate and stroke volume

The heart rate in the sitting position decreases with age, while the heart rate in the supine position at rest does not alter significantly. However, the most significant changes are seen during exercise.

The cardiovascular response to exercise is markedly different in the older heart than in younger subjects. Maximum oxygen consumption (VO_2 max) is decreased in older people; the extent of this decrease is dependent not only on age but also other factors such as smoking status and physical conditioning. There is also a decrease in the maximum heart rate attainable through exercise with age, which results in a decrease in cardiac output. Stroke volume is maintained through the Frank–Starling mechanism, except during vigorous exercise when there is a limited increase in stroke volume. Unlike in younger individuals, early diastolic filling does not change on acute exercise in older people.

Heart rate variability is closely related to cardiac autonomic function. The ageing heart becomes less responsive to catecholamines – often associated with a reduction in diurnal heart rate variability.

As heart rate decreases with age, stroke volume must compensate if cardiac output is to be maintained. In men, cardiac output is maintained with an increased stroke volume. However, women seem less able to compensate in this manner, thus have a slightly decreased cardiac output. This may be explained by higher levels of physical activity in men than in women.

Cardiac output

At rest, ejection fraction is essentially unchanged with age. However, the heart must adapt to maintain this in the context of the increasing afterload – a product of increased arterial stiffness. This is accomplished through preservation of end diastolic volume and/or prolonged contraction time.

End diastolic volume is preserved in the healthy older person lying supine and, indeed, it increases in men. Due to stiffening and decreased compliance of the left-ventricular wall, the left ventricle is less able to relax during diastole, leading to a decrease in early diastolic filling. Between the ages of 20 and 80 years old, the rate of early diastolic filling drops by 50%. To maintain end diastolic volume, a larger contribution is made by contraction of the left atrium in late diastole.

Contraction of the heart muscle is prolonged in older people, in part due to the changes in calcium signalling and the action potential already detailed. This may help to cope with the increase in arterial stiffness to preserve ejection fraction.

THE VASCULAR SYSTEM

Anatomical and physiological changes

In the vasculature, the arterial wall undergoes thickening, dilatation and fibrosis resulting in increased arterial stiffness and pulse wave velocity.

Vascular endothelial cells become flatter and larger and, as in the myocardium, deposition of collagen and increased collagen cross-linking occur in the vasculature. These processes take place particularly in the intima of large arteries, for example, the carotids. This is coupled with calcification of the arteries and a decrease in the concentration and cross-linking of elastin in the intima.

Although intimal thickening with age has sometimes been seen as a form of subclinical atherosclerosis, studies suggest that age-associated thickening can occur independently of atherosclerosis.

Decrease in arterial compliance with age is proposed to contribute to a loss of baroreceptor reflex sensitivity. The reflex relies on stretch-sensitive nerve endings, which, in older stiffer arteries, may require a greater blood pressure change to elicit a response than in more compliant vessels.

Gene expression in vascular endothelial cells undergoes a number of changes as they age. This includes up-regulation of endothelial adhesion molecules and components of the renin–angiotensin signalling pathway, for example, angiotensin I.

Studies in rats suggest that vascular ageing processes such as elastin fragmentation are modulated by cytokines like transforming growth factor-beta, which in turn affect the action of enzymes such as the matrix metalloproteinases. In particular, matrix metalloproteinase-2 has been shown to play a key role in vascular elastin changes.

Increased levels of these molecules create a metabolically active environment, which provides a base for endothelial dysfunction and the development of cardiovascular disease (e.g. atherosclerosis).

As with myocardial cells, the endothelial cells of the circulation cope less well with damage as they age and become less responsive to nitric oxide (which regulates vascular tone). There is also less potential for angiogenesis in the ageing vasculature with decreased expression of factors such as vascular endothelial growth factor.

Effects on blood pressure

The vasculature stiffens with age. Pulse wave velocity is a directly related measure of vascular stiffness and increases with age. When the heart muscle contracts, a forward pulse wave travels through the vasculature and, at points of bifurcation, wave reflection occurs. In healthy vasculature, this reflected wave arrives back at the heart in diastole (*see* Figure 6.1[A]). However, with increased arterial stiffness, the wave is reflected back more quickly and arrives in systole (*see* Figure 6.1[B]). This results in augmentation of the systolic blood pressure that leads to an increase in systolic hypertension with age. Systolic blood pressure rises from the age of 40 years, with a peak during the eighth decade. Along with increased vascular stiffness, diastolic pressure falls, leading to an increase in pulse pressure. It has been argued that a wide pulse pressure is a surrogate marker for vascular stiffness.

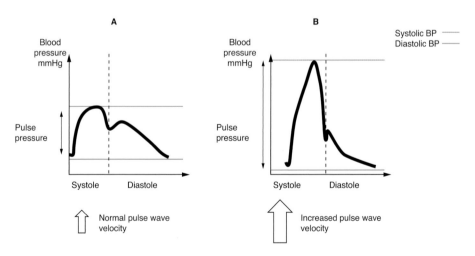

A Young arteries: normal compliance, pulse wave reflection occurs in diastole.
B Ageing arteries: decreased compliance with late systolic peak in blood pressure due to arrival of the reflected pulse wave during systole.

FIGURE 6.1 The relationship between aortic pressure, arterial compliance and pulse wave velocity. (A) Young arteries: normal compliance; pulse wave reflection occurs in diastole. (B) Ageing arteries: decreased compliance with late systolic peak in blood pressure due to the arrival of the reflected pulse wave during systole

CLINICAL IMPLICATIONS

Impact on disease management

Due to these anatomical, physiological and molecular changes, the prevalence of cardiovascular disease increases markedly with age. British Heart Foundation (BHF) statistics show that in the UK in 2008, 35% of all deaths in the aged 65 years or over age group were due to cardiovascular disease. Approximately 13% of men and women over the age of 75 have heart failure and 12% of women and 17% of men in the same age category suffer from angina. In addition, over 65% of those over 75 years of age have hypertension.

The principles of treating heart failure and ischaemic heart disease in older people are similar to those in younger patients. However, the changes that occur in the cardiovascular system with age do have an impact on the management of cardiovascular disease. In particular, orthostatic hypotension and dosing and drug response should be considered.

Orthostatic hypotension

'Orthostatic hypotension' is defined as a drop of 20 mmHg in systolic pressure or of 10 mmHg in diastolic on changing from a supine to an upright position. Blunted baroreceptor responses, decreased cardiac response to sympathetic stimulation, diuretic use and age-related changes in renal function all contribute to the high prevalence of orthostatic hypotension in older people.

In the healthy well-hydrated older patient, cardiac output is maintained on standing. However, dehydration and use of vasodilating drugs can affect this.

Supine hypertension and orthostatic hypotension may coexist. Indeed, long-standing hypertension contributes to the blunting of baroreceptor reflexes. When considering treatment for hypertension, the risk of worsening hypotension in older patients must be taken into account.

Dosing and drug response

Cardiovascular drugs are some of the most commonly prescribed medications in older people. However, the physiological changes with age and the resultant alterations in pharmacokinetics and pharmacodynamics lead to an increased risk of adverse reactions to them. Studies on adverse drug reactions in hospitalised older people have revealed a incidence rate varying from 5% to 31%. Cardiovascular medications are implicated in many of these – 2.4 times as many as other groups of medications.

DIURETICS

Although older patients are more susceptible to the side effects of diuretics (e.g. postural hypotension), they remain key to the management of heart failure in an older population. Due to the age-associated decrease in renal function, doses of loop diuretics may often need to be higher to achieve the same effect as in younger subjects (*see* Chapter 10, 'The kidneys'). However, due to the potential for electrolyte disturbance and renal impairment, the dose should be carefully titrated to the minimum effective level, with close monitoring of fluid balance and electrolytes. Indapamide, a thiazide-like diuretic, has been shown to be of benefit in those aged over 80 years for hypertension and prevention of heart failure. As with thiazide diuretics, it can cause hypokalaemia but has limited effects on glucose and lipid levels.

ANGIOTENSIN-CONVERTING ENZYME (ACE) INHIBITORS AND ANGIOTENSIN II RECEPTOR BLOCKERS

A number of trials have shown reduction in mortality from the use of ACE inhibitors for heart failure in older patients. Angiotensin II receptor blockers are of use in patients for whom ACE-inhibitor side effects are intolerable. Older patients are more susceptible to first-dose hypotension, so it is important to start with a low dose, titrating up slowly. Trial data suggest that ACE inhibitors are generally well tolerated in older people, with a low incidence of postural hypotension. Renal artery stenosis due to atherosclerosis is not uncommon in the older population and ACE inhibitors may precipitate acute renal failure in the case of bilateral renal artery stenosis.

CALCIUM CHANNEL BLOCKERS

There is good evidence for the use of calcium channel blockers, particularly in isolated systolic hypertension in older people. Their use may be limited by side effects, which include peripheral oedema, constipation, postural hypotension and – in the case of non-dihydropyridines such as verapamil – negative inotropic effects. The dihydropyridines, therefore, have restricted use in older people with severely impaired left-ventricular systolic function.

DIGOXIN VERSUS BETA BLOCKERS IN OLDER PEOPLE

Digoxin and beta blockers are some of the most commonly prescribed cardiovascular medications in older people in the treatment of both chronic heart failure and atrial fibrillation (AF).

Digoxin is of most use in patients with both heart failure and AF (a common precipitant of heart failure in older people), in which it is a rate-controlling agent.

Due to renal insufficiency, increased volume of distribution and hypokalaemia, older people have a higher susceptibility to digoxin toxicity for a given dose and its use is associated with an increase in hospital admissions among older patients. Avoiding adverse reactions requires lower maintenance doses and monitoring of serum levels. Digoxin is also subject to a wide array of drug interactions, often with other cardiovascular medications, for example amiodarone and calcium channel blockers, which predispose patients to drug toxicity. Despite this, there is still good evidence for the symptomatic benefit of digoxin for heart failure in older people, although there is no proven mortality benefit.

In contrast, beta blockers have a significant mortality benefit in systolic heart failure in older patients and are generally well tolerated. They are of particular use in the treatment of coronary heart disease through reduction of myocardial oxygen demand and in rate control of AF in active patients.

However, older patients (with an increased prevalence of left-ventricular dysfunction and conduction defects) are more predisposed to adverse effects, which include vasoconstriction, bronchospasm and alterations in glucose and lipid metabolism. This is particularly true in those patients with multiple co-morbidities – for example, peripheral vascular disease, chronic obstructive pulmonary disease and diabetes mellitus – in which beta blockers must be used with caution. Due to the potential for side effects, cardioselective beta blockers such as nebivolol are preferred and have been shown to be well tolerated in older people.

Heart failure

The decreased cardiac response to stress and the changes in left-ventricular filling in diastole predispose the ageing heart to failure. The Framingham Study found a heart failure prevalence of 66 per 1000 in men aged 80–89 years old and 79 per 1000 in women in the same age range. Of those with heart failure, approximately 50% of patients over 70 years old have heart failure with preserved systolic function (or diastolic heart failure). The aetiology of heart failure in older people is, as with younger patients, most commonly due to ischaemia, hypertension or valvular disorders. However, cardiac amyloidosis, calcific aortic stenosis, mitral annulus calcification and mucoid degeneration of the mitral valve are more often seen in older patients and these may contribute to development of heart failure.

An important distinction in older patients is between diastolic heart failure and systolic impairment. 'Diastolic heart failure' (or heart failure with preserved ejection fraction) is defined as symptoms and signs of heart failure coupled with preserved ejection fraction (>50%) and diastolic dysfunction.

Around 30%–40% of patients aged 60–70 years old with heart failure have preserved systolic function and this percentage increases with age. Age-associated change in diastolic function may well explain why fewer younger heart failure patients present with preserved ejection fraction.

Clinically, it may be difficult to distinguish between systolic and diastolic impairment and the definitive investigation is echocardiography. However, studies suggest diastolic heart failure is often found in older hypertensive females and may respond poorly to classical pharmacological therapy.

In heart failure with systolic dysfunction, beta blockers, aldosterone antagonists, ACE inhibitors, angiotensin II receptor blockers, and combined hydralazine and nitrates have been shown to be of prognostic benefit.

In contrast, no pharmacological therapy has been shown to improve clinical outcomes in older patients with diastolic heart failure. However, it is recommended that coexistent hypertension, AF, pulmonary oedema and coronary ischaemia related to diastolic dysfunction be treated.

Conflicting evidence exists regarding the prognosis of diastolic heart failure in older people. Some studies showing significantly better prognosis when compared to systolic failure and others finding no significant difference.

Valvular disease and management

Mitral valve disease in older people is predominantly due to the effects of ischaemia and degeneration of the valve. Calcification of the mitral annulus is seen with age (more often in women) and may contribute to the development of mitral regurgitation. With age, the aortic valve becomes calcified. Degenerative disease of the aortic valve is also associated with smoking, hypertension and male sex and may manifest as aortic stenosis. In The Helsinki Aging Study (1993), a 5% prevalence of moderate to severe aortic stenosis was found in those aged between 75 and 86 years old. Medical treatment for valvular disorders is largely as in younger patients. Aortic valve replacement has low mortality in older people and provides excellent symptomatic relief from aortic stenosis. Bioprosthesis may be preferred as in general these valves do not require long-term anticoagulation.

Transcatheter aortic valve implantation (TAVI) offers a less invasive method of valve replacement for those patients with severe aortic stenosis who are deemed unsuitable for surgical replacement and has shown promising results when compared with medical therapy. The Placement of Aortic Transcatheter Valves trial (PARTNER, 2011) showed that, compared with surgical valve replacement, major vascular complications were more common with TAVI but new AF and bleeding complications were less frequent. This may change with improving techniques. Survival at 1 year for both techniques in severe symptomatic aortic stenosis is similar.

Coronary heart disease

Coronary heart disease accounted for 59 978 deaths in the aged over 75 years population in the UK in 2008 (BHF statistics) and continues to present a huge economic burden. Diastolic dysfunction, decreased response to catecholamines and the stress put upon it by increased arterial stiffness may predispose the ageing heart to ischaemia and infarction.

Clinical presentations in older patients are often atypical, without the classical combination of chest pain, electrocardiography (ECG) and cardiac enzyme changes. The Rotterdam Study (2006) reported the incidence of 'silent' or unrecognised MI in those aged over 55 years old as 3.8 per 1000 person years (the incidence of clinically recognised MI being 5 per 1000 person years).

Worsening diastolic function and afterload increase in older people increases oxygen demand and predisposes patients with ischaemia to develop dyspnoea, which is a common presenting feature of MI. Patients may have a wide range of other presenting features, including atypical chest pains, nausea and neurological symptoms. Older people are also more prone to complications following MI and have a higher mortality following MI than younger patients.

Coronary artery calcification

The pathological significance of the increase in coronary artery calcification seen with age has been the subject of much debate. Despite the strong association between calcification and age, there is marked heterogeneity in degree of calcification among older people; in some individuals it is negligible. In younger people, the degree of coronary calcification is heavily influenced by other cardiovascular risk factors (e.g. smoking), however, this effect may be attenuated in older populations.

Studies have shown that the presence of coronary artery calcification is a highly sensitive but moderately specific predictor of significant atherosclerotic stenosis. This can be improved using age-specific threshold scores. Although much of the evidence supporting this comes from studies in younger people, research looking specifically at the older population supports the idea that coronary artery calcification remains an independent indicator of prognosis, even in older age groups.

Management of coronary artery disease

THROMBOLYSIS

The side effects of bleeding and intracranial haemorrhage tend to be more prevalent in older patients than in younger with thrombolysis, although the risk is low overall.

PERCUTANEOUS CORONARY INTERVENTION (PCI) IN OLDER PEOPLE

PCI is often avoided in older people, perhaps due to perceived technical difficulties with increasingly tortuous, non-compliant vessels. However, evidence suggests that it can be beneficial in this group.

Several trials have found that PCI in eligible older patients has more favourable outcomes than fibrinolytic therapies, including decreased 30-day mortality, re-infarction rate and stroke incidence in patients with ST elevation MI. Three large randomised controlled trials have favoured an early invasive strategy (i.e. angiography and PCI if appropriate) over best medical management and subsequent angiography if this had failed. However, a mortality benefit in these cases has not been demonstrated as yet.

Cardiac arrhythmias

Fibrosis of the conduction system and loss of sino-atrial node cells predisposes the ageing heart to cardiac arrhythmia. ECG monitoring of older patients has revealed an increase in the number of ectopic beats seen with age and a prolongation of the PR interval. As with ischaemia, presentation may be quite vague. However, the management of arrhythmias is similar to that in younger patients.

AF and anticoagulation

AF is one of the most common arrhythmias seen in older people (over 5% of those aged over 75 years old). The Atrial Fibrillation Follow-up Investigation of Rhythm Management (AFFIRM) trial found no benefit of rhythm control over rate control strategies, with both groups requiring anticoagulation. Rate control tends to be preferred in older people due to poor tolerance of cardioverting drugs and high risk of recurrence after DC cardioversion. Beta blockers, calcium channel blockers and digoxin are all options for rate control, with digoxin providing less control of ventricular rate during exercise. Those with refractory symptoms may respond to pacing.

Older patients have the greatest absolute benefit from oral anticoagulation in AF, despite the risk of haemorrhage. The recent Birmingham Atrial Fibrillation Treatment of the Aged Study (BAFTA) in patients aged 75 years or older, showed fewer major strokes, intracranial haemorrhages or systemic emboli in those in AF randomised to warfarin than in those randomised to aspirin. Warfarin is superior to aspirin in the absence of contraindications. However, older patients are prone to over-anticoagulation with warfarin, often with poor dietary intake of vitamin K, concomitant liver disease or the use of antiplatelet agents.

Newer oral anticoagulants such as dabigatran, an oral direct thrombin inhibitor, have shown promise in the prevention of stroke in older patients. These drugs have a good side-effect profile in older people, but they are not as easily monitored as warfarin and the potential for over-anticoagulation may be high, especially in those with renal impairment, and long-term side effects will need to be followed up.

Hypertension

BHF statistics for 2008 reported that 68% of men and 73% of women aged over 75 years old have hypertension, an important risk factor for stroke and MI. Increasing arterial stiffness and endothelial dysfunction leads to an increase in systolic blood pressure in older people. This often manifests as isolated systolic hypertension, although systolic/diastolic hypertension does often exist.

The HYVET trial (2008) provided evidence that blood pressure reduction continues to have mortality and morbidity benefit in those aged 80 years and older, although there is still some debate about appropriate blood pressure targets.

Hypertension in older people is often the result of the interactions between a variety of risk factors, for example high salt diets and obesity. These should be modified where possible. Exercise has been found to decrease the rate of decline in arterial compliance.

Anti-hypertensives have also been shown to slow the decline in compliance. Current National Institute for Health and Clinical Excellence guidance (2011) recommends calcium channel blockers as first-line treatment in those aged over 55 years old, with the addition of an ACE inhibitor or angiotensin receptor blocker if hypertension remains uncontrolled. If the patient remains hypertensive, addition of a thiazide-like diuretic is advised. Thiazide-like diuretics (e.g. indapamide) should be considered for those at high risk or with evidence of heart failure. A study of indapamide showed it to be more selective for the reduction of systolic blood pressure, with relatively little effect on the diastolic in comparison to calcium channel blockers and ACE inhibitors, thus minimising the risk of hypotension.

Choice of anti-hypertensive should be guided by individual patients' characteristics including co-morbidities and other medications, which may often be extensive in older patients. Combinations of anti-hypertensives are often required.

Beta blockers should be considered in those with a history of MI. However, relative to other anti-hypertensives, there is an increased risk of stroke. Unlike calcium channel blockers and ACE inhibitors, they have no effect on reflection of the systolic pulse wave that contributes to systolic hypertension in older people.

CARDIOVASCULAR RISK FACTORS AND MECHANISMS IN OLDER PEOPLE

The changes seen with age in the cardiovascular system are subject to modification by the presence of cardiovascular risk factors. The effects of both modifiable and non-modifiable risk and protective factors on cardiovascular ageing are outlined in Table 6.1.

TABLE 6.1 Effects of modifiable and non-modifiable risk and protective factors on cardiovascular ageing

Cardiovascular risk/ protective factor	Effect(s) on cardiovascular ageing and disease
Sex	Females on hormone replacement – increase in prevalence of MI and stroke
	Androgen deficiency or excess increases cardiovascular morbidity
Race	Afro-Caribbean people have accelerated arterial ageing, aortic stiffness, left-ventricular wall thickness and higher stroke risk
Smoking	Decreased arterial compliance
Dietary factors	Low sodium and fish oils improve endothelial function and increase arterial compliance

Cardiovascular risk/ protective factor	Effect(s) on cardiovascular ageing and disease
Obesity	Increased arterial stiffness
Alcohol	Moderate intake – decreased arterial stiffness, lower cardiovascular risk
	High intake – hypertension
Exercise	Protects against oxidative stress in endothelial wall and myocardium
	Improves baroreceptor reflexes
	Increases VO$_2$ max
	Induces angiogenesis
	Increases arterial compliance
	Slows development of left-ventricular diastolic dysfunction

CONCLUSION

Age is a key risk factor for cardiac disease. Changes seen in the heart as part of the 'normal' ageing process provide a background upon which pathological dysfunction can develop. The more we can understand about the complexities of ageing and the interactions between age and other cardiac risk factors, the more we may be able to begin to view age as a potentially modifiable risk factor in the development of disease.

FURTHER READING

AFFIRM: Olshansky B, Rosenfeld LE, Warner AL *et al.*, AFFIRM investigators. The Atrial Fibrillation Follow-up Investigation of Rhythm Management (AFFIRM) study: approaches to control rate in atrial fibrillation. *J Am Coll Cardiol.* 2004; **43**(7): 1201–8.

BAFTA: Mant J, Hobbs FD, Fletcher K *et al.*, BAFTA investigators. Warfarin versus aspirin for stroke prevention in an elderly community population with atrial fibrillation (the Birmingham Atrial Fibrillation Treatment of the Aged Study, BAFTA): a randomised controlled trial. *Lancet.* 2007; **370**(9586): 493–503.

Fleg JL, Strait J. Age-associated changes in cardiovascular structure and function: a fertile milieu for future disease. *Heart Fail Rev.* 2011; **17**(4–5): 545–54.

Framingham Heart Study: Cheng S, Xanthakis V, Sullivan LM *et al.* Correlates of echocardiographic indices of cardiac remodeling over the adult life course: longitudinal observations from the Framingham Heart Study. *Circulation.* 2010; **122**(6): 570–8.

HYVET: Beckett NS, Peters R, Fletcher AE *et al.* Treatment of hypertension in patients 80 years of age or older. *N Engl J Med.* 2008; **358**(18): 1887–98.

Lakatta EG, Levy D. Arterial and cardiac aging: major shareholders in cardiovascular disease enterprises. Part II: the aging heart in health: links to heart disease. *Circulation.* 2003; **107**(2): 346–54.

Lindroos M, Kupari M, Heikkilä J *et al.* Prevalence of aortic valve abnormalities in the elderly: an echocardiographic study of a random population sample. *J Am Coll Cardiol.* 1993; **21**(5): 1220–5.

National Institute for Health and Clinical Excellence. *Hypertension: clinical management of primary hypertension in adults.* NICE guideline 127. London: NIHCE; 2011.

Scarborough P, Bhatnagar P, Wickramasinghe K *et al. Coronary Heart Disease Statistics 2010 Edition.* London: British Heart Foundation; 2010.

PARTNER Trial: Smith CR, Leon MB, Mack MJ, PARTNER Trial Investigators. Transcatheter versus surgical aortic-valve replacement in high-risk patients. *N Engl J Med.* 2011; **364**(23): 2187.

The Rotterdam Study: de Torbal A, Boersma E, Kors JA *et al.* Incidence of recognized and unrecognized myocardial infarction in men and women aged 55 and older: the Rotterdam Study. *Eur Heart J.* 2006; **27**(6): 729–36.

QUESTIONS: THE CARDIOVASCULAR SYSTEM

1 A number of physiological changes occur in the ageing heart. Which one of the following is not true of normal ageing?

A decreased heart rate variability with standing
B increased early diastolic filling of the left ventricle
C increased late diastolic filling
D systolic blood pressure continues to rise from the age of 50 years
E the pulse pressure increases with ageing.

Answer: B

2 With regard to the management of hypertension in older people, which one of the following statements is correct?

A ACE inhibitors are first-line management for hypertension in older people
B blood pressure reduction has no mortality benefit in those over 80 years old
C calcium channel blockers are recommended for hypertension in patients with evidence of heart failure
D hypertension does not contribute to the development of orthostatic hypotension
E regular aerobic exercise contributes towards blood pressure lowering in older people.

Answer: E

3 Heart failure in older patients is associated with a decline in physical function. Which one of the following statements regarding heart failure is true?

A age-related changes in diastolic function do not predispose to heart failure
B heart failure with preserved ejection fraction is more common in older hypertensive men
C the 5-year mortality in patients with ejection fraction less than 25% is now less than 15% due to improvements in heart failure management
D the aetiology of heart failure in older people is most commonly ischaemia, valvular disease or hypertension
E the majority of patients aged over 65 years with heart failure have preserved ejection fraction (>50%).

Answer: D

4 With regard to exercise, which has a number of beneficial effects in older people, which one of the following statements is false?

A early diastolic filling does not change on acute exercise
B exercise improves baroreceptor reflex function
C exercise induces oxidative stress in the myocardium
D exercise slows age-related decline in left-ventricular diastolic function
E with age, there is a decrease in maximum heart rate with exercise.

Answer: C

5 Cardiac medications are associated with a number of adverse effects in older people. Which one of the following statements is not true?

A beta blockers do not affect the systolic pulse wave
B despite side effects, oral anticoagulants have the greatest absolute benefit in older patients
C due to renal impairment, older patients often require a decreased dose of loop diuretics to achieve good diuresis
D no pharmacological therapy has been shown to be of prognostic benefit in heart failure with preserved ejection fraction
E older patients are more susceptible to first-dose hypotension when commenced on ACE inhibitors.

Answer: C

CHAPTER 7

The respiratory system

MARTIN R MILLER

INTRODUCTION

There is considerable discussion around what constitutes normal ageing and how the effects of ageing on humans differ from those due to disease. For example, how much atherosclerosis in the arterial tree can be considered to be due to normal ageing or is it all due to disease? The lungs are exposed to atmospheric conditions from the moment of birth and there is considerable evidence relating occupational and environmental airborne exposure to lung disease. The species *Homo sapiens* has successfully manipulated their environment so that they are alone as a species in having doubled their life expectancy. Is it then reasonable to consider some of the deleterious effects of these manipulations as diseases when they have extended life expectancy? For instance, using an open fire inside caves to produce warmth would have exposed the occupants to smoke from biomass fuel and possibly harmed the lungs.

In the twenty-first century, many humans are able to protect themselves from the deleterious effects of exposure to many environmental pollutants but others cannot. No one can live in a perfectly controlled atmosphere and so everyone will to some extent be exposed to noxious elements in the atmosphere and their lungs may be adversely affected. We have no record of normal human beings living in a completely clean atmosphere, so we do not know whether lungs would age more slowly under these conditions. Data from animals raised and maintained in a clean environment show no change in the alveoli with age, which is contrary to findings in humans. This led to the hypothesis that lung ageing is due to environmental exposures. It is known that patients with the genetically defined lung disease due to deficiency in alpha-1 antitrypsin, an enzyme that protects against harmful circulating proteases, have a better prognosis if they are not exposed to tobacco smoke and live in a relatively smoke-free environment.

The primary function of the lungs is gas exchange, in which air is brought in very close proximity to blood to allow the transfer of O_2 into the blood and the removal of carbon dioxide (CO_2) from the blood. The lungs are not only exposed to noxious elements in the inspired air, but they also receive the whole cardiac output, so are exposed to any circulating agents that might be harmful. In fact, the lungs have a metabolic role in clearing a number of substances from the circulation. It is known that trauma releases noxious substances into the blood that can lead to oxidative stress for the lungs. In severe cases, this causes adult respiratory distress syndrome. How much minor everyday trauma might contribute in this way to lung function decline is not known.

The number of older subjects in the population is ever increasing because of our extended life expectancy. Therefore, it is clinically important to be able to distinguish changes in lung function that result from 'natural' ageing from those due to disease processes so that accurate diagnosis and prognosis is possible and disease monitoring and therapeutic interventions can be reliably undertaken.

We know that lung function declines with age and this chapter will outline what we know of the processes involved, by considering how ageing affects the alveoli, the conducting airways, the chest wall, gas exchange and, finally, breathing control.

ALVEOLI

The principal observed change in the lungs with age is an increase in alveolar size without any inflammation or alveolar wall destruction. This change is different from emphysema, in which the increase in alveolar size is also associated with alveolar wall destruction. Skin ageing is associated with a loss of elastin support in the dermis, so it is intuitively attractive to think the same is happening in the lungs, especially as diseases such as emphysema are thought to involve changes in elastin within the lungs. However, this loss of recoil is not related to any change in elastin, with the amount of elastin and collagen in the lung parenchyma not appearing to change with age.

The elastic recoil of the lungs is reduced with ageing, as shown in Figure 7.1. This loss of recoil appears to be due to a reduction in the surface tension forces from all the alveoli, since their individual diameters have been increased. Alveoli act like small bubbles with a thin layer of fluid over their surfaces. Laplace's law means that the surface tension force from this surface of fluid is much greater for a small bubble compared with a larger one. Thus, an increase in alveolar size reduces the surface tension force and so reduces lung recoil. Early experiments measured recoil pressure in air-inflated lungs and then compared this with fluid-filled lungs. They showed that most of the so-called elastic recoil force from the lungs was due to the surface tension forces in the surfactant. What little is known about changes in the surfactant with age suggests there are no significant changes in its properties, but these findings will need further confirmation. Several researchers who have studied the pathology of lungs in older people have demonstrated the increased airspace diameter of the alveoli with age. They have showed an increased distance between airspace walls (called the 'mean linear intercept') with age. As lungs inflate, the helical fibre network uncoils around the alveolar ducts and adjacent alveoli, thus maintaining an even tension on the alveolar walls so that they do not crinkle or collapse as the lung inflates and deflates. It is still not clearly understood why alveolar spaces increase with age, but it is likely that changes in the coiling structure of the helical fibre network around the alveolar ducts lead to a larger alveolus and alveolar ducts. This causes an evenly distributed increase in the size of all alveoli with age with no destruction of alveolar walls.

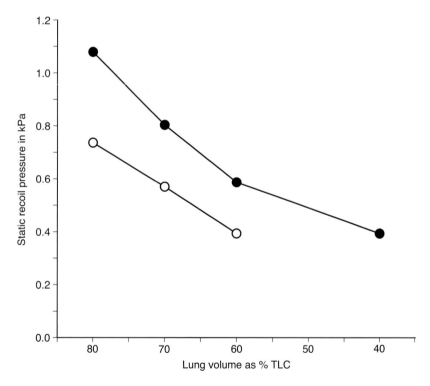

FIGURE 7.1 Static recoil pressure plotted against lung volume as a percentage of total lung capacity (TLC) for men aged 35–45 years (closed circles) and men aged 65–75 years (open circles). Adapted from Babb TG, Rodarte JR. Mechanism of reduced maximal expiratory flow with aging. *J Appl Physiol.* 2000; **89**(2): 505–11

As an alveolus increases in size, its surface area becomes larger, but that area, as a proportion of the volume of the alveolus, is now smaller, so gas exchange from ventilating this volume is less effective. The proportion of all the air in the lungs that is in the alveoli reduces with age, while the proportion in the alveolar ducts and respiratory bronchioles increases to a greater extent, thus increasing the inter-alveolar distances.

CONDUCTING AIRWAYS

For a large part of the maximum forced expiratory manoeuvre the exhaled flow is not effort dependent but depends on the elastic recoil at the given lung volume as driving pressure. Therefore, any reduction in the elastic recoil should have an influence on the expiratory airflow and this has been confirmed as the cause of reduced expiratory flow with age. A more compliant airway can collapse more easily during expiration, which would also lead to a reduced maximum flow. Figure 7.2 shows that, for any given recoil pressure, the maximum flow in older subjects is the same as that in younger subjects, so changes in airway resistance are not the reason for reduced airflow with ageing.

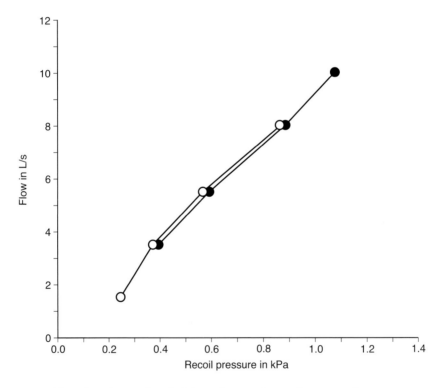

FIGURE 7.2 Plot of expiratory flow in L/s against static recoil pressure in young men aged 35–45 years (closed circles) and older men aged 65–75 years (open circles). Adapted from Verbeken EK *et al.* The senile lung. 2. Functional aspects. *Chest.* 1992; **101**(3): 800–9

'Closing volume' (CV) is the volume of gas that can still be exhaled, starting from the point of sharp change in alveolar concentration of nitrogen or tracer gas after the alveolar plateau, during a long slow exhalation; this point indicates that some basal airways have just closed. The sum of residual volume and CV is called the 'closing capacity' (CC) and this can be expressed as a percentage of total lung capacity (TLC). In young adults, CC is about 10% of TLC or cannot be detected. The CC increases linearly with age to be about 30% of TLC at the age of 70 years. This airway closure may arise because with less elastic recoil the airways are less well supported and collapse. The CC in normal subjects usually remains well below functional residual capacity (FRC), even in old age, thus this airway collapse does not usually cause problems with gas exchange (*see* pp. 87–8). However, with age the airways close off progressively earlier during an expiratory manoeuvre, so the residual volume (RV) in the lungs increases with age. In disease states such as chronic obstructive pulmonary disease and emphysema the CC can be above the FRC. This impinges on tidal breathing, cutting off areas of the lungs from gas exchange, thus causing hypoxia.

CHEST WALL

The alveolar ventilation required for gas exchange is achieved by the action of the diaphragm and respiratory muscles to expand the thorax causing air to be inhaled into the lungs. Age-related changes in the respiratory muscles and the characteristics of the chest wall affect ventilation.

With age, there are alterations in the three-dimensional shape of the thorax that are due to the age-related tendency to stoop and develop kyphosis. This is partly due to loss of vertebral height with age and partly due to muscular changes. These changes cause an increase in the anteroposterior diameter of the chest. However, a longitudinal study of patients with marked and mild scoliosis found there was no excessive decrement in lung function over more than 10 years except in those with the most extreme kyphosis (kyphosis angles >100 degrees). Therefore, the normal slight tendency to stoop with age does not seem to cause a significant effect on lung function. However, loss of height with age may lead to an underestimation of the relation between height and predicted lung function – so, when making predictions about such a subject's lung function it may be better to use the height recorded at an earlier age or use arm span as a surrogate for height.

The thoracic cage becomes less compliant with age; that is, it requires a greater force to deform or change its shape. The 'functional residual capacity' is the natural resting position of the respiratory system when all muscles are relaxed. At FRC, the chest wall is trying to expand back to its natural resting position but is checked from doing so by the inward elastic recoil of the lungs. Thus, the outward force from the chest wall is balanced by the elastic recoil from the lungs. With age, not only is the lung elastic recoil reduced (*see* Figure 7.1) but the chest wall also resists deformation more forcefully than in younger subjects, so the FRC tends to increase with age, as does RV. Figure 7.3 shows the changes between the ages of 30 and 70 for a man 1.77 m tall taken from the cross-sectional equations commonly used to predict lung function. This shows how RV and FRC tend to increase with age whereas forced vital capacity (FVC) and forced expiratory volume in 1 second (FEV$_1$) fall.

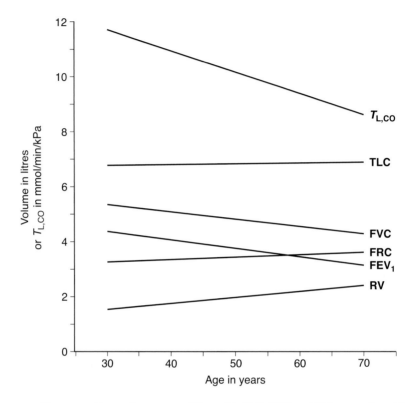

FIGURE 7.3 Changes with age for a man 1.77 m tall in TLC, FRC and RV, as predicted from the equations of Crapo RO *et al. Bull Europ Physiopath Resp.* 1982; **18**: 419–25, FVC and forced expiratory volume in 1 second (FEV$_1$), as predicted from the equations of Hankinson JL *et al. Am J Crit Care Med Respir.* 1999; **159**(1): 179–87, and lung transfer factor ($T_{L,CO}$), as predicted from the equations of Miller A *et al. Am Rev Respir Dis.* 1983; **127**: 270–7

General muscle strength is known to decline with age and the degree of this muscle weakness is independently a predictor of future disability. Age-related decline in respiratory muscle strength means diaphragm strength is up to 25% lower in the seventh decade than in subjects in their second decade. A subject's TLC is measured at the point of maximum inflation, which is determined by the strength of respiratory muscles that have to work against the summed force of the elastic recoil of the lungs and the chest wall's resistance to expansion. Therefore, the reduced elastic recoil with age should mean a significant increase in TLC, but as this is mitigated by the age-related increased stiffness of the chest wall and reduced muscle strength, the TLC does not greatly increase with age (*see* Figure 7.3).

These effects are summarised in Figure 7.4 as principal effects and their consequences.

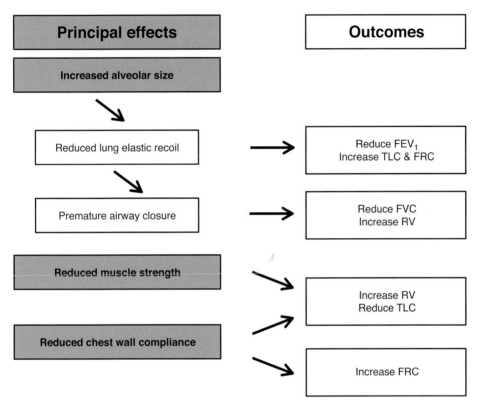

FIGURE 7.4 Outline of the principal effects of ageing on the lungs and the outcome these have on lung function

GAS EXCHANGE

Figure 7.3 shows that the transfer factor for lungs is known to reduce with age. Resting arterial O_2 tension falls slightly with age but is stable after the age of 70 years. Although the alveolar surface area increases with age, the surface area in relation to alveolar ventilation is reduced and the blood supply to these alveoli does not match the increase in surface area. This means gas exchange is impaired. The distribution of ventilation ($\dot{V}_A$) and perfusion ($\dot{Q}$) across the lungs changes with age. In young subjects in the upright position, the distribution of $\dot{V}_A/\dot{Q}$ is relatively uniform, but in older subjects the scatter of the distribution of both $\dot{V}_A$ and $\dot{Q}$ is increased. Therefore, there are proportionally more lung units with high $\dot{V}_A/\dot{Q}$ and more lung units with low $\dot{V}_A/\dot{Q}$ in older subjects than in young. Those areas with a high $\dot{V}_A/\dot{Q}$ have wasted ventilation and those units with low $\dot{V}_A/\dot{Q}$ result in hypoxia. Both these effects mean gas exchange is impaired. A study in subjects up to the age of 70 years old found the dispersion of $\dot{V}_A/\dot{Q}$ increased by about 25% between the ages of 20 and 60 years, which was found to account for the observed alveolar arterial O_2 difference in older subjects. The slight increase in CV in older subjects (*see* p. 84) was shown not to contribute to the age-related changes in dispersion of $\dot{V}_A/\dot{Q}$.

CONTROL OF VENTILATION

Age-related changes in the control of ventilation might influence the response to exercise in older subjects and might affect the propensity to develop sleep-related disordered breathing. A 6-year longitudinal study of exceptionally fit and active people aged over 60 years showed the expected decline in measures of expiratory flow, increase in CV and decline in exercise performance, with an 11% drop in maximum O_2 consumption over the duration of the study, which was associated with higher exercise ventilation. A major part of this reduction is due to age-related reduction in cardiac performance rather than changes in the respiratory system. However, older subjects have a greater increase in ventilation ($\Delta\dot{V}_E$) to exercise, higher CO_2 production and higher O_2 consumption at all levels of work. In older people at rest, the ventilatory sensitivity to changes in arterial partial pressure of carbon dioxide in the blood ($PaCO_2$) – $\Delta PaCO_2$ – has been found to be not as great as in the young, but this sensitivity increases considerably during exercise. As the slope of $\Delta\dot{V}_E$ to $\Delta PaCO_2$ in older people is much higher during exercise, this enhanced ventilatory response helps counter the less good gas exchange from increased $\dot{V}_A/\dot{Q}$ dispersion, maintaining isocapnia during exercise.

During sleep, the ventilatory response to changes in $PaCO_2$ decreases in all subjects. However, as central sleep apnoeas are more common in older people, it was thought possible that the response to changes in $PaCO_2$ might decline with age. A study of steady-state ventilatory responses to $PaCO_2$ in a group of older normal subjects in their seventh to ninth decade found responses were similar in both awake and sleeping states in comparison to those for subjects in their third to fourth decade. Both age groups showed the same degree of reduced response on falling asleep. Thus, there appears to be no change in CO_2 responses with age to account for the observed increase in central apnoeas with age. This means that they presumably relate to unknown changes in the central controlling mechanism.

PREDICTING LUNG FUNCTION IN OLDER PEOPLE

When assessing a patient, it is common for the patient's lung function to be judged against an expected value for that patient to determine if they have evidence of unusual change in lung function that might reflect a disease process. Performing lung function tests is a complex task and may not be possible in older patients with confusion or dementia. Being unable to perform satisfactory lung function tests has been shown to be an independent predictor of poor subsequent patient survival.

To prepare prediction equations for lung function data, very large surveys of the normal population who are free of disease or any other factors that might adversely affect lung function need to be carried out. Such studies are expensive and difficult to perform, and obtaining representative samples of subjects over the age of 70 is problematic. For example, the prediction equations used for FVC and FEV_1 in Figure 7.3 were only derived from subjects up to the age of 70 years old. Using these equations for older subjects means extrapolating the data without any confidence that the predictions are valid. In the near future, new equations pertaining to people up to the age of 95 years should be available from the Global Lungs Initiative (*see* 'Further reading'), which should be a tremendous help. Most equations for lung function have predictions based on age, sex and height; however, as already noted, in older people there is a reduction in height due to loss of height in the vertebral column and changes in posture. These changes are unlikely to have an impact on the lung size within the thorax, so using an inappropriately low height for a subject due to these age-related changes may lead to underestimation of the predicted lung function. This may mean that any true changes in function are also underestimated. Thus, if an older subject knows what their true height was, say, when aged 40, this might be a more appropriate height to use in the prediction equation.

Having obtained a predicted value, the next question is how to relate this to the patient's value. As absolute values for FEV_1 and FVC fall with age, the commonly applied method of 'percent of predicted' means small deviations from predicted give disproportionate changes in percent of predicted compared with younger subjects who have higher predicted values. Thus, an 80% predicted rule introduces an age bias, meaning older subjects are more likely to be deemed abnormal when their lung function is actually within the normal 90% confidence limits adopted for lung function indices. Therefore, it is especially important not to apply the percent of predicted method to lung function data in older people. Instead, the method of standardised residuals (SRs), which are the same as z-scores, should be employed, with SR = (observed value – predicted value)/RSD, where 'RSD' is the residual standard deviation from the prediction equation (which is also called the standard error of the estimate and is a measure of the scatter in the normal population). An SR value of -1.645 is an estimate of the lower 90% confidence limit. With respect to survival, it is not how far a subject's value is above or below their predicted that matters, but how far their lung function is from the 'bottom line'. Since lung function values are affected by sex and height, it has been shown that FEV_1 and FVC divided by the cube of height are the best predictors of subsequent survival.

All current prediction equations have been derived from cross-sectional studies; thus subjects aged 70 years old in any such study would have had a different life experience in terms of nutrition and upbringing than subjects aged

30. This cohort effect means that the estimated annual change in lung function from cross-sectional studies may overestimate the true annual decline in a subject. Thus, the best we can do is to use the available equations, realising their potential limitations. The advent of the new Global Lungs Initiative equations should be of tremendous benefit to those involved in assessing older patients.

CLINICAL IMPLICATIONS

With age there is an expected reduction in exercise capacity, which is mainly related to changes in cardiovascular performance and not due to any reduction the gas-exchanging properties of the lungs. In Westernised and affluent societies, obesity is an increasing problem, especially in older subjects due to a failure to reduce food intake as both exercise activity and metabolic rate decrease with age. Obesity per se will affect chest wall mechanics and reduce lung function – it is important to attribute these changes to the clinical problem of obesity and not to the natural ageing of the lungs.

Do the age-related changes in lungs predispose older people to developing pulmonary disease? Older people are especially prone to pneumonia, which is a common cause of death in this age group. The major reasons for this susceptibility relate to reduced protection of the airway as a consequence of loss of muscle strength and a reduction in cough effectiveness. Moreover, poorer dental and oral hygiene and an increased incidence of spontaneous aspiration while asleep lead to increased exposure of the lungs to pathogens. Immune defences, including splenic function, are impaired, so the clearance of pneumococci from the bloodstream is less effective and means that when infections occur they can be much more devastating than in younger subjects.

The age-related changes in lung function described in this chapter actually play only a small part in increasing risk of disease. However, as lung function declines with age, if the absolute values of spirometry indices, such as the FVC or FEV_1, fall as low as 0.5 L, then the ability to maintain adequate ventilation becomes impaired and mortality increases dramatically. Lung function is one of the most important predictors of long-term survival at any age. In a study of 95-year-olds, lung function has been found to be still an important predictor of survival and was second only to dementia, which was the most important predictor. It is likely that low function means that intercurrent events, such as pneumonia, stroke or an accident, become lethal events because lung function is now insufficient to cope with the changed clinical circumstances.

There is a large range of values found in the normal population for any given age and height. What determines where a particular subject lies in this distribution will relate to genes inherited from their parents and their lung growth, which begins *in utero* and continues through childhood. It can thus be appreciated that subjects aged 90 in the year 2012 will have grown up in the 1920s when nutrition and environmental circumstances, which can affect lung growth, were very different from those of today. If a subject entered adult-hood in the lower range of normal function due to problems affecting their lung growth, then the expected annual decrements in function might lead to lung function reaching critical levels in old age which might not occur in more advantaged (genetically and environmentally) subjects.

CONCLUSION

Age has a marked effect on lung function but in a relatively predictable way. This chapter has given an overview of this, explaining the main age-related changes affecting the lungs. The changes with age presented in Figure 7.3 are taken from equations predicting lung function from cross-sectional surveys. It is known that these data include cohort effects, that is the subjects aged 70 years provide lung function data having had a completely different child-hood and young adult experience to those aged 30, which may have affected lung growth. In fact, true longitudinal change tends to be less than that shown from cross-sectional data. However, reasonable predictions can be made for subjects that take into account the expected changes due to age. When assess-ing older patients and determining if they truly have any effect from disease on their lungs, it is essential that clinicians understand and take into account the age-related changes in lung function discussed here.

FURTHER READING

Babb TG, Rodarte JR. Mechanism of reduced maximal expiratory flow with aging. *J Appl Physiol.* 2000; **89**(2): 505–11.

Global Lungs Initiative. www.lungfunction.org

Janssens JP, Pache JC, Nicod LP. Physiological changes in respiratory function associated with ageing. *Eur Respir J.* 1999; **13**(1): 197–205.

Kirkwood TB. Understanding the odd science of aging. *Cell.* 2005; **120**(4): 437–47.

McClaran SR, Babcock MA, Pegelow DF, *et al.* Longitudinal effects of aging on lung func-tion at rest and exercise in healthy active fit elderly adults. *J Appl Physiol.* 1995; **78**: 1957–68.

Verbeken EK, Cauberghs M, Mertens I *et al.* The senile lung: comparison with normal and emphysematous lungs. 1. Structural aspects. *Chest.* 1992; **101**(3): 793–9.

——. The senile lung: comparison with normal and emphysematous lungs. 2. Functional aspects. *Chest.* 1992; **101**(3): 800–9.

LIST OF ABBREVIATIONS

$\dot{V}_A$	alveolar ventilation per minute
Δ	change in an index (delta)
$\Delta\dot{V}_E$	change in ventilation per minute
CC	closing capacity
CO_2	carbon dioxide
CV	closing volume
$\dot{V}_E$	expiratory ventilation per minute
FEV_1	forced expiratory volume in 1 second
FRC	functional residual capacity
FVC	forced vital capacity
O_2	oxygen
$\dot{Q}$	perfusion per minute
$\dot{V}_A/\dot{Q}$	ratio of alveolar ventilation to perfusion
RV	residual volume
TLC	total lung capacity

QUESTIONS: THE RESPIRATORY SYSTEM

1 The resting ventilatory position (FRC) is increased with age due to:
 A increased chest wall compliance
 B increased residual volume
 C premature airway closure
 D reduced lung elastic recoil
 E reduced respiratory muscle strength.

Answer: D

Comment: *Elastic recoil is reduced with age, so the force tending to collapse the lungs around the resting ventilatory position is reduced and chest wall expansion stretches the lungs to a higher FRC. Chest wall compliance is reduced in age. Premature airway closure affects RV not FRC. Muscle strength is not pertinent around the resting ventilatory position, in which all muscles are relaxed. FRC can vary independently of RV.*

2 Reduced respiratory muscle strength significantly contributes to age-related:
 A arterial hypoxia
 B increased closing volume
 C increased residual volume
 D increased total lung capacity
 E reduced exercise capacity.

Answer: C

Comment: *Poorer muscle function means the chest wall cannot be forced into as low as volume as before, especially since the chest wall is less compliant. Arterial hypoxia relates to $\dot{V}_A/\dot{Q}$ changes. CV is increased due to less elastic recoil and so less airway support. Increased muscle strength would be needed to increase TLC. Lower exercise capacity is largely due to cardiac performance changes.*

3 Compared with younger subjects, for a given level of exercise in older people:
 A arterial oxygen falls
 B CO_2 production is increased
 C closing volume is reduced
 D O_2 consumption is reduced
 E the ventilatory response is reduced.

Answer: B

Comment: *CO_2 production, O_2 consumption and the ventilatory response are all increased. There is no hypoxia, and CV would tend to increase as breathing frequency increases.*

4 Arterial partial pressure of O_2 is slightly lower in older people due to:
   A   reduced alveolar ventilation
   B   reduced muscle strength
   C   reduced ventilatory response to CO_2
   D   reduced ventilatory response to hypoxia
   E   ventilation to perfusion distribution abnormalities.

Answer: E

Comment: *While O_2 and CO_2 responses may be slightly reduced at rest, they do not contribute to resting O_2 levels. Muscle strength does not affect resting ventilation levels or cause alveolar hypoventilation in older people.*

5 Pneumonia in older people is more of a problem due to:
   A   increased closing volume
   B   pre-existing ventilation perfusion abnormalities
   C   reduced lung compliance
   D   reduced muscle strength
   E   reduced ventilatory response to CO_2.

Answer: D

Comment: *Reduced cough effectiveness and lack of deep inhalation to ventilate basal areas due to reduced muscle strength predisposes individuals to pneumonia and increases the chances of a poor outcome. CO_2 responses and increasing CV are not relevant and existing $\dot{V}_A/\dot{Q}$ abnormalities are trivial when compared with those resulting from types of pneumonia.*

CHAPTER 8

The gastrointestinal system

HASAN HABOUBI, TANVIR AHMED AND NADIM HABOUBI

INTRODUCTION

Although the physiological changes in the ageing gastrointestinal (GI) tract can be subtle, these effects can place an older person at increased risk during illness. Such changes include: the physiological anorexia of ageing, which predisposes older people to malnutrition, especially when acutely ill; presbyoesphagus, a condition characterised by alteration in motor function of the oesophagus as a result of degenerative changes occurring with advancing age, which may lead to increased reflux disease, dysphagia and aspiration pneumonia; and atrophic gastritis, which can cause decreased absorption of calcium, iron and vitamin B_{12}. Furthermore, changes in small-bowel motor pattern may be associated with dyspepsia, small bowel overgrowth and irritable bowel syndrome. In the large bowel, thickening of the colon wall can lead to increased forced contractions causing diverticula. A common occurrence in older people is change in intestinal motility, often leading to constipation and, at times, faecal incontinence.

This chapter provides an understanding of the biological and physiological changes of the GI tract in older people and their clinical consequences.

GUT HORMONES AND CHANGES WITH AGEING

Cholecystokinin (CCK) is released in the proximal bowel in response to nutrients from the antrum, particularly lipids and proteins. Its predominant functions are to stimulate the release of pancreatic enzymes to assist with digestion and to produce bile, with gall bladder contraction and sphincter of Oddi relaxation, resulting in bile release into the duodenum, emulsifying fats. However, CCK has been shown to cause increased satiety, predominantly through a mechanism of reduced gastric emptying, although central effects may also be contributory. Elevated levels of CCK have been demonstrated in older people and have been correlated with increased satiety and reduced hunger.

Pancreatic polypeptide (PP), and its peptide family members peptide YY (PYY) and neuropeptide Y (NPY), have also been shown to have an effect on the hunger–satiety equilibrium. Despite similarities in their chemical structures, their actions and locations of release are quite distinct: the pancreas secretes PP, PYY is released in the distal intestine in the presence of nutrients in the lumen and NPY is a neurotransmitter found in both the central and peripheral nervous systems.

PP, released following a meal, has a multitude of local effects. It is thought to reduce gall bladder contraction and bowel motility and also has inhibitory effects on pancreatic exocrine function. PYY also exerts its effects through slower gut motility and inhibits NPY, causing satiety. Both CCK and PYY are enteric peptides involved in GI motility in response to eating. High levels of fasting and postprandial CCK and PYY may cause prolonged satiety by slowing antral emptying.

The hypothalamus controls hunger and satiety. The nucleus arcuatus has neurons that release NPY and agouti-related peptide, which mediate hunger, inhibit satiety and increase food intake. Pro-opiomelanocortin, produced in the nucleus arcuatus, stimulates satiety.

Leptin is a hormone produced by adipose cells and its pivotal role is maintaining energy balance by indicating levels of energy storage to the central body system. A low leptin level signals loss of body fat and a need for energy intake, while a high leptin level implies adequate body fat and no further need for food intake. Studies have shown older people tend to have higher levels of leptin.

Insulin regulates glucose metabolism. It is a satiety hormone. It works by enhancing the leptin signal to the hypothalamus and inhibiting ghrelin (which is produced by the stomach), the only peripheral hormone known to stimulate appetite. Ageing is associated with reduced glucose tolerance and elevated insulin levels. This may amplify the leptin signal and inhibit ghrelin, inducing a false sensation of increased satiety.

THE GUT NEUROENDOCRINE SYSTEM (NES)

The NES of the gut consists of the endocrine and paracrine cells in the mucosa and the enteric nervous system (ENS), both of which secrete bioactive peptides and amines. Endocrine and paracrine cells are found between epithelial cells and are often flask or basket shaped with a broad base, while the apical part reaches the gut lumen. Some of the cells have long, slender cytoplasmic processes projecting to neighbouring cells, making their paracrine action more efficient. The ENS consists of neurons with their cell bodies located in the gut wall. There are two main nerve plexuses: (1) the myenteric plexus (Auerbach's), located between the longitudinal and circular muscle layers of the entire GI tract, containing neurons involved in motility and gastric acid control; and (2) the submucosal plexus (Meissner's), located between the submucosa and the circular muscle, involved in the control of fluid transport and vasodilator reflexes. The ganglia of the two plexuses are connected to a continuous meshwork; that of the myenteric plexus is more regular. The ENS receives some input from the central nervous system (CNS), but most input comes from other enteric neurons.

The ENS (*see* Figure 8.1) has been described as a 'second brain' for several reasons. It can operate autonomously and it normally communicates with the CNS through the parasympathetic (e.g. via the vagus nerve) and sympathetic (e.g. via the prevertebral ganglia) nervous systems. However, studies show when the vagus nerve is severed, the ENS continues to function independently.

The ENS includes efferent, afferent and interneurons, all of which make the ENS capable of carrying reflexes and acting as an integrating centre in the absence of CNS input. There are more nerve cells in the ENS than in the entire spinal cord. The sensory neurons report on mechanical and chemical conditions. Through intestinal muscles, the motor neurons control peristalsis

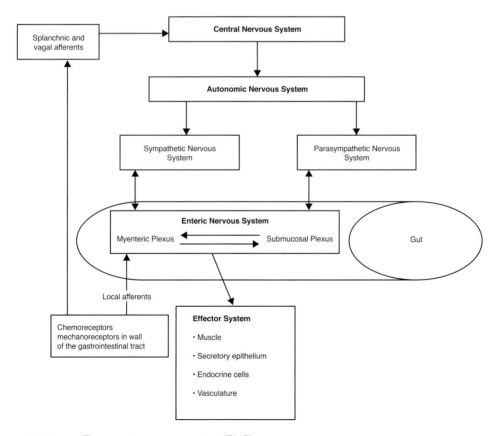

FIGURE 8.1 The enteric nervous system (ENS)

and the churning of intestinal contents. Other neurons control the secretion of enzymes. The ENS makes use of more than 30 neurotransmitters, most of which are identical to those found in the CNS, such as acetylcholine, dopamine and serotonin. More than 90% of the body's serotonin lies in the gut, as well as 50% of the body's dopamine.

The effects of ageing on the neuroendocrine system

The myenteric plexus is primarily involved in the initiation and control of smooth-muscle motor patterns such as peristalsis. Animal studies have demonstrated age-related loss of neurons in the GI tract, with the greatest loss of neurons occurring in the large intestine, followed by the small intestine and, to a lesser degree, in the stomach. Both small and large intestine neuronal loss follow a consistent temporal progression. Neurodegeneration begins in adulthood and, once initiated, continues throughout middle and old age. Studies examining the submucosal plexus, important for coordination reflexes such as secretion and absorption as well as motor control of smooth muscle, are more limited.

Enteric neurons can be distinguished on the basis of their chemical coding. Nitrergic neurons and cholinergic neurons represent two separate subpopulations. They collectively account for the entire population of the myenteric plexus. Nitrergic neurons use nitric oxide synthesised by nitric oxide synthase and are inhibitory neurons that innervate the smooth muscle. Studies have shown that their axons become swollen with ageing and have decreased nitric oxide expression.

Cholinergic neurons use acetylcholine and have multiple functions; they include interneurons, intrinsic sensory neurons and excitatory motor neurons that innervate smooth muscle. Studies have demonstrated cholinergic neurons also decrease with age. Cholinergic neurons can be further subdivided based on their expression of calcium-binding proteins. Calcium-binding proteins are important for the regulation of a calcium pool, critical in establishing synaptic plasticity. Calretinin forms much of the larger proportion of myenteric neurons compared to calbindin neurons. Calcium-binding proteins are particularly sensitive to the insult of age. As yet, no cause has been identified, but it is believed that an increased level of free oxygen species could be contributory and that caloric reduction of foods containing antioxidants may enhance age-related loss of myenteric neurons.

Enteric glia are predominately located within the ganglia of both the myenteric and sub-myenteric plexus, where they interdigitate with neurons. Apart from providing structural support, they have been shown to have metabolic and trophic functions and to offer protective support to neurons. Enteric glia decrease with age, which parallels the decrease in neurons. Similarly, sympathetic innervations of the myenteric plexus and sub-myenteric plexus deteriorate with age. However, visceral afferents do not appear to be as severely affected.

Changes in the neuroendocrine system can be either primary or secondary. Secondary changes are compensatory to preceding changes in receptors or effector organs – for example, CCK-level increases due to reduced CCK-receptor density in the gall bladder. Increased CCK levels prolong gastric emptying.

The number of serotonin cells decreases in the intestine with age; this is thought to be due to degeneration of the ENS. Serotonin is important for peristalsis. Even though these changes are secondary, they could lead to GI dysmotility and subsequent dysfunction.

The number of somatostatin cells also decreases with age. Somatostatin inhibits gastrin secretion, thus raised gastrin levels lead to increased gastric acid secretion with increasing age. This, coupled with the raised CCK levels (which slow gastric emptying and gut transit time) and an increase in substance P (which reduces lower oesophageal sphincter pressure), results in gastro-oesophageal reflux seen commonly in older individuals.

PHYSIOLOGICAL AND ANATOMICAL CHANGES WITH AGEING
The oral cavity and taste

Enjoyment of food is dependent not only on taste and the sensations of touch, temperature and pain, but also on chemicals released from food in the mouth that stimulate odour receptors in the nasal epithelium. All these sensations are integrated in the orbitofrontal cortex. Approximately 50% of the population aged over 65 years has impaired olfaction and this increases to 75% of the population aged over 80 years. This is greater in patients with Alzheimer's disease. There is continuous damage to the nasal epithelium leading to a loss of olfactory receptors at the rate of 10% per decade. In the cerebral cortex, there is a small decrease in the dentrites and spines in the piriform cortex layer Ia, resulting in reduction of olfactory and event-related potentials. In Alzheimer's disease, there is a reduction in the size of olfactory tracts and their myelination, which is associated with a high presence of amyloid plaques and neurofibrillary tangles in the areas of the brain receiving projection from the olfactory bulbs.

There are five basic taste sensations: sweet, salt, bitter, sour and umami, a taste of savouriness due to protein building blocks such as glutamate. A variety of compounds such as peptides, catechins, polyphenols and caffeine activate bitter taste receptors. Alterations in taste-receptor sensation are related to genetic status, previous exposure, cultural beliefs and learned evasion.

Taste and smell detection is dependent on the activation of G-protein-coupled receptors in taste buds. There are about 800 olfactory receptors and there are major families of receptors that detect odours: the olfactory receptor, the trace amine-associated receptor and two vomeronasal receptor families – V1R and V2R. Over half of the human olfactory receptor genes are inactive. The effect of age on these receptors is unknown. Similar protein-coupled taste receptors have been identified throughout the GI mucosa. They play a role in regulating which substances are absorbed and which potentially toxic substances are excluded from absorption. In addition, they appear to have a role in activating neural pathways and in the release of GI peptide hormones. There is no evidence that age alters these taste receptors and their intracellular transduction mechanisms.

Studies have shown that the greatest variation in taste sensitivity is seen with salty and umami tastes. Men appear to have greater age-related decline in taste threshold sensitivity than women. Older individuals perceive tastants dissolved in water as less intense than younger persons. However, when tastants are mixed within a product, this appears to be only true for salty and sweet tastes. There is a huge variation in taste bud-receptor density and, in certain anatomical areas, such as the epiglottis, this declines with age. It is thought, however, that the physiological decline in taste sensitivity is primarily due to altered membrane function rather than change in receptor number. Alteration in saliva due to xerostomia via increased salt content, poor mouth hygiene, periodontal disease, medications and cigarette smoking may all play a greater role in altered taste sensation. Furthermore, zinc deficiency leading to hypo- or dysgeusia – the distortion of sense of taste – can be caused by diabetes mellitus, cancer, liver disease and diuretics.

The effect of changes in taste sensation on food intake with ageing is controversial. In general, it is believed that taste plays a minor role in total food intake but a more important role in food choice. It has been estimated that changes in olfaction account in a decline of 100 calories per day in food intake between the ages of 20 and 80 years. Studies have demonstrated that food variety delays satiation and therefore increases food intake in older people. In addition, using taste enhancers in older people has been shown to increase food intake.

Swallowing is a highly complex process involving over 40 muscle pairs working in concert over less than a second. There are three phases of swallowing: oral, pharyngeal and oesophageal. Age-related alterations in dentition, combined with a decrease in saliva production, affect the formation of food bolus.

Oral transit time is increased with ageing and there is impairment of tongue function. Older individuals have decreased peristaltic amplitude and velocity in the pharynx, which leads to an increase in duration of pharyngeal swallow time. In older persons, there is an absence of hypopharyngeal bolus acceleration due to an increased trans-sphincteric pressure gradient. Moreover, the upper oesophageal sphincter diameter is smaller and there is a delay in its relaxation and opening with age.

Similar impairment is seen in the laryngeal reflex. There is a decrease in the contractile function of the suprahyoid muscles. Older people have a smaller excursion of the anterior hyoid and larynx during swallowing. One-third of older people have cricopharyngeal bars, which are associated with a decrease in the opening size of the upper oesophagus. Overall, these findings, coupled with reduced cough reflex in older people, increase the risk of aspiration. Poor oral hygiene further increases the incidence of aspiration pneumonia due to the colonisation of pathogenic bacteria in the oropharynx.

The pharyngeal tracheal epithelium is heavily innervated by substance P-containing nerves. Substance P depletion results in a decrease in cough response and swallowing reflex. Moreover, it appears that reduction in substance P-induced reflexes plays an important role in silent aspiration. Angiotensin-converting enzyme (ACE) inhibitors block the breakdown of substance P, increase the cough reflex and enhance the swallow reflex.

The oesophagus

Older people in their 80s and 90s have significantly decreased amplitude, but not duration and velocity, of peristaltic pressures. There is also an increased frequency of non-propulsive, often repetitive, contractions.

Morphological studies have shown an age-related loss of enteric neurons in the human oesophagus. The number of neurons decreases after the age of 70 years, which is accompanied by an increase in the size of neurons, especially in the upper third of the oesophagus at the junction with the pharynx. There is also evidence of reduced contractions in the lower oesophagus of older people, resulting in impaired acid clearance. Episodes of reflux are of longer duration in older people, although the frequency does not significantly vary with age.

The stomach and proximal bowel

Hyperproliferation occurs in the epithelial cells of the stomach, the small intestine and the large intestine of stable-fed, aged rodents when compared with young mature rodents. The number of gastric and colonic mucosal cells undergoing apoptosis was found to be lower in older animals. Furthermore, abnormalities of proliferative and differentiation responses become evident when GI tissues are stimulated by injury, or by starvation and re-feeding. These observations suggest that nutritional modulation of mucosal cell proliferation is affected by ageing.

Age-associated changes in GI mucosal cell proliferation could also be secondary to alterations in hormonal influences, especially in the gastric mucosa. It has been reported that responsiveness of the gastric mucosa to different peptides, such as gastrin, bombesin and epidermal growth factor, changes at different stages of life. Age-related decline in gastrin secretion could partly be attributed to a higher ratio of somatostatin to gastrin cells in the antral mucosa. There is also a progressive loss of gastric mucosal responsiveness to both the acid secretory and growth-promoting actions of gastrin. One explanation for this could be loss of the functional receptors of gastrin with age.

Earlier studies have reported a significant reduction in gastric acid secretion with age. However, the majority of these studies were retrospective and did not take into account the presence of possible gastric atrophic lesions. Recent studies including patients aged 80 years and older without gastric atrophic lesions showed that gastric acid secretion remained normal with age, with 90% of patients having normal acid secretion.

Normal gastric acid secretion has been demonstrated in *Helicobacter pylori*-negative patients, while it decreased with age in *H. pylori*-positive patients. The decline in gastric acid secretion in *H. pylori*-positive patients depended on both increasing prevalence of fundic atrophic gastritis and inflammatory cytokines such as interleukin-1β and tumour necrosis factor-α, which are known to inhibit parietal cells.

Epidemiological studies have shown atrophic gastritis is present in 50%–70% of patients aged over 80 years old. A series of studies has focused on the long-term effects of *H. pylori* infection and its role in the development of the histological changes that occur with ageing. In a large multi-centre trial, both atrophic gastritis and intestinal metaplasia were strongly associated with *H. Pylori* infection and not with ageing.

As a result of atrophic gastritis, there is decreased acid secretion. This may lead to two consequences in older people: 1. bacterial overgrowth in the proximal intestinal tract, and 2. gastrointestinal malabsorption.

A study to determine the prevalence of small-bowel bacterial overgrowth in older adults using a hydrogen breath test was 15.6%. The use of proton pump inhibitors (PPIs) contributed significantly to the high prevalence of a positive breath test in older adults, which was associated with lower body weight, lower body mass index, lower plasma albumin concentration and higher prevalence of diarrhoea.

Gastric malabsorption may be another consequence of reduced gastric acid secretion. In fact, malabsorption of food-bound cobalamin in older people may be due to reduced gastric acid production in older people combined with bacterial overgrowth. Decreased gastric acid production may lead to a reduction in the release of free vitamin B_{12} from food protein. Hypochlorhydria also causes intestinal bacterial overgrowth, which in turn interferes with vitamin B_{12} absorption. Atrophic gastritis may also affect ferric iron and calcium absorption. Both calcium and ferric iron are kept soluble and, hence, absorbable in the intestinal milieu through the acidifying effects of gastric acid, with ferric iron becoming insoluble above pH 5.

Chronic inflammation in the gastric mucosa may have several consequences such as an increased production of reactive oxygen species (ROS). There is increasing evidence that ROS play a key role in the processes of tissue damage and ageing. In the stomach mucosa, ROS might directly damage or kill epithelial cells and thereby contribute to atrophy. However, more complex mechanisms of action are conceivable. ROS may lead to a heightened sensitivity of the ageing stomach to pro-inflammatory stimuli and may damage DNA, thereby leading to mutations and cancer genesis. The molecular sources of ROS that contribute to the ageing process are still a matter of debate. ROS generation by mitochondria has been implicated but more recently the role of the nitrous oxide (NOX) family of superoxide-generating nicotinamide adenine dinucleotide phosphate (NADPH) oxidases is receiving increased attention. Previous studies on expression of NADPH oxidases in gastric mucosa have mainly been performed in guinea pigs. In these animal models, NOX1 (an NADPH oxidase with its main localisation in the colon) was found and proposed to be involved in the regulation of the inflammatory response and/or cell proliferation.

Chronic inflammation in the gastric mucosa may also affect expression of gastric satiety-inducible peptides such as leptin or ghrelin, which play a role in the regulation of food intake. Recent evidence supports the view that leptin is secreted not only from adipose tissues but also from the gut in humans and rats. Studies reported that gastric inflammation induced by *H. pylori* infection raised gastric leptin expression, which in turn induced satiety and lowered body mass index.

Ghrelin is a peptide produced mainly in the stomach that has been implicated in the control of food intake and energy homeostasis in both humans and rodents. A recent study reported that cure of *H. pylori* infection increased plasma ghrelin, which in turn may lead to increased appetite and weight gain. Thus, chronic gastric inflammation may induce variations of expression of both leptin and ghrelin and play a role in the physiopathology of anorexia in older patients.

The large bowel

Normal stool output is approximately 200 g daily. Activity of the proximal colon determines the consistency and volume of delivery of contents to the rectum. As rectal filling gradually proceeds, anorectal sampling permits subconscious perception of the consistency of the content. An intact internal anal sphincter maintains continence. Autonomic neurons relay anorectal sensation of rectal contents. Activation of these afferents results in relaxation of recto-anal inhibitory reflexes to begin relaxation of the internal anal sphincter. Reflex voluntary contraction of the external sphincter maintains continence until voluntary defaecation is possible.

Defaecation starts with rectal sensory awareness of a critical level of filling and a message is relayed to the cerebral cortex as the perception of the need to evacuate the rectum. The volume that triggers perception depends on the condition of the rectum and the character of its contents. When an individual is in the squatting position it causes straightening of the anorectal angle allowing more effective defaecation. The external anal sphincter and puborectalis muscle relax. Rectal contents relax the internal anal sphincter. Abdominal pressure rises and relaxation of pelvic floor allows the stool to enter the lower rectum. Sensory input is maintained until the rectum is fully voided. This reflex is mediated at the level of the spinal cord. As stools pass through the anal canal, it stretches the external anal sphincter and creates on it a traction force. After the last bolus of stool has passed, the closing reflex of the external anal sphincter is stimulated by the release of traction.

Age-related anatomical changes in the lower GI tract might contribute to delayed transit time and delayed stool water content. Such changes may include intestinal wall atrophy, reduced tone, reduced blood supply and intrinsic neuronal changes.

Gut transit time and colonic motility are similar in healthy older people and younger subjects. However, older people with chronic illness who report constipation have a prolonged gut transit time of 4 to 9 days (normal is less than 3 days), with evacuation delayed through the lowest part of the large bowel and rectum. Those in nursing homes have even longer transit times of up to 3 weeks, with immobility, causing constipation and subsequent faecal incontinence due to overflow. Colonic function appears to be influenced by factors associated with ageing, such as chronic disease, immobility and medication, rather than ageing itself.

OTHER PATHOPHYSIOLOGICAL CHANGES

Anorexia of ageing

With advancing age, appetite declines and food intake is reduced. Healthy older people feel fuller before meals, hence are less hungry, which leads to the consumption of smaller meals. Furthermore, they have been shown to eat more slowly, have fewer snacks between meals and become satiated after meals more rapidly following a standard meal than younger individuals. The average daily intake decreases by up to 30% between the ages of 20 and 80 years. Most of the age-related decrease in energy is a response to the decline in energy expenditure with age. However, in many older people, the decrease in energy intake is greater than the decrease in energy expenditure. Therefore, body weight as a whole is reduced.

Older people commonly complain of increased fullness and early satiation during meals. This may be caused by changes in the GI sensory function; with age there is reduced sensitivity to GI distension. Ageing is associated with impairment in receptive relaxation of the gastric fundus, causing rapid antral filling and distension and earlier satiety. The decline in fundal compliance appears to be secondary to a decrease in nitric synthase activity.

Ageing and GI carcinogenesis

Increasing age is associated with higher incidence of malignancy, including gastric and colorectal cancers. The risk of developing GI cancers increases, with peak incidence occurring in the seventh decade. Many reasons, including altered carcinogen metabolism and long-term exposure to cancer-causing agents, have been suggested responsible for the age-dependent rise in malignancies. Carcinogenesis results from the accumulation of mutations during progression from normal epithelium to carcinoma. For colon cancer, studies have reported that the loss or inactivation of the tumour-suppressor gene *APC* (adenomatous polyposis coli) initiates genomic instability, which results in the phenotypic appearance of an adenoma. With the inactivation of the tumour-suppressor *APC*, additional alterations in tumour-suppressor *p53* and *DCC* (deleted in colon cancer) oncogenes may accumulate and lead to the development of an adenomatous polyp and eventually carcinoma. A higher incidence of mutations of these tumour-suppressor genes, *APC*, *DCC* and *p53*, has been found in the gastric mucosa of older patients.

COMMON PROBLEMS IN THE OLDER PATIENT
Postprandial hypotension

Postprandial hypotension occurs commonly in older people and those with diabetes mellitus. It is associated with an increase in falls, syncope, stroke, myocardial infarction and general mortality. It occurs most often in response to carbohydrate intake but can also be seen in response to protein and fat. It is caused by the release of a vasodilatory peptide, most probably calcitonin gene-related peptide, which causes peripheral vasodilatation. Slowing gastric emptying results in a decrease in postprandial hypotension, mediated through stimulating the release of glucagon-like peptide-1 (GLP-1) from intestinal cells. The $\alpha 1$ glucosidase inhibitors acarbose and miglitol all increase GLP-1 levels in conjunction with meals, forming an effective therapeutic strategy. Acarbose has been shown to attenuate postprandial hypotension.

Gastro–oesophageal reflux disease (GORD)

GORD is common in older people and places a significant burden on medical resources since it is a chronic disease with complications including oesophagitis, stricture formation and Barrett's oesophagus.

It is caused by spontaneous complete relaxation of a normal lower oesophageal sphincter, the main anti-reflux barrier, which is augmented by extrinsic compression from the diaphragm. Physiological reflux can occur due to transient relaxation of the lower oesophageal sphincter. Symptoms of reflux disease are typical and exacerbated by meals and recumbency. Oesophagitis is associated with GORD and is more common in older people due to the breakdown of various protective mechanisms combined with risk factors such as medications including aspirin and bisphosphonates. Treatment includes a long-term management plan involving lifestyle modification and the use of antacids and PPIs. Surgical options are available using open or laparoscopic fundoplication but are not always appropriate in an older age group.

Disease severity and symptoms are poorly correlated, especially in older people, and the condition may first manifest as an acute emergency such as a GI bleed. Strictures occur in approximately 10% of patients with GORD and are responsive to periodic dilatation and use of PPIs. In those where it is a persistent problem, malignant transformation can occur. Barrett's oesophagus results from metaplastic changes in the oesophageal mucosa due to chronic reflux. It is an important predisposing factor for developing adenocarcinoma of the oesophagus.

Coeliac disease

Coeliac disease in the older patient is an important cause of malabsorption and poor nutrition. Numerous studies have demonstrated that this condition is under-diagnosed in older people.

There is a female preponderance of coeliac disease in younger adults, but in the older population, men are more likely affected. Diagnostic difficulty is experienced, primarily owing to coexisting pathologies; symptoms are non-specific and can include non-intestinal features. Diarrhoea is common but constipation is also recognised. Glossitis, aphthous ulcers, bone pain and neurological features like ataxia can occur and are related to underlying nutritional deficiencies.

Numerous conditions are associated with coeliac disease, including dermatitis herpetiformis – of which 10% of these cases occur in people aged over 60 years, as well as other autoimmune-type conditions such as diabetes mellitus, thyroid disease and inflammatory bowel disease, through shared histocompatibility antigens. It has also been found that diabetic control is difficult in gluten-sensitive patients and improves on a gluten-free diet.

Diagnosis of coeliac disease is made by serological screening tests and villous atrophy on duodenal biopsy, which is reversed on a gluten-free diet. The detection of immunoglobulin (Ig) A and IgG anti-tissue transglutaminase antibodies, which are highly sensitive and specific for coeliac disease, can form part of a screening test. Adherence to a gluten-free diet remains the cornerstone of treatment; in addition, replacement of vital nutrients, vitamins and minerals is often required. There is an increased tendency to small bowel lymphoma in old age. This risk is reduced by prompt treatment through dietary manipulation by means of a gluten-free diet.

Constipation

Constipation is a common problem in older people and increases with age. It can present as an acute illness or as a chronic condition. Constipation has been defined as having a bowel motion fewer than three times per week, although, more recently, the Rome III criteria (*see* Box 8.1) have been used to help in differentiating chronic functional constipation from other causes.

There are two mechanisms involved in the pathophysiology of constipation: colonic motility dysfunction and pelvic floor dysfunction.

Colonic motility dysfunction is a failure of coordinated motor activity to move stool throughout the colon. Three types of colonic delay have been identified: right colonic, left colonic and rectosigmoid. Mechanisms of delay include

---

BOX 8.1 Rome III criteria for constipation

1 Must include two or more of the following:
   - straining during at least 25% of defaecations*
   - lumpy or hard stools in at least 25% of defaecations*
   - sensation of incomplete evacuation for at least 25% of defaecations*
   - sensation of anorectal obstruction/blockage for at least 25% of defaecations*
   - manual manoeuvres to facilitate at least 25% of defaecations, e.g. digital evacuation, support of the pelvic floor*
   - fewer than three defaecations per week.
2 Loose stools rarely present without the use of laxatives.
3 Insufficient criteria for irritable bowel syndrome.

Criteria fulfilled for the last 3 months with symptom onset at least 6 months prior to diagnosis.

Longstreth GF, Thompson WG, Chey WD *et al.* Functional bowel disorders. *Gastroenterology.* 2006; **130**(5): 1480–91.

---

autonomic system dysfunction, disruption of the ENS, disruption of the neuroendocrine system and colonic myopathy. Interstitial cells of Cajal (ICCs) are important for colonic motor activity. In slow-transit constipation, there is a significant decrease in the number of ICCs within the colonic wall, including the external muscle layer. This causes weak or absent colonic electrical activity, which leads to constipation. Nerve fibres in the colonic circular muscle may be abnormal in slow-transit constipation. A reduction in the density of excitatory nerve fibres with tachykinin and enkephalin immunoreactivity has been found in the colonic circular muscle of patients with slow-transit constipation, whereas the innervation of all other layers appears normal.

Gut hormones (cholecystokinin, PYY, somatostatin, enteroglucagon, pancreatic peptides) are thought to have potent effects on GI motility. Plasma cholecystokinin and PYY have not been found altered in patients with slow-transit constipation. However, specific abnormalities in circulating gut hormones have been identified, including higher levels of circulating somatostatin, lower levels of somatostatin integrated with an incremental meal response and decreased levels of enteroglucagon 30–60 minutes after a meal. Significantly fewer enteroglucagon and serotonin immunoreactive cells were also found in patients with slow-transit constipation. However, how changes in these hormones contribute to the pathogenesis of slow-transit constipation has not yet fully been elicited.

When constipation is accompanied by an immobile perineum, patients have impaired balloon expulsion, impaired and delayed artificial stool expulsion, decreased straightening of the anorectal angle, decreased descent of the pelvic floor with defaecation and prolonged rectosigmoid transit times. All are thought to be signs of pelvic floor dysfunction rather than delayed transit time.

Constipation is thought to be a natural part of ageing, but ageing itself does not cause the disorder. Changes in the GI tract associated with ageing may predispose individuals to constipation. The disorder usually has a multifactorial aetiology and may continue through the patient's lifetime (*see* Table 8.1).

TABLE 8.1 Causes of constipation

Endocrine and metabolic disease	Diabetes mellitus hypothyroidism
Neurological disease	Autonomic neuropathy, Parkinson's disease Multiple sclerosis, spinal cord injury
Psychological conditions	Anxiety, depression
Structural abnormalities	Fissures, haemorrhoids, rectal prolapse, rectocele obstructive lesions
Lifestyle	Dehydration, low calorie diet, low fibre diet Immobility
Iatrogenic	Medications including opiates

Disordered defaecation can occur as a result of injury to the pudendal nerve. The incidence of increased pudendal nerve terminal motor latency, an indicator of pudendal nerve dysfunction, is increased in older females. Injury to the pudendal nerves can lead to abnormal perineal descent, which can affect rectal emptying by causing partial prolapse of the anal canal by the anterior rectal mucosa.

Several types of anorectal abnormalities occur in older people with constipation, including dyschezia and pelvic dyssynergia. Dyschezia is characterised by reduced tone, increased compliance and impaired sensation, such that a greater degree of rectal distension is required to induce the defaecatory mechanism. It is seen most commonly in frail older individuals, who subsequently succumb to recurrent rectal impactions, a frequent consequence of which is faecal soiling. Although faecal soiling as a symptom itself affects up to 28% of older people, it is a problem not readily assessed by doctors or nurses. Pelvic dyssynergia, also termed 'anismus', involves a failure to relax the pelvic floor and external anal sphincter muscles during defaecation.

Diarrhoea

Diarrhoea can be an important symptom of small bowel disease and may be acute or chronic. It is characterised by an increased stool volume and is usually associated with increases in liquidity and frequency.

Older people are more vulnerable to diarrhoea due to factors like hypochlorhydria or achlorhydria, exposure to enteropathogens, luminal stasis, decreased mucosal immunity and the use of drugs such as antibiotics.

Acute diarrhoea is usually infectious and is more likely to occur with increasing severity in older infirm patients, with a consequent increased mortality of up to 35%. Bloody diarrhoea can occur in conditions such as bowel ischaemia and inflammatory bowel disease. Chronic diarrhoea may be secretory (which often results from the secretion of water and electrolytes into the bowel as a result of hormonal stimulation) or osmotic (secondary to food solutes or drugs such as laxatives and antacids).

Drug-induced causes of diarrhoea are important in older people and the mechanisms of causation are diverse. Disruption of GI tract defences (such as that caused by PPIs, which alter gastric acid secretion; anticholinergics, which affect intestinal motility; or even antibiotics, which deplete intestinal flora) is one manner in which drugs can cause diarrhoea. Others include damage to the mucosal surface (microscopic colitis) and impaired fluid absorption and secretion due to drug-induced effects on the absorbing surface, transport mechanisms and gut motility. Older people are more susceptible to dehydration and systemic toxicity as a result. Hence, it is imperative to treat diarrhoea more aggressively with fluid replacement. Age affects the intestinal microflora, with a decrease in anaerobes and *Bifidobacterium* spp. and an increase in enterobacteria. These changes, coupled with a reduced gut immune response, make many older people susceptible to infectious diarrhoea.

The liberal use of antibiotics in hospitals and in the community has resulted in an increased incidence of antibiotic-associated diarrhoea and *Clostridium difficile*-associated diarrhoea, with its consequent morbidity and mortality, not to mention increased healthcare costs. In addition to standard treatment with metronidazole and vancomycin, newer approaches to treatment of this condition include the use of probiotics, which have been shown in various studies and recent meta-analyses to have beneficial results. Both *Lactobacillus* spp. and the yeast *Saccharomyces boulardii* have been found to be more beneficial than placebo in the prevention of diarrhoea. Their acceptance into clinical practice, together with changes to antibiotic policies and infection control procedures, has the potential to significantly reduce the incidence of *Clostridium difficile*.

Diverticular disease

Diverticular disease is highly prevalent in older patients. It results from asymmetric contraction of the bowel wall, leading to segmentation and development of pulsion outpouchings in areas of weakness. Around a third of people with the condition are aged over 60 years and two-thirds are 80 years and over; the disease affects more women than men and contributes significantly to healthcare costs. Although predominantly a disease of the West, where it occurs on the left side, it is also seen in Asia, where the condition is located more frequently on the right side of the colon and tends to affect middle-aged patients.

Diverticular disease is related to a reduced-fibre diet, and iatrogenic factors may also contribute to flare-ups in disease activity. Non-steroidal anti-inflammatory drugs can exacerbate colonic diverticulitis; a greater incidence of perforation has been noted in this setting, necessitating surgical treatment. Furthermore, the disease is possibly related to the use of opiates in the older patient and there is a greater risk of developing *Clostridium difficile*-associated pseudomembranous colitis after antibiotic use.

Presentation varies from mild episodes of inflammation with pain, fever and lower GI bleeding to more severe features of abscess formation and perforation. However, there can be a paucity of signs in older people.

Diagnosis rests on the use of colonoscopy and imaging and it is important to rule out the presence of colonic neoplasms, which share many presenting features. A computed tomography (CT) scan with contrast is the preferred test in older people, as an alternative to a barium enema, as it may allow for simultaneous percutaneous drainage of a diverticular abscess. Bowel rest and antibiotics remain the mainstay of treatment of diverticulitis; if no improvement occurs within 48 hours, a CT scan is mandatory and a surgical opinion should be sought. Lifestyle modification, such as increasing exercise, reducing fat intake and increasing dietary fibre, can prevent attacks of diverticulitis. Despite recent advances in the treatment of various abdominal symptoms like pain, bloating and constipation, the morbidity and cost implications of diverticular disease in older people continue to be important.

Colorectal cancer

Colorectal cancer predominantly affects older people; 90% of colon cancers occur in people aged over 50 years and 20%–40% are seen in men and women aged 80 years or older. The causes and risk factors are diverse and include dietary, geographical and genetic factors. Indeed, there is a two- to threefold increase in the risk of cancer in first-degree relatives of affected cases compared with those without a family history. Most cancers arise from pre-existing adenomatous polyps and, given the familial tendency, screening is merited.

The current recommendations for screening are tailored to early detection; colonoscopy should start at 50 years in those with average risk but at 40 years for those with a family history of colorectal cancer. A combination of faecal occult blood testing, flexible sigmoidoscopy and, in certain cases, double-contrast barium enema is associated with good detection rates and correlates with improved survival outcomes.

Increasingly, CT colonography is now used instead, particularly in older people, when pain, bowel stenosis or strictures are limiting factors and difficulties are expected with colonoscopy. Helical CT examination, in which the air-distended colon is evaluated by three-dimensional imaging for the presence of polyps and cancer, uses a dry bowel preparation with oral barium as contrast, permitting better visualisation of the bowel wall. Although it has a high accuracy, recent studies have shown a reduced sensitivity in detection of polyps less than 10 mm in size, in comparison with colonoscopy (59% versus 98%, $P = 0.0001$). It can be a useful adjunct to colonoscopy; the segmental unblinding technique uses endoscopic visualisation of a bowel segment to evaluate false-positive lesions detected by scanning.

Survival figures are poor in older people. In addition to disease mortality, the risks of treatment are also high, thus there is sometimes a reluctance to institute treatment options. Increasing age is an independent predictor of short- and long-term mortality after surgery for both rectal and colon cancer, and surgical resection for advanced bowel cancer is not a commonly exercised option. Part of the problem in older people is that a significant number of cases present acutely (20%); consequently, there is a tendency for emergency surgery in this group, with its inherent complications, leading to increased post-operative mortality.

The advent of advanced surgical techniques has been of particular benefit to the older patient with bowel cancer. In one study, patients treated by laparoscopic colonic resection recovered faster and had reduced morbidity. The procedure was associated with decreased post-operative pain, early return to normal bowel function, lower cardiopulmonary risk and shorter hospital stay. There is some concern, however, about a limited surgical field, port-site metastasis and long-term outcomes of minimally invasive operations. The need for open laparotomy conversion, currently occurring in 11%–22% of cases, is also an issue of debate, although this is often the result of delays in diagnosis owing to unusual presentations. Despite these concerns, the use of laparoscopy remains a safe and effective surgical technique in older patients. Stenting may be a temporary measure in acute malignant obstruction (where it allows bowel preparation and elective surgery), or even used as a palliative procedure for unresectable tumours. Studies have shown a clinical success rate of 84%–100% and a complication rate of 14%–42%.

Chemotherapy has an important role in the treatment of colorectal cancer in older people. Studies have demonstrated an improved survival in those aged over 65 years old (70%) compared with younger counterparts (56%) ($P = 0.085$) when used as an adjunct to surgery. Standard regimens of 5-fluorouracil in combination with levamisole or folinic acid are useful in both locally advanced and metastatic disease. Radiotherapy is also a useful treatment option when used in conjunction with chemotherapy for Duke stage B and stage C rectal tumours. It has been shown to reduce local recurrence and improve survival.

FURTHER READING

Bhutto A, Morley JE. The clinical significance of gastrointestinal changes with aging. *Curr Opin Clin Nutr Metab Care.* 2008; **11**(5): 651–60.

D'Souza AL. Aging and the gut. *Postgrad Med J.* 2007; **83**(975): 44–53.

McCrea GL, Miaskowski C, Stotts NA *et al.* Pathophysiology of constipation in the older adult. *World J Gastroenterol.* 2008; **14**(17): 2631–8.

Phillips RJ, Powley TL. Innervation of the gastrointestinal tract: patterns of aging. *Auton Neurosci.* 2007; **136**(1–2): 1–19.

Sandström O, El-Salhy M. Age-related changes in neuroendocrine system of the gut: a possible role in the pathogenesis of gastrointestinal disorders in the elderly; minireview based on a doctoral thesis. *Ups J Med Sci.* 2001; **106**(2): 81–97.

QUESTIONS: THE GASTROINTESTINAL SYSTEM

1 An 82-year-old woman was reviewed by her general practitioner and noted to have lost 2 kg over the last 3 years. She admitted to symptoms of increased satiety, but felt well otherwise. Which one of the following statements is false?
A a diagnosis of gastric cancer is unlikely in this age group
B a physiological change in her PP levels may account for a change in satiety
C her CCK levels are likely to be elevated
D leptin levels may be high in physiological age-related satiety
E thyroid function tests are an important component of the initial workup.

Answer: A

Comment: *All patients with weight loss and increased satiety should be investigated for the possibility of a malignant process.*

2 A 77-year-old man with severe symptoms of acid reflux had an upper GI endoscopy that revealed a 2 cm segment of Barrett's oesophagus within a small hiatus hernia. Oesophageal biopsies confirmed Barrett's with low-grade dysplasia. His medications included aspirin, simvastatin, ramipril and ranitidine. Which one of the following is the best management option?
A endoscopic mucosal resection
B long-term PPI therapy with repeat endoscopy and biopsy
C Nissen fundoplication, with the intention of reversing his Barrett's
D no change in management
E oesophagectomy.

Answer: B

Comment: *The presence of low-grade dysplasia warrants further endoscopy as part of a surveillance programme, but there is no indication for more invasive management. PPIs may be of some benefit, but there is no benefit from H2 antagonists aside from symptomatic relief from reflux. High-grade dysplasia requires further treatment, either endoscopic or surgical.*

3 Which one of the following best describes the role of leptin?
A is a hormone produced by adipose cells that maintains energy balance by giving the central body system a sign of energy storage
B is produced in the small bowel
C older people have lower levels of leptin
D reduces gall bladder contraction and gut motility
E stimulates the release of pancreatic enzymes to assist with digestion.

Answer: A

Comment: *Leptin is produced by adipose tissue and its main role is in maintaining energy balance by giving the central body system a sign of energy storage. A low leptin level signals loss of body fat and a need for energy intake, while a high leptin level implies adequate body fat and no need for further food intake. Older people tend to have higher levels of leptin.*

4 Which one of the following best describes the effect of ageing on the GI neuro-endocrine system?

A CCK levels decrease with age, which leads to prolonged gastric emptying
B cholinergic neurons increase with age
C the greatest loss of neurons occurs in the stomach
D neurodegeneration begins late in life, after the seventh decade
E serotonin cells decrease with age, which could lead to gastric dysfunction.

Answer: D

Comment: *Neurodegeneration begins in adulthood and continues throughout middle and old age. The greatest loss of neurons occurs in the large bowel followed by the small bowel and, to a lesser degree, in the stomach. Cholinergic neurons decrease with age. Serotonin cells, important for peristalsis, decrease with age, which can lead to gastric dysfunction. CCK levels increase with age due to decreased CCK-receptor density in the gall bladder. Increased levels of CCK prolong gastric emptying.*

5 An 83-year-old woman was seen in clinic with change in bowel habit, passing of blood in her stools and weight loss. She had a medical history of atrial fibrillation, and transient ischaemic attack. Her medication included bisoprolol and warfarin. Physical examination was unremarkable.

Investigations:

Haemoglobin concentration (Hb)	9.2 g/L (115–165)
Mean corpuscular volume (MCV)	68.9 fL (80–96)
White-cell count (WCC)	3.4 × 10^9/L (4.0–11.0)
Platelet count	512 × 10^9/L (150–400)
International normalised ratio (INR)	3.2 (<1.4)
Serum total protein	54 g/L (61–76)
Serum albumin	30 g/L (37–49)
Serum alanine aminotransferase	38 U/L (5–35)
Serum alkaline phosphatase	102 U/L (45–105)
Serum total bilirubin	22 μmol/L (1–22)
Serum ferritin	12 μg/L (15–300)

Her general practitioner organised a colonoscopy, but she was not keen on endoscopic investigation. What is the next most appropriate investigation?

A barium enema
B capsule endoscopy
C CT pneumocolon

D faecal occult blood

E serum carcino-embryonic antigen.

Answer: C

Comment: *CT pneumocolon provides an excellent alternative to colonoscopy. Faecal occult blood testing will not be of any additional use in light of an already known history of rectal bleeding. Tumour markers are useful but will not provide a diagnosis. Barium enemas can be used if access to CT pneumocolon is not readily available. Capsule endoscopy is contraindicated in case a stricture lesion obstructs the passage of the capsule.*

CHAPTER 9

The liver

THARANI THIRUGNANACHANDRAN, MARISSA MINNS
AND OLIVER J CORRADO

INTRODUCTION

Changes to the liver with advancing age are less marked than in many other organ systems, however, the ageing liver has many important clinical implications that will be addressed in this chapter.

ANATOMICAL AND HISTOLOGICAL CHANGES OF THE LIVER

The liver is responsible for a variety of body functions; central to many of these is the blood supply the liver receives directly from the portal system, with up to a quarter of the cardiac output passing to the liver via the portal vein (75%) and hepatic artery (25%). This provides liver cells with access to nutrients as well as toxins and microbes absorbed from the intestine. In addition, it facilitates the processing and synthesis of metabolic fuels and the detoxification of absorbed compounds by the acinus, the functional unit of the liver (*see* Figure 9.1). The acinus is where terminal portal veins meet exiting hepatic venules, the two being connected by specialised fenestrated capillaries called 'sinusoids'. The sinusoids form a network that runs through the plates of hepatocytes and biliary canaliculi, enabling the passage of larger molecules such as lipoproteins through fenestrations in their lining endothelial cells. The endothelial cells play a vital role in removing waste products (endocytosis). Hepatic macrophages (Kupffer cells) lie within the sinusoids and at their surface is the extravascular space of Disse, which contains lymphocytes and fat-storing stellate cells.

Several important changes occur to this microanatomy with age that help to explain the effect of age on liver function.

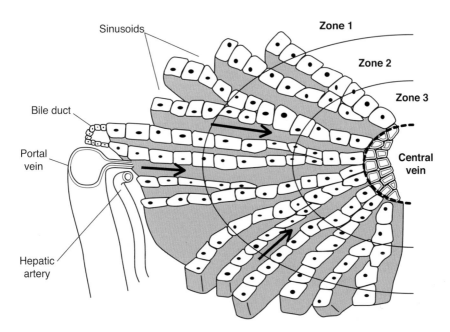

FIGURE 9.1 The hepatic acinus. Reproduced with kind permission from Brosnan ME, Brosnan JT. Hepatic glutamate metabolism: a tale of 2 hepatocytes. *Am J Clin Nutr.* 2009; 90(3): 857S–61S

The gross anatomy of the liver changes with age. As a result of an age-related reduction in hepatic blood supply, liver volume decreases by approximately 35% in people aged over 65 years when compared to those aged under 40 years. Decreased hepatic size and blood flow reduce sinusoidal perfusion, which in turn decreases the hepatic clearance of substrates and drugs; this will be discussed in more detail further on in this chapter.

Histological changes that occur with ageing may also affect liver function in older people. The number of hepatocytes appears to increase with age and these have more nuclei and nucleoli around the terminal hepatic veins. There is also an age-related accumulation of pigmented lipofuscin (highly oxidised insoluble proteins) within hepatocytes, resulting in a microscopically darker brown colour to the liver with age. It is believed the presence of these proteins interferes with cellular pathways and facilitates free radical formation. In addition, there is a decrease in the surface area of the smooth endoplasmic reticulum, with a reduction in microsomal enzyme activity.

With advancing age, changes occur in most parts of the hepatic acinus, but perhaps the most important of these, termed 'pseudocapillarisation', occurs in the liver sinusoidal endothelial cells. This can reduce sinusoidal endothelial fenestrations by as much as 50%, causing these normally unique capillaries to resemble those found elsewhere in the body. This defenestration has clinical implications for the passage of lipoproteins (specifically, chylomicron remnants) from the bloodstream to hepatocytes. Many age-related diseases such as atherosclerosis, diabetes mellitus and dementia have been linked with an age-related reduction in endocytic function of liver sinusoidal endothelial cells causing an increased risk of extra-hepatic deposition and harm from circulating waste products.

There is also an increase in the number and activity of Kupffer cells within the sinusoids with age, which is thought to be due to the general age-related increase in systemic markers of inflammation. Despite these changes, the uptake of substrates, effects on endocytic activity and ability to mount an effective immune response may be impaired in ageing Kupffer cells. This may at least partly explain why individuals are more susceptible to developing acquired liver disease with increasing age as their ability to tolerate a hepatic insult falls with each cumulative decade.

The ageing process also has an important effect on stellate cells that are located in the extracellular space of Disse. Their primary function is fat storage, but they also have a role in regulating sinusoidal blood flow. One of the most important aspects of ageing is the inability to regenerate tissues, particularly in response to injury. In the younger liver, stellate cells are activated in response to injury (such as hepatic fibrosis) by releasing fat droplets. It is likely that this response is impaired with increasing age, as electron microscopy has shown increased numbers of fat-engorged non-activated stellate cells. This may explain the significant age-related decrease in the regenerative capacity of the liver. The swollen stellate cells have been shown to protrude into the sinusoidal lumen and, in theory, could potentially further reduce sinusoidal blood flow.

CHANGES IN METABOLIC PROCESSES

Many biochemical functions and metabolic processes occur in the liver (*see* Table 9.1). The liver plays an important role in the metabolism of carbohydrates, amino acids, proteins, lipids and lipoproteins.

The synthesis of albumin is an important function of the liver. There is conflicting evidence on whether ageing affects this process and it is not clear if hepatic albumin biosynthesis does decrease with age as some animal studies have suggested. It has been postulated that the decrease in serum albumin concentration that occurs with age may be related to reduced expression of the albumin gene or to the decline in rough endoplasmic reticulum with age. Other studies have shown an increase in extracellular proteins such as albumin and a decrease in intracellular proteins in the ageing liver, which has been attributed to an increase in liver content of albumin mRNA. It is generally accepted that albumin levels may fall with age, especially in the context of illness, and this has important implications for the handling of protein-bound medication in older people; this will be discussed further on in this chapter.

TABLE 9.1 Summary of changes in metabolic processes in the older person

	Synthesis	Metabolism/ Breakdown	Storage	Changes with ageing
Lipids	Cholesterol	Lipogenesis		Increased cholesterol and triglyceride levels Increased biliary cholesterol secretion
Carbohydrates	Gluconeogenesis	Glycogenolysis Glycogenesis	Glucose (as glycogen)	Decreased glucose tolerance
Proteins	Amino acids Albumin	Ammonia to urea		Decreased albumin levels
Hormones	Thrombopoietin Insulin-like growth factor 1 Angiotensinogen	Insulin		Increased insulin resistance
Others	Coagulation Factors (I, II, V, VII, IX, X, XI) Proteins C and S Antithrombin Bile synthesis	Numerous drugs (e.g. anticonvulsants, non-steroidal anti-inflammatory drugs [NSAIDs], alcohol) Glucuronidation of bilirubin	Vitamins A, D and B_{12} Copper Iron	Decreased biliary salt excretion

Several changes in lipid metabolism occur with age and these may contribute to the increase in coronary artery disease of the ageing population. Perhaps the most clinically important is an increase in hepatic and serum cholesterol and triglyceride levels and marked postprandial hypertriglyceridaemia. Pseudocapillarisation, described earlier, is thought to contribute significantly to this dislipidaemia. Another aspect of lipid metabolism thought to be influenced by age is the function of the peroxisome. Peroxisomes are respiratory organelles involved in cellular oxygen consumption and the production and removal of reactive oxygen species. In the liver, they are involved in gluconeogenesis and lipid metabolism. Conditions such as diabetes, thyroid disease and partial hepatectomy can cause peroxisome proliferation. Although there is limited information on the relationship between peroxisomal metabolism and age, it is believed peroxisomal function decreases with age.

As well as the increase in cholesterol formation already described, there is an increase in biliary secretion of cholesterol and reduced bile-salt secretion. The consequent precipitation of supersaturated bile and cholesterol crystallisation predisposes older people to gallstone formation.

CLINICAL IMPLICATIONS

Liver biochemistry and other synthetic functions (serum bilirubin, transaminases, alkaline phosphatase, albumin and coagulation) should be checked when assessing liver disease in older people. Biochemical markers of liver function are unaffected by the ageing process and any change in these parameters should be considered abnormal and investigated accordingly. As liver function tests are often done routinely in clinical practice, their abnormality is often the first indicator of the possibility of underlying liver or biliary tract disease. It must also be remembered, particularly in the older patient, who is more likely to have multiple co-morbidities, that derangement of liver function tests may be due to the impact of other organ dysfunction on the liver, such as congestive cardiac failure, sepsis, thyroid disease and rheumatological conditions including polymyalgia rheumatica and active rheumatoid arthritis. In such cases, treatment of the underlying condition will result in improvement or resolution of liver biochemistry.

Impact of ageing on common liver diseases

With the increase in life expectancy in developed countries, common conditions that cause chronic liver disease (including hepatitis C, alcohol, non-alcoholic fatty liver disease and hepatitis B infection) are becoming an increasingly important cause of morbidity and mortality in older people.

Viral hepatitis

Acute viral hepatitis is uncommon in older people; however, the prevalence of hepatitis B and C in the older population will increase over the next 20–30 years. In hepatitis A infection, older people are at greater risk of acute liver failure and have a higher mortality than younger people. The cause for this is multifactorial and includes the increased prevalence of co-morbid illness, slower regenerative capacity of the liver and a reduced immune function with age. Hepatitis B is rare after the age of 65 years, but there is an increased risk of progression to chronic infection and hepatocellular carcinoma with age. The same is true for hepatitis C infection, in which an older age at the time of infection is a risk factor for the progression of chronic infection and fibrosis. Despite the low prevalence of infective hepatitis in the older population, it is still advisable to provide vaccination to those at risk of hepatitis A and B, as the consequences of disease can be serious.

Biliary tract infections

Bacterial infection of the biliary tree may occur due to achlorhydria, which is common in older people (in up to 80% of those aged over 80 years) due to atrophic gastritis. Bacterial infection can lead to an acute cholangitis as a result of colonisation of the small bowel with coliform organisms, leading to bile contamination. Older people with biliary tract infections tend to present in a more atypical fashion, often without fever or abdominal pain. In one study of older patients with acute cholecystitis, over 10% had normal liver enzymes and 5% had no pain on presentation. Endoscopic retrograde cholangiopancreatography (ERCP) is an effective therapeutic intervention for older people that has a success rate of up to 98% in ductal stone clearance and no significant difference in mortality or complication rates between young patients and those aged over 80 years.

Autoimmune liver disease

Autoimmune hepatitis (AIH) can be classified as type 1 or 2. In contrast to type 2 AIH, which is predominantly a disease of the young, type 1 AIH has bimodal peaks of presentation occurring at ages 10–30 years and a later peak between 50 and 70 years. It is characterised by the presence of anti-smooth muscle and antinuclear antibodies. Although AIH generally has an excellent prognosis if remission is induced, in older people diagnosis may often be delayed due to an insidious presentation and a reluctance to perform liver biopsy in this age group. These factors may further delay initiation of treatment, which can result in more severe disease in the older person. As discussed earlier, the reduced endocytic activity of ageing Kupffer cells may play a role in the development of autoimmune disease in older people and, in addition, age-related defenestration may be a factor by impairing the interaction between hepatocytes and native T lymphocytes, which are thought to induce immunotolerance.

Malignancy

The incidence of cholangiocarcinoma is greater in those aged over 65 years, with approximately 65% of biliary tumours occurring in this age group. Of these, 95% are adenocarcinomas; in older people, these commonly present at a more advanced stage with signs of biliary obstruction. In comparison, intrahepatic cholangiocarcinomas may initially present with more systemic features such as general malaise or weight loss, hence incidental discovery on radiographic examination is not uncommon. In contrast, the incidence of hepatocellular carcinoma peaks between 40 and 60 years of age; however, with demographic change, more cases are likely to be seen in older people in the future. Hepatic resection for hepatocellular carcinoma can be undertaken in older people, but hepatic regeneration is impaired with age and post-operative mortality is also greater in older people, so the potential benefits need to be carefully balanced against the risks in this age group. A percutaneous or ablative approach is an alternative method and may have a better outcome in older people.

Drug and toxic injury

Drug-induced liver disease is an important and not uncommon problem in older people. The most common offenders include antibiotics, anti-epileptic drugs and NSAIDs. Presentation of drug-induced liver disease is non-specific and can range from mild abnormalities in liver function tests to fulminant hepatic failure. The diagnosis is made by excluding other causes of liver disease, a temporal relationship with the introduction of a drug and improvement, and resolution following drug withdrawal. In older people, alcohol hepatitis is unusual and alcohol-related liver disease is more likely to present as cirrhosis.

AGEING AND DRUG HANDLING BY THE LIVER

Medications are frequently prescribed for older people: up to 45% of prescriptions dispensed in the UK are for people aged over 65 years. The incidence of adverse reactions in older people is almost three times that of younger people because of age-associated pharmacokinetic changes. Changes in hepatic drug metabolism play an important part, as do more general factors that occur with age, including reduced serum albumin, total body water and lean body mass, and increased body fat stores.

Drug metabolism and clearance by the liver are dependent on a combination of hepatic blood flow, protein binding and intrinsic clearance, the latter encompassing enzyme activity (biotransformation) and hepatic mass. Highly extracted drugs are absorbed from the gut and transported to the liver by the portal vein where they are metabolised before reaching the systemic circulation. This is known as 'first-pass metabolism'. First-pass drug metabolism is therefore dependent on hepatic blood flow, which, as mentioned earlier, can fall by up to 40% in older people. When the concentration of a drug surpasses the ability of the liver to extract and metabolise it, any small increase in drug dosage will result in a large increase in systemic drug concentration. Thus, reduced hepatic blood flow can result in the reduced clearance of high-extraction drugs such as nitrates, verapamil and propranolol, with subsequent increase in systemic bioavailability. The decline in hepatic drug metabolism of low-extraction drugs is thought to be influenced by the decrease in liver mass associated with ageing. Therefore, intrinsic clearance and, to a lesser extent, protein binding are important in the metabolism of low-extraction drugs such as phenytoin, alcohol and theophylline.

Hepatic drug biotransformation is categorised into Phase I and Phase II reactions (*see* Table 9.2). Phase I reactions include oxidation, reduction, demethylation and hydrolysis. These reactions mainly detoxify or inactivate the bioactive molecule but, at times, can enhance the molecule to an active prodrug. They are among the most widely studied group of reactions and are catalysed in the hepatocyte smooth endoplasmic reticulum by the cytochrome P_{450} (CYP_{450}) system. Phase II reactions on the other hand involve conjugation of certain ionised groups to the drug molecule by glucuronidation, sulphation, methylation or acetylation amongst others. Phase II reactions inactivate drugs or the active metabolites formed from Phase I reactions and allow drug excretion in the urine or bile (depending on the molecular weight) by making it water-soluble. Data on the hepatic metabolism of drugs in ageing humans are limited and largely inferred from animal models. *In vitro* studies of hepatocytes isolated from humans and rats found no difference in the rates of Phase I and II reactions with age. However, *in vivo* animal studies have shown that while increasing age has very little impact on Phase II pathways, Phase I oxidative metabolism may be impaired. It has been suggested that the difference found in oxidative metabolism between *in vitro* and *in vivo* studies may be explained by reduced hepatocyte oxygen supply in older animals as a result of the pseudocapillarisation of hepatic sinusoids acting as a barrier to diffusion. Pseudocapillarisation leads to relative hypoxia and lower adenosine triphosphate–adenosine diphosphate ratios in older rats in comparison to younger rats. This may impair the clearance of drugs that undergo oxidative metabolism such as theophylline. Furthermore, over the age of 70 years, it is believed there are reduced cytochrome P_{450} levels in the liver, with an associated 30% decline in hepatic drug metabolism, which can be compounded by the use of drugs that induce or inhibit cytochrome enzymes. The majority of drug interactions and adverse reactions in older people are related to hepatic biotransformation of drugs that involve this enzyme family. However, it should be remembered that there is marked genetic variability in rates of CYP_{450} metabolism within both normal healthy young and older populations.

TABLE 9.2 Summary of biotransformation reactions occurring in the liver

Hepatic biotransformation	Type of reaction	Action	Effect in older people
Phase I	Oxidation Reduction Demethylation Hydrolysis Mostly cytochrome enzyme related	Mainly detoxify or inactivate drug	Oxidative metabolism may be impaired by reduced hepatocyte oxygen supply and reduced cytochrome activity (30%)
Phase II	Glucuronidation Sulphation Methylation Acetylation	Increase drug excretion in urine or bile	Very little effect on pathway

Drug binding can also be affected by age. As the pharmacological effect of a drug is determined by the amount bound to plasma proteins, reduced total protein levels in older people play an important role in drug bioavailability. Basic drugs are bound by α1-acid glycoprotein, which, with age, is believed to be either unaltered or increased because of a greater predominance of age-associated inflammatory disease. However, most drugs are acidic and are bound to serum albumin. Serum albumin falls by up to 10% with age and drug-binding capacity decreases to a similar extent resulting in a higher free fraction of drug. This often necessitates dose reduction of protein-bound drugs, including warfarin and phenytoin, to reduce the risk of adverse effects in older people.

As the liver ages, the duration and extent of both therapeutic and adverse effects can be increased. The liver is a major site of drug clearance, with hepatic drug elimination reduced by up to 50% in older people. The effect of liver ageing on some specific commonly prescribed drugs and the mechanism involved is described below (*see* Table 9.3).

TABLE 9.3 Drugs affected by altered hepatic drug handling in the older person

Drug metabolism	Age-related changes	Drugs affected
First-pass metabolism	Decreased hepatic blood flow	Amitriptyline Aspirin Nitrates Propranolol Verapamil
Phase I hepatic biotransformation (catalysed by CYP$_{450}$)	Reduction in drug clearance	Amitriptyline Chlordiazepoxide Codeine Diazepam Diltiazem Ibuprofen Piroxicam Propranolol Theophylline Tramadol Verapamil
Phase II hepatic biotransformation	Unchanged	Lorazepam Temazepam
Drug binding	Reduced binding secondary to a fall in albumin levels	Diazepam Phenytoin Warfarin

SPECIFIC DRUG GROUPS AFFECTED BY THE AGEING LIVER
Alcohol
In the older person, increased blood concentrations and toxic effects of ethanol occur at lower doses due to a combination of age-related reduction in water distribution volume and the reduced activity of enzymes such as acetaldehyde dehydrogenase involved in ethanol metabolism.

Analgesics and NSAIDs

Paracetamol is metabolised by conjugation to glucuronide and sulphate metabolites, thereby detoxifying the reactive metabolite. In a healthy older population, intrinsic conjugation is preserved, but this may be reduced by frailty and malnutrition. Therefore, reduced paracetamol dosage is recommended in the treatment of frail older people.

NSAIDs are subject to hepatic clearance and conversion to inactive metabolites. NSAIDs such as ibuprofen and piroxicam that are metabolised by Phase I reactions have longer plasma half-lives in older people. Aspirin has significant first-pass metabolism; thus, in the older person, it can accumulate in the ageing liver due to the impaired first-pass response and result in toxicity.

Weak opioids, codeine and tramadol are metabolised to active metabolites by cytochrome enzymes. The effectiveness of codeine is primarily dependent on its metabolism in the liver to the activated metabolite morphine, and it is thought that up to 10% of the population are unable to metabolise codeine into morphine due to differences in cytochrome enzyme activity. Morphine is extensively metabolised in the liver via glucuronidation to the active metabolites morphine-3-glucuronide and morphine-6-glucuronide. Both metabolites penetrate the blood–brain barrier, but it is thought that morphine-3-glucuronide is responsible for the neurotoxic effects of morphine, which can be more marked in older people.

Anti-epileptic drugs

Older people are sensitive to the side effects of anti-epileptic drugs, even at lower doses. Drugs such as phenytoin, carbamazepine and lamotrigine can accumulate due to reduced hepatic metabolism. Many anti-epileptic drugs cause cognitive disturbance through inhibitory effects on the central nervous system. Moreover, with increasing age and the reduction in hepatic reserve, older people are more sensitive to the hepatic induction or inhibition of anti-epileptic drugs and associated drug interactions.

Benzodiazepines

With increasing age there is increased sensitivity to the effects of benzodiazepines on the central nervous system. Benzodiazepines such as lorazepam and temazepam are subject only to Phase II metabolism and therefore do not exhibit the prolonged elimination times that are seen in older people with chlordiazepoxide or diazepam. In contrast, these latter drugs are subject to both Phase I and Phase II reactions. Chlordiazepoxide or diazepam can cause prolonged sedation in older people due to the impaired Phase I reactions previously discussed.

Calcium channel antagonists

These drugs are predominantly metabolised in the liver and, as a rule, dosage should be reduced in older people and titrated to clinical response. The clearance of verapamil is reduced with ageing due to decreased hepatic blood flow and age-related changes in Phase I drug metabolism. Diltiazem, however, does not undergo extensive first-pass metabolism and reduced clearance of the drug is only associated with changes in Phase I hepatic metabolism. Although clearance of amlodipine is also diminished in the older person, it is generally an effective and well-tolerated anti-hypertensive in the older population, with reduction in blood pressure comparable to that seen in younger people.

Warfarin

Warfarin has a narrower therapeutic range in older people for a variety of reasons. There is greater inhibition of vitamin K-dependent clotting factors, with similar plasma concentrations of warfarin in older people than in younger people. Warfarin is highly bound to albumin and the binding capacity of warfarin is reduced in older people because of the lower protein levels found in this group. Concomitant use of warfarin and aspirin can increase the risk of bleeding due to increased displacement of warfarin from plasma albumin by aspirin. With aspirin, warfarin displacement of 1%–2% can double or triple the concentration of active plasma anticoagulant.

It has been suggested that genetic, environmental and person-specific factors such as smoking have a greater impact on hepatic drug metabolism than ageing per se. Although physiological changes associated with ageing are important, an individual's characteristics must also be taken into consideration. However, as a general rule, it is advisable to reduce the dosage of drugs metabolised by the liver in older people, as it can be anticipated that hepatic clearance will be reduced.

CONCLUSION

The liver has many functions and it is not surprising that liver dysfunction has major implications for disease management in older people. When managing liver disease in older people, it should be remembered that the ability of the liver to regenerate after toxic injury diminishes with age. In this chapter, we have outlined the changes that occur in the liver with age that we feel are the most important, clinically relevant and significant.

FURTHER READING

Anantharaju A, Feller A, Chedid A. Aging liver: a review. *Gerontology*. 2002; 48(6): 343–53.
Bressler R, Bahl JJ. Principles of drug therapy for the elderly patient. *Mayo Clin Proc*. 2003; 78(12): 1564–77.

Junaidi O, Di Bisceglie AM. Aging liver and hepatitis. *Clin Geriatr Med.* 2007; **23**(4): 889–903.

Le Couteur DG, Warren A, Cogger VC *et al.* Old age and the hepatic sinusoid. *Anat Rec (Hoboken).* 2008; **291**(6): 672–83.

McLean AJ, Le Couteur DG. Aging biology and geriatric clinical pharmacology. *Pharmacol Rev.* 2004; **56**(2): 163–84.

QUESTIONS: THE LIVER

1 Which one of the following changes occurs within the hepatic sinusoid with ageing?

A an increase in the surface area of the smooth endoplasmic reticulum correlating with decreased enzyme activity of microsomal enzymes

B an increase in number and activity of stellate cells, which are associated with age-related increase in systemic markers of inflammation

C increased transfer of lipoproteins across the liver sinusoidal endothelial cells

D Kupffer cells are activated in response to injury releasing fat droplets

E pseudocapillarisation of the hepatic sinusoids leads to reduced sinusoidal perfusion.

Answer: E

2 The effect of age on the hepatic sinusoids affects the passage of lipoproteins from the bloodstream. What is this change called?

A defenestration

B fibrosis

C glucuronidation

D oxidation

E steatosis.

Answer: A

3 Which one of the following is an expected finding in healthy older people?

A an increased incidence of hepatitis A infection

B elevation in serum alkaline phosphatase

C impaired metabolism of metoclopramide

D postprandial hypertriglyceridaemia

E preserved capability of hepatocytes to recover from a toxic insult.

Answer: D

4 Drugs are metabolised and cleared by the liver in different ways. Which one of these drugs undergoes Phase II hepatic biotransformation?

A amitriptyline

B aspirin

C propranolol

D temazepam

E warfarin.

Answer: D

5 Liver volume decreases with age. What is the proportionate reduction in liver volume in people aged over 65 compared with those aged under 40 years?

A 15%

B 35%

C 45%

D 65%

E 75%.

Answer: B

CHAPTER 10

The kidneys

AZA ABDULLA AND WILLIAM OGBURN

INTRODUCTION

The kidneys are the most powerful regulators of the body's internal environment. Healthy kidneys are vital to maintain conditions in which all of the body's other processes can function optimally. This includes acid/base and electrolyte homeostasis, regulation of blood volume and pressure, removal of waste products, regulation of red cell mass and synthesis of vitamin D.

In the absence of disease, the kidneys will continue to function normally into the third decade of life but then the function will slowly decline. This chapter discusses this natural process. Terms such as 'chronic renal failure' or 'insufficiency' are often used, but they are unhelpful as they describe a pathological process rather than the physiological decline of renal senescence. It is also important to appreciate that separating the two can be very difficult due to the large number of common chronic medical problems that older people may accrue during life, which have an impact on renal function.

Senescent kidneys are able to maintain homeostatic equilibrium when not affected by acute illness, but this fine balance may be rapidly lost when the individual is placed under stress. It is this loss of physiological reserve that is important to be aware of when managing older patients and can affect many aspects of their care – from determining which drugs to prescribe to how to best replace fluid and electrolytes.

ANATOMICAL CHANGES IN THE KIDNEYS WITH AGE

Trying to define the anatomical changes in the kidney with advancing age can be very difficult. Much of the published literature of the last century arrived at varying conclusions on changes in renal size and morphology. This is because many studies did not differentiate between the consequences of age and chronic disease. Even those that attempted this had difficulties due to the shifting definitions of diseases such as hypertension or used post-mortem specimens with limited clinical information. However, it does appear that now opinion is reaching consensus.

From birth, renal weight increases up until the fourth or fifth decade, reaching a peak of 250–270 g. Weight then gradually declines to 180–200 g by the seventh to ninth decades. Most descriptions of the gross anatomy of senescent kidneys come from post-mortem specimens. Approximately 50% show a fine granularity or smooth mottled surface and up to 14% are grossly scarred. Senescent scarring is widely distributed at all sites, whereas pyelonephritic scarring, which causes calyceal deformity that is absent from purely aged kidneys, is usually only found at the poles. The literature describing the volume loss with age varies depending on the modality used. Post-mortem findings have described the loss as 20% between the ages of 50 and 80 years, but intravenous urography has indicated volume loss of 40% and reduction in kidney length of 2 cm. Computed tomography (CT) scans show even greater change, with a decrease in transverse area of 30%–33% after the age of 70 years. The loss of renal mass predominantly affects the cortex with relative sparing of the medulla. There is also an increase in the amount of fat deposition in the renal sinuses, which can account for 17% of the renal mass at post-mortem.

Approximately one-half of all people over 40 years have one or more simple cysts in the kidneys. These degenerative cysts are typically unilocular and contain clear fluid resembling interstitial fluid. Simple cysts are thought to arise from dilated tubules, glomeruli or even tubular diverticula that have become cut off from the tubule.

VASCULAR CHANGES

Ageing is also associated with changes in the renal vasculature. There is progressive thickening of the intima of small interlobular arteries at the expense of elastic tissue and loss of the media. This is termed 'collagenous fibrosis' or 'intimal fibroplasia'. This process is patchy and may be the underlying cause of the heterogeneous loss of nephrons. The arteries themselves become distorted and spiralled. In smaller afferent arterioles, the changes are caused by hyaline arteriosclerosis with thickening of the intimal layer due to deposition of hyaline and collagen fibres. There is some debate still as to whether arteriosclerosis of the smaller renal vessels is truly a consequence of normal ageing; the current view is that the changes are part of the natural ageing process and are accelerated by hypertension. In vessels larger than arterioles, it is accepted that this process is part of normal vascular ageing and precedes the changes in the smaller vessels.

Multiple studies have shown that increasing age is associated with a decrease in renal blood flow. Furthermore, significant increases in filtration fraction and renal vascular resistance with ageing have been found in every human study in which they have been measured. Total renal blood flow is preserved up until the fourth decade of life; thereafter, a progressive decline of approximately 10% per decade occurs. This may be due to the concomitant loss of renal mass and the decrease in blood flow may be proportionate or the flow per unit mass may even increase. There is also evidence that autoregulation may be lost or altered with ageing and that both the sensitivity and responsiveness of the renal arterioles may be affected.

The decrease in renal blood flow is most profound in the cortex with relative sparing of the deeper medullary areas. This may explain the increase, as the juxtamedullary glomeruli have a greater filtration fraction.

GLOMERULAR AND INTERSTITIAL CHANGES WITH AGEING

The estimates of total numbers of glomeruli in adults have varied in the literature, from 0.6×10^6 to 120×10^6, but some of the studies included patients who died of disease that affected renal function and half to two-thirds of subjects were over 70 years of age. The number varies across race and sex, and has been shown to have a linearly proportional relationship to birthweight. In the young, the glomerular volume does not vary in different zones of the kidney; however, in the fifth and sixth decades, the superficial glomeruli are significantly larger. There is a general consensus that the number of glomeruli decreases with age. Glomeruli are lost through the process of glomerulosclerosis. The glomerular basement membrane becomes thickened and the mesangial area increases. The cross-sectional area of the glomerulus also decreases. The capillary tuft in the centre of the glomerulus loses complexity, which leads to a reduction in filtering surface. The filtering membrane becomes wrinkled and more permeable to large molecules such as proteins, which then appear in the urine. Given the reduced glomerular blood flow, this leads to a reduction in glomerular filtration. The percentage of sclerotic glomeruli increases with age, is higher in men and they start to appear in the third decade of life. Up to 30% of glomeruli are sclerotic by the eighth decade of life.

In the senescent kidney, the tubules degenerate and atrophy. There is a decrease in number and individual tubules show reduced length, decrease in volume and increased diverticula. On a cellular level, there may be wrinkling, with thinning of the tubular basement membranes, simplification of the tubular epithelium or dilatation of tubules with regular hyaline casts. The interstitium also undergoes changes with ageing. The proportion of interstitial tissue made up of glomeruli and tubules decreases fourfold; an increasing volume is now made up of areas of scarring, fibrosis and tubular atrophy. There is also variable infiltrate of mononuclear cells, which may be a result of renal damage but may also be part of the process of attempted repair.

Therefore, the whole of the kidney undergoes age-related changes, which have varying effects on function. Table 10.1 provides a summary of these changes.

TABLE 10.1 Summary of morphological changes that occur in the ageing kidney

Structure	Individual component	Change
Gross anatomy	Renal mass	↓
	Scarring	↑
	Cysts	↑
Vascular	Vascular resistance	↑
	Intimal thickness	↑
	Total renal blood flow	↓
	Homeostatic responsiveness	↓
	Tortuosity	↑
Glomerular and interstitial tissue	Number of glomeruli	↓
	Cross-sectional area of glomeruli	↓

↑= increase; ↓= decrease

PHYSIOLOGICAL CHANGES WITH AGE

Glomerular filtration rate (GFR)

The time-honoured gold standard for measuring GFR is by inulin clearance (Cin). Inulin is a polysaccharide freely filtered by the glomerulus and neither reabsorbed nor secreted by the tubules. However, in everyday clinical practice, assessment of GFR is done through measurement of creatinine clearance (CrCl), which is endogenously produced from muscle creatine and filtered through the glomerulus. Since creatinine is normally secreted by the renal tubule, CrCl overestimates GFR by about 22%.

Studies, both cross-sectional and longitudinal, have been consistent in demonstrating a steady decline in GFR with age starting from the fourth decade, with an accelerated rate of decline by the seventh decade. The average decline in GFR that has been reported is 0.96 mL/min/year or about 10 mL/min/decade; in one study involving 548 normal subjects, the CrCl fell from 140 mL/min/1.73 m^2 at age 30 years to about 97 mL/min/1.73 m^2 at age 80. In another more recent study, the rate of decline in CrCl slowly accelerated to reach a peak value of –3.25 mL/min/year after the age of 80. In this study, the average rate of decline in CrCl was –0.75 mL/min/year. However, the universality of this process has been questioned by two studies: the first demonstrated that older people on high a protein diet maintained a normal GFR and the second reported that in around a third of older people there was no demonstrable decrease in GFR with age. The latter study, however, was short-lived (lasting only 5 years) and has not been substantiated, while the first observation may be explained as the phenomenon of renal reserve (the capacity of the kidney to increase its basal GFR by at least 20% after a protein load), which is preserved in healthy older people, albeit at a reduced magnitude.

The decline in GFR appears to be a normal process of ageing and, importantly, independent of hypertension or other co-morbid conditions. It is a consequence of the progressive loss of glomeruli through global glomerulosclerosis and changes in the renal vascular tree, and perhaps related to the effect of oxidative stress and telomere shortening, or linked to an action of angiotensin II.

Tubulo-interstitial functional changes

The proximal tubule is where the majority of organic solutes (glucose, amino acids and inorganic phosphate), small proteins, bicarbonate and approximately two-thirds of the sodium and water are reabsorbed. The handling functions of these chemicals have not been shown to change between younger and older age, but the maximum rate of reabsorption, tubular maximum (Tm), is decreased. The Tm of glucose, for example, diminishes in tandem with the GFR. The proximal tubules also have important metabolic functions such as the removal of insulin. Insulin is filtered by the glomerulus then absorbed by renal tubular cells that then degrade it. As this function declines with age, insulin clearance decreases.

The proximal tubule leads next into the loop of Henle. The main function of this segment of the tubule is to create a concentration gradient in the medulla of the kidney. This allows for the production of concentrated urine. In simple terms, the descending limb of the loop of Henle has a low permeability to ions but a high permeability to water, whereas the ascending limb has the opposite, creating a countercurrent multiplier.

With age, the ability of the ascending limb to reabsorb sodium is decreased, leading to a higher osmotic load on the distal sections of the tubular system. The collecting ducts only reabsorb approximately 3% of the sodium in the glomerular filtrate, which leads to a state of overall sodium loss. Furthermore, the kinetics of sodium handling is also affected by ageing. In one study, the ability to conserve sodium following acute dietary salt restriction in older individuals, assessed by determining the half-time taken for proportionate reduction in sodium excretion, was almost twice that of younger people (31 versus 17 hours). Conversely, due to the generally lower GFR of older subjects, sodium loading takes longer to be cleared; thus, normal older subjects can be described as 'salt sensitive'. Not only is excretory capacity for sodium impaired, but there is also a circadian variation, with older people excreting sodium at higher rates at night than younger persons.

The sluggish adaptive response in older people to abrupt changes in salt intake may have major consequences – for example, following surgery or acute illness – resulting in reduction in extracellular fluid compartment and effective circulatory volume.

Fluid balance and the ability to concentrate or dilute urine

The maintenance of fluid balance is controlled by a number of factors. These include thirst, posterior pituitary function and the ability of the kidneys to respond by producing either dilute or concentrated urine. As people age, the thirst response becomes less effective and general fluid intake decreases. The normal physiological responses to dehydration in older people are all present and some aspects – for example, vasopressin secretion – are actually higher than in younger subjects. However, these physiological responses still fail to elicit a thirst response in some cases. The reasons for this are unclear but several factors have been suggested, including decreased sensitivity to dryness of the mouth and loss of taste sensation.

Total body water in older people is lower, at about 54% of total body mass, than in younger people (66% of total body mass). This is due to a higher proportion of body mass comprising fat. The loss of fluid seems to be predominantly intracellular, as the total plasma volume is preserved in men and significantly increased in women, as some studies have shown.

It is also well recognised that the ability to concentrate urine declines with age. The reasons for this are still not entirely clear. Initially, this was attributed to the decline in GFR but studies have failed to confirm this. Other studies postulated that it is due to increased medullary blood flow leading to 'washout' of the medullary concentrating gradient. In support of this is the fact that older subjects have been shown to have a higher fractional excretion rate of urea, which is an important contributor to maintaining this gradient.

The declining ability to conserve water is not of any real clinical significance in the context of the healthy older subject with free access to fluids but can be a significant issue when the subject is suffering from intercurrent illness or has difficulty accessing hydration (*see* 'Clinical implications', p. 139)

The study evidence for the effects of ageing on the kidneys' ability to produce dilute urine is sparse. Most studies have been performed in rats, so the findings have to be applied with care. The general consensus seems to be that the ability to produce dilute urine in response to water loading is diminished but the change is mild. It must also be remembered that many medicines commonly prescribed for older people impair water excretion, such as non-steroidal anti-inflammatory drugs (NSAIDs), morphine and tricyclic antidepressants.

Reduced renal blood flow, gradual loss of nephrons and decreased GFR reduce the ability of the kidneys to maintain the levels of major electrolytes. Sodium handling has already been described, but senescence also affects potassium, calcium and chloride handling. Total body potassium is 15% lower in older subjects, and the decrease is more marked in women. This may be due to the lower fraction of body weight made up of muscle in older subjects. Older subjects also tend to eat a diet lower in potassium; despite these factors, the plasma potassium level is unchanged from that of the young. The basal urinary secretion of potassium in older subjects is also decreased. This has been attributed to a relatively low serum aldosterone and aldosterone resistance in healthy older people.

Calcium is an important ion in many bodily functions, from cardiac action potential to the clotting cascade. The kidneys reabsorb 98% of filtered calcium and this appears unchanged in the older population, although this only applies to a healthy older subject with adequate calcium intake, sun exposure and parathyroid hormone (PTH) levels. The mechanism for maintaining a normal calcium concentration is a complex multi-organ system involving bone, gut and kidney. The study evidence for changes in chloride handling is lacking but is felt to mirror sodium.

The kidney is doubly important, since not only does it control excretion via urine, but it is also responsible for the hydroxylation of vitamin D to its active form – this will be further on in the chapter.

Acid–base balance

The kidneys are the most important organs in acid/base homeostasis. The lungs are also important, as rapid correction of pH can be mediated by changes in respiratory rate and levels of CO_2, but only the kidneys can directly remove acidic/basic molecules from the circulation. In normal healthy individuals, there is no difference in resting pH but the response and time to resolution of acid loading is greater in older individuals. Unfortunately, there are very few studies looking at this subject and the few that there are, are difficult to compare. This is due to the differing protocols used in the studies, including subject position (supine or upright) and the baseline renal function and electrolytes of the subjects. Given the limited evidence available, the consensus seems to be that renal acid/base handling is unchanged between young and older subjects. In fact, in some older individuals, acid excretion may even be increased. The main difference is a lag in response to acid/base loading. In older subjects, acid/base loading takes longer to resolve and there may be a more exaggerated movement away from baseline for the same amount of load. This is due to the corrective mechanisms, such as bicarbonate and ammonium ion excretion, taking longer to respond.

Renin–angiotensin system (RAS)

The RAS is a renal hormone-based system that is vital in blood pressure and fluid balance autoregulation. When circulating volume is low, the juxtaglomerular cells produce renin directly into the circulation. The liver produces angiotensinogen, which is converted by circulating renin to angiotensin I. In turn, angiotensin I is converted to angiotensin II by the angiotensin-converting enzyme (ACE) in the lungs. Angiotensin II is a potent vasoconstrictor causing increased blood pressure. It also stimulates the adrenal cortex to produce aldosterone. This causes the renal tubules to retain sodium and water leading to expansion of plasma volume and facilitates tubular excretion of potassium.

The level of activity of this system in the ageing population has been well studied in rats and humans. It appears to decline with age in both baseline and stimulated states. In the stimulated state, the decline appears to be even more marked. It is estimated that plasma rennin activity in older people is 40%–60% lower than in the younger population. Similarly, there is a progressive age-related decrease in basal aldosterone as well as aldosterone response to upright posture and volume depletion.

The sluggish renin–aldosterone response to acute stimuli may explain the reduced capacity for sodium retention and reduced potassium excretion.

Erythropoiesis

Erythropoiesis involves several organ systems including the liver, bone marrow and kidneys. The role of the kidney is to produce erythropoietin (EPO), a single-chain glycoprotein made up of 166 amino acids. It is a specific growth factor for the erythroid cell line with a minor stimulating effect on the megakaryocyte-platelet cell line. Its production is modulated by cell oxygen availability monitored by a renal oxygen sensor using a haem protein. To increase production, more cells are recruited to start production, as there are no intracellular stores of EPO, and hypoxia stimulates production at the mRNA level. The effect of ageing on this system is not well documented. In various epidemiological studies, anaemia has been shown to be increasingly common as a population ages, but this is not considered to be a normal physiological decline in red blood cell production. Given the multi-systemic nature of the maintenance of red blood cell mass, there are many different disease processes that could affect it and lead to anaemia. Thus, it is a real challenge to try to document and study the normal physiology of ageing in this context. The kidney's role in this process is to produce EPO. EPO levels have actually been found to be higher in the older population in the absence of renal disease, which is felt to be due to the need for higher levels to maintain a normal red cell mass. This may be due to end-organ resistance or senescent failure of bone marrow.

Vitamin D

Vitamin D_3 (cholecalciferol), either formed in the skin from 7-dehydocholesterol by ultraviolet light or absorbed through the intestine, is biologically inactive and needs to undergo a two-stage hydroxylation to be metabolised into 1,25-dihydroxyvitamin D_3 [1,25$(OH)_2D_3$], the active form of vitamin D. The initial step occurs in the liver hepatocytes, where cholecalciferol is converted to 25-hydroxyvitamin D [25$(OH)D$] by cytochrome enzymes. The second step occurs in the kidney.

The proximal tubule cells of the kidney are the site of the second hydroxylation. The main enzyme responsible is 1-alpha-hydroxylase. Although alternative pathways do exist for hydroxylation of 25(OH)D, such as 24-hydroxylase, these are much less effective.

1,25(OH)$_2$D is regarded as the primary metabolite responsible for the biological actions of vitamin D and acts as an endocrine modulator of calcium and phosphate homeostasis. Low dietary calcium and phosphate result in enhanced activity of 1-alpha-hydroxylase. Elevated PTH, resulting from hypocalcaemia, is a primary signal, mediating the induction of 1,25(OH)$_2$D$_3$ synthesis in the kidney. It is secreted into the circulation and it is transported, bound to vitamin D-binding protein, to tissues involved in the regulation of calcium and phosphorus – namely, the intestine, bone, parathyroid glands and the kidneys themselves.

Levels of 25(OH)D reflect the supply and nutritional status of vitamin D, whereas those of 1,25(OH)$_2$D$_3$ reflect the biological and functional status of the vitamin. In contrast to 25(OH)D, the half-life of 1,25(OH)$_2$D$_3$ in the circulation is very short (around 4–6 hours versus 2–3 weeks, respectively).

Serum levels of 1,25(OH)$_2$D$_3$ are affected by age. In rats, it has been demonstrated that the activity of the enzyme 1-alpha-hydroxylase is reduced with age. In humans, an increase in 1,25(OH)$_2$D$_3$ levels following infusion of PTH, an inducing agent for the enzyme 1-alpha-hydroxylase, correlated inversely with age. An increase in clearance of 1,25(OH)$_2$D$_3$ with ageing has also been reported. Thus, the activity of the 1-alpha-hydroxylase enzyme is inversely correlated to age.

In contrast, studies have shown that levels of 25(OH)D are unaffected by age per se, despite the reduction in cutaneous vitamin D synthesis with age. This is probably explained by the decline in renal function with age and reduction in 1-alpha-hydroxylase activity resulting in reduced clearance of 25(OH)D in old age. These effects, therefore, cancel each other out, so that ageing has no effect on 25(OH)D levels. However, there is an inverse correlation between PTH and 25(OH)D in older people, suggesting that although older adults are efficient in maintaining 25(OH)D, they need more vitamin D than younger individuals to produce the higher 25(OH)D concentrations required to overcome the hyperparathyroidism associated with their diminishing renal function.

The combined effect of a decline in the ability of the kidney to synthesise 1,25(OH)$_2$D$_3$ and an increase in the renal metabolism of 1,25(OH)$_2$D$_3$ may contribute to age-related bone loss.

Table 10.2 summarises the physiological changes that occur in the kidney with ageing.

TABLE 10.2 Summary of the physiological changes that occur in the kidney with ageing

Function	Component	Change
Glomeruli	Membrane permeability	↑
	GFR	↓
Tubulo-interstitial	Electrolyte homeostasis	↓
	Metabolic functions	↓
	Response to dehydration	↓
Fluid balance	Urine concentrating ability	↓
	Vasopressin secretion	↑
	Total body water	↓
	Homeostatic responsiveness	↓
Acid–base balance	Homeostatic responsiveness	↓
Renin–angiotensin system	Activity	↓
	Postural response	↓
Erythropoiesis	Incidence of anaemia	↑
	EPO levels	↑
Vitamin D	Alpha-hydroxylation	↓
	Renal metabolism	↑

↑= increase; ↓= decrease

CLINICAL IMPLICATIONS

Estimating GFR: uses and limitations

Measuring GFR, by Cin or radioactive markers like ^{51}Cr-EDTA or iothalamate is impractical for routine clinical practice. An alternative test is CrCl and, although still in common use, it requires timed urine collection, which may be quite laborious and prone to collection error in older people.

To overcome these problems, formulas for estimating CrCl from serum creatinine have become commonplace in clinical practice. One such formula is the Cockcroft–Gault (CG) formula, which predicts CrCl from serum creatinine, age, weight and sex. However, several studies have questioned its clinical utility in older people, as it significantly underestimates GFR in this group.

More recently, a second formula, from the Modification of Diet in Renal Disease (MDRD) study, has gained popularity. In this method, the estimated value of GFR (eGFR in mL/min/1.73 m^2) is calculated from the serum creatinine concentration using the modifier variables of age in years, sex and race (black versus non-black) as surrogates for endogenous creatinine production and excretion. The MDRD formula is more accurate than the CG formula but is not without its limitations.

The formulas for estimating GFR by the two methods are shown following.

MDRD: eGFR (mL/min/1.73 m²) = 186 × (creatinine/88.4) − 1.154 × (age) − 0.203 × 0.742 (if subject is female)

CG: eGFR (mL/min) = (140 − age [years]) × weight (kg)/(0.814 × creatinine) × 0.85 (if subject is female)

The MDRD eGFR formula is not very accurate for assessing GFR above 60 mL/min/1.73 m² and requires additional modifications for different ancestries (e.g. Chinese). Moreover, it may not be applicable to subjects with regular diets different from those used to derive the formula (e.g. strict vegetarians).

Many hospitals currently use the MDRD to report eGFR routinely with every serum creatinine measurement. The report gives the actual calculated eGFR if it is less than 60 mL/min/1.73 m² or, if higher than this, states that the eGFR is greater than 60 mL/min/1.73 m² without providing the precise value.

There are important issues when interpreting eGFR in older people using this formula. First, the MDRD study population was recruited from persons under 70 years of age diagnosed with chronic kidney disease (CKD; mean serum creatinine 200 µmol/L) and the formula has not been widely validated in a community-based older population. Second, the MDRD equation has been reported to be less accurate in populations without CKD. Compared with direct GFR measurement in population studies with average GFR estimates of less than 90 mL/min/1.73 m², the MDRD formula may underestimate the GFR by up to (−)30 mL/min. This difference may lead to a false-positive diagnosis of CKD in persons who do not have the disease but have a mild reduction in GFR, a situation not uncommon in older people.

The diagnosis or labelling of CKD is the result of the recent classification of CKD by the National Kidney Foundation, the Kidney Disease Outcomes Quality Initiative (KDOQI), which uses an arbitrary cut-off of GFR less than 60 mL/min/1.73 m² to define Stage 3 CKD and above (*see* Table 10.3).

TABLE 10.3 The National Kidney Foundation KDOQI stages of CKD classification system

Stage	eGFR (mL/min/1.73 m²)	Severity of kidney disease
1	>90	Damage (with normal eGFR)
2	60–89	Mild
3	30–59	Moderate
4	15–29	Severe
5	<15	Kidney failure

The classification has led to the inappropriate labelling of many older people with normal renal function, commonly older females, as having CKD, often causing unnecessary anxiety in the patient and possibly inappropriate management.

Thus, eGFR should always be interpreted with caution in older people. Despite these limitations, eGFR does provide important information regarding suitability of prescribing and dosing of drugs.

A salient example to illustrate this point is the use of NSAIDs. These drugs block the synthesis of cyclo-oxygenase products and disrupt renal prostaglandin synthesis. The role of prostaglandins in maintaining renal perfusion in healthy states is debatable. However, it becomes important in conditions where renal blood flow is compromised and GFR is adversely affected. In these situations, NSAIDs can lead to fluid retention and oedema, hypertension and hyperkalaemia. One study showed that in patients with congestive heart failure on diuretics, the use of NSAIDs increased the risk of hospitalisation twofold. Similarly, the co-prescription of a NSAID and an ACE inhibitor has also been reported to worsen renal function and lead to acute renal failure. These effects are usually reversible on discontinuing the NSAID.

When managing older patients, it is important to have an overview of what can be considered 'normal ageing'. Although many patients will have pre-existing renal disease, patients who are considered to have normal renal function on testing cannot be treated in the same way as young 'normal patients'. This has to be taken in to account when prescribing drugs and replacing fluid and/or electrolytes. A good cautionary example is the use of intravenous contrast agents in CT imaging. Usually, a patient cannot have contrast agents administered if there is evidence of renal dysfunction. The standard tests used to assess renal function, such as urea or creatinine levels, do not give a true picture of the functional state of the kidney, so damaging contrast agents may be given leading to further decline in renal function. A normal value of serum creatinine should always be interpreted with care in the older individual. Creatinine is a breakdown product of creatine in muscle and also from meat in the diet. Older subjects generally have a smaller muscle mass and may have a lower meat intake than younger subjects. This may lead to falsely low levels of serum creatinine in the presence of significant renal disease. It should also be appreciated that the capacity of the kidneys for removal of creatinine is large; thus, for serum creatinine levels to rise, the subject's GFR must already be significantly impaired. The kidneys' ability to remove toxic metabolic waste products is also highly dependent on fluid balance. Studies of the effects of dehydration have shown that CrCl can drop from 130 mL/min to 96 mL/min and increase up to 160 mL/min with adequate rehydration. This may be due to increased tubular water secretion, decreased resorption or both. This is significant because, due to poor thirst drive and medications like diuretics, older people tend to be chronically dehydrated.

Drug clearance

Normal creatinine levels in the blood do not necessarily mean that the renal clearance of drugs will be the same as in younger subjects, as GFR is reduced in the vast majority of older subjects. This means that even in the absence of disease or evidence of renal insufficiency, drug regimens must be adjusted in older patients. A general principle to adopt is the 'start low and go slow' approach. The only exception, however, is with diuretics.

Diuretics in older people

The diuretic class of drugs is commonly used in older people. They are employed to offload fluid in patients with anything from mild pedal oedema to severe congestive cardiac failure. With the exception of spironolactone, diuretics exert the desired effect by inhibiting tubular sodium reabsorption from the luminal side of the tubule. Except for mannitol, which is filtered through the glomerulus, they reach the tubular lumen through active secretion at the proximal tubule site; the higher the concentration of the diuretic in the filtrate, the greater the diuresis. In turn, the capacity of the nephrons to secrete diuretics to their site of action is proportional to the amount of drug reaching the transport sites of the nephrons. This is a function of the renal blood flow. In conditions where renal perfusion is compromised, it follows that the delivery of the diuretic to the site of action is reduced and the effect is diminished. Therefore, diuretics will also be less effective in older patients due to the lower GFR. Studies have shown that, on average, older people deliver around half as much of a loop diuretic into the urine as younger adults. Consequently, to produce a similar effect, older people require double the dose of a diuretic given in younger people with normal renal function.

As already discussed, fluid and electrolyte handling in the kidneys is impaired in older people. Homeostasis can be maintained in a state of health but response to stress is blunted significantly. Sudden fluid and electrolyte depletion cannot be tolerated as well in older subjects and is much more likely to lead to serious complications such as hypotension and collapse.

Problems arising from reduced concentrating ability

The declining ability to concentrate urine and conserve water may in certain cases accentuate dehydration, especially in summer months during unexpected sudden surges in temperature – such as the occurrence of a heatwave. This is more marked in patients with pre-existing diseases or those on diuretics. At the other end of the spectrum, the diminished ability of the senescent kidney to produce dilute urine in response to water or saline load may become problematic in older people, leading to fluid overload, as well as clinically relevant in those with underlying compromised cardiac function.

These physiologic changes lead to a greater tendency to both hyper- and hyponatraemia in older people. They often cause the course of acute illness to become complicated by deranging fluid and electrolyte homeostasis, which may lead to delayed recovery.

The blunted aldosterone response in association with a reduced GFR in older people increases the risk of hyperkalaemia. The problem is further compounded by certain drugs that have the potential to impair potassium handling, such as potassium-sparing diuretics, NSAIDs and beta blockers, which are commonly prescribed in older people.

Simple cysts

These cysts are slow growing, usually asymptomatic and found incidentally on imaging of the kidneys, usually in the lower pole. However, large cysts of over 20 cm in diameter have been described and may be a cause of discomfort or dull ache in the renal angle. Very rarely, large cysts may cause calyceal obstruction, haematuria and resistant hypertension due to arterial compression leading to segmental ischaemia.

Given their generally benign nature, simple cysts in older people should not distract from more important diagnoses.

Renal diseases associated with ageing

It is important to appreciate that urinalysis is normal in healthy older people; there is no haematuria or proteinuria. Proteinuria is an indicator of progressive renal impairment in ageing.

Certain renal diseases are seen more commonly in older people. For example, there is an increased prevalence of certain types of glomerulonephritis, namely crescenteric (fourfold increase) and membranous (two- to threefold increase), in older people. The latter may be related to its association with malignancies.

Both hypertension and diabetes mellitus, widely prevalent in older people, accelerate renal ageing in addition to producing specific disease-related changes in the kidneys. Atheromatous renal artery stenosis is frequently associated with hypertension and end-stage renal disease in older people.

Asymptomatic bacteriuria is much more common in older people. It is at least three times more common in community-dwelling women than men over the age of 70 years. Infection, especially ascending infection, predisposed by obstructive uropathy is also more common. Bacteriuria in older people is associated with reduced survival.

Ageing and renal transplant

The high success rate of renal transplantation has encouraged its use in older people, with documented success. However, older recipients have significantly higher rates of complications post-transplant than young patients. The age of the host is important with regard to age-related rejection of graft. Furthermore, cardiovascular events and infections are the two leading causes of death among older transplant patients. Infection accounts for 50% of deaths in older transplant recipients compared with 15% in younger patients. Given the underlying immune senescence state in older people, immunosuppression should be used cautiously.

CONCLUSION

The changes in the kidney with ageing are wide and varied. Although most subjects who reach advanced age will have at least one disease process that will impact on renal function it is important to understand what the 'normal' changes associated with senescence are and how they will affect management. Even subjects with normal measured renal function cannot be considered to be the same as matched younger subjects when prescribing drugs or managing fluid balance, and older subjects will also behave differently in the presence of acute illness. With the growing elderly population and increasing life expectancy an understanding of these changes is becoming more and more vital.

It should also be stated that more research is needed to examine this process as much of the evidence is poor. Many studies use disease definitions that would now be considered out of date, much of the evidence is only in animal models that would have to be applied with caution and very little new research uses elderly subjects. This is understandable as study design using elderly subjects is bound to be more complex due to the likelihood of pre-existing illness, which can confound findings.

FURTHER READING

Macías-Núñez JF, Cameron JS, Oreopoulos DG, editors. *The Aging Kidney in Health and Disease*. New York: Springer; 2008.

Martin JE, Sheaff ME. Renal ageing. *J Pathol*. 2007; **211**(2): 198–205.

Musso CG, Oreopoulos DG. Ageing and physiological changes of the kidneys including changes in glomerular filtration rate. *Nephron Physiol*. 2011; **119**(Suppl. 1): S1–5.

Stevens LA, Coresh J, Greene T *et al*. Assessing kidney function: measured and estimated glomerular filtration rate. *N Engl J Med*. 2006; **354**(23): 2473–83.

Zhou XJ, Rakheja D, Yu X *et al*. The ageing kidney. *Kidney Int*. 2008; **74**(6): 710–20.

QUESTIONS: RENAL SENESCENCE

1 Which statement best describes the physiology of senescent kidneys?
   A EPO is a vital link in erythropoiesis and the incidence of anaemia increases with age, despite higher levels of EPO in older people
   B study evidence has shown no difference in acid/base handling between young and old subjects
   C the ability of the kidney to produce $1,25(OH)_2D_3$ is unaffected by age, so age-related bone loss should be considered to be independent of renal senescence
   D the age-related changes in the tubular system are inclined towards sodium retention and a predisposition to hypernatraemia
   E the RAS tends to be hyperactive and shows an exaggerated response to changes in posture.

   Answer: A

2 In glomerular ageing, which of the following statements is true?
   A by the fifth decade, up to 30% of glomeruli have been lost through glomerular necrosis
   B glomerular number shows little variation between sex and race
   C glomeruli are lost by glomerulosclerosis and the rate of loss with age is higher in men
   D in the young, there is a wide variation in glomerular size, but this decreases with age due to the hypertrophy of smaller glomeruli
   E there is a general consensus on the total number of glomeruli and its decline with age.

   Answer: C

3 Regarding fluid balance in older people:
   A the percentage of total body water is actually higher in older people due to loss of muscle bulk
   B the normal physiological response to dehydration is maintained and may even show higher activity
   C the senescent kidneys have a decreased ability to concentrate urine due to decreased medullary blood flow
   D there is a decreased ability to conserve water due to reduced vasopressin secretion in response to dehydration
   E thirst response is an accurate measure of dehydration.

   Answer: B

4 Which one of the following statements best describes the gross anatomical changes in the normal senescent kidney?

A   as the kidneys shrink with age, less of their mass is made up of fat than in younger subjects

B   imaging studies show consistent reduction in size, irrespective of the modality used

C   most individuals over the age of 40 years will have multiple multi-locular cysts in both kidneys

D   renal mass increases until the four or fifth decade then decreases, and a minority will show generalised scarring

E   the kidneys diminish in size from the third decade onwards and will mostly show scarring at the poles.

Answer: D

5 The importance of renal senescence is characterised by:

A   even in healthy older people with normal measured renal function, subjects should be considered to have a degree of renal failure

B   in the absence of disease and with normal measured renal function, drugs can be prescribed in the same doses as younger patients

C   in the absence of renal disease, older subjects should be considered to be no different than younger subjects when prescribing vitamin D

D   senescent kidneys are able to maintain homeostasis in a state of health, but this balance can be rapidly lost under physiological stress

E   when indicated, a lower dose of diuretic should be prescribed in older patients than in younger.

Answer: D

CHAPTER 11

The urogenital system

MUNIR AHMED

INTRODUCTION

The structure and function of urogenital organs change with age as a result of hormonal, non-hormonal (e.g. vascular, musculoskeletal) and iatrogenic factors. However, the effect of age on the functions of the urogenital system (micturition, sexual potency and fertility) goes beyond physiological and anatomical changes. Psychological, social, cultural and adaptability factors modify expressions of urogenital function that are accepted as part of normal ageing. Urogenital function is very sensitive to these external factors. The effect of ageing on body organs is mostly through atrophy and loss of elasticity. Similar effects are seen in the urogenital system, mostly in response to hormonal factors. However, in men, the prostate is unique in that it enlarges with age, resulting in major changes in the lower and upper urinary tracts.

Lower urinary tract function declines with advancing age in a gradual, progressive and linear manner. Although structural changes in men and women in the lower urinary tract may follow different courses, the clinical effect in both sexes is lower urinary tract symptoms (LUTS).

This chapter will outline the changes in the urogenital system and their impact on aspects of urinary, sexual and fertility function.

AGE-RELATED CHANGES IN THE LOWER URINARY TRACT IN MEN

The major change with age in males is enlargement of the prostate, which is termed 'benign prostatic hyperplasia' (BPH). In BPH, changes include an increase in the volume of the prostate with an associated rise in prostate-specific antigen (PSA), nodule formation and changes in the zonal anatomy.

Microscopically, BPH affects approximately 50% of men aged 50–60 years old, 75% of men aged 60–69 years old and up to 90% of men over the age of 80.

Other age-related changes include decline in detrusor contractility, decline in bladder capacity, reduced ability to withhold voiding, decline in maximal urethral closure pressure and length, increase in post-voiding residual urine and hyper-methylation in prostatic DNA, leading to an increased chance of cancer. In addition, there are changes in the circadian sleep–wake pattern of urine output, in the antidiuretic and atrial natriuretic hormones, and renin–aldosterone system. These changes lead to LUTS and a predisposition to urinary incontinence, which are often associated with an impact on quality of life.

Risk factors for the development of LUTS are the same as for erectile dysfunction (ED) signalling pathways, as the mechanisms of smooth-muscle contraction in the penis are comparable with those for smooth-muscle contraction in the bladder neck, prostate and urethra.

Therefore LUTS and ED are probably interrelated. Four theories that support this relationship are: (1) decrease/alteration in nitric oxide synthase/nitric oxide levels in the prostate and penile smooth muscle; (2) autonomic hyperactivity effects on LUTS, prostate growth and ED; (3) increased Rho-kinase activation/endothelin activity; and (4) prostate and penile ischaemia.

AGE-RELATED CHANGES IN THE LOWER URINARY TRACT IN WOMEN

The female genitourinary tract is primarily dependent on circulating oestrogens: the changes in genital tissues associated with ageing reflect the progressive decline in gonadal-endocrine stimulation. However, musculoskeletal, neurological and other factors significantly contribute to the age-related changes in the lower urinary tract in women.

Pelvic prolapse

The genitals, urinary bladder, urethra and rectum are closely related anatomically and functionally and rely heavily on pelvic floor support for proper functioning. Prolapse of pelvic organs is common in ageing women. Although the precise cause of pelvic prolapse is unknown, it is suggested that a number of factors may contribute to its development, including damage during childbirth, striated muscle weakness or neuromuscular disorder caused by disease, trauma, ageing and loss of tissue elasticity and turgor due to a fall in oestrogen levels.

Urinary leakage

Approximately 30% of community-dwelling older women and over 50% of institutionalised older women have involuntary urinary leakage, primarily due to the age-related decrease in urethral closure pressure resulting from histological changes seen in urethral striated muscle, blood vessels and connective tissues, and overactive bladder. In a sample of nulliparous women aged between 21 and 70 years old, maximal urethral closure pressure in the senescent urethra was 40% of that in the young urethra; increasing age did not affect clinical measures of pelvic organ support, urethral support or levator function.

LUTS AND GENDER

The term 'lower urinary tract symptoms' was introduced to dissociate male urinary symptoms from any implied site of symptom origin, such as the prostate. However, the conceptual pathophysiological model of increasing prostate size causing bladder outflow obstruction with secondary changes in bladder function has been refuted by epidemiological studies, which suggest that it is misleading to attribute individual symptoms to sex differences or to a specific organ.

LUTS are a non-sex-specific, non-organ-specific group of symptoms, which are age-related, progressive and show a strong association with co-morbidities. The symptoms are equally common in both sexes and unrelated to any specific organ in the urinary system. Symptoms primarily concern voiding in men and storage in women.

The possible causes and mechanisms remain unclear. Possible contributing factors that warrant further investigation include age-related reduction in bladder capacity, uninhibited contractions, decreased urinary flow rate and a diminished urethral pressure profile in women and increased post-void residual volume.

THE MALE REPRODUCTIVE SYSTEM

Unlike in women, changes in men are slow and progressive. Testicular mass decreases gradually, but the male hormone level declines very little. Fertility and sexual function are two important aspects of male genital function.

Semen parameters and fertility

Testicular volume decreases with age and sperm production declines, along with sperm motility and structure. The testicles continue to produce sperm until a very advanced age. Seminal fluid volume and transmission of sperm and semen tubes may be affected by loss of elasticity (sclerosis) in the epididymis and the vas deferens.

The major effect of age is on sperm motility, with intermediate effects on semen volume and the smallest effects on sperm numbers. For men aged 50 years old, there is an approximate predicted 80% probability of clinically abnormal motility, 35% probability of abnormally low semen volume and 15% probability of abnormally low sperm count; these probabilities increase to approximately 100%, 80% and 50%, respectively, for men aged 80 years old.

This age-related decline in spermatogenesis may lead to a moderate decline in male fertility.

Genetic defects in sperm increase with age, possibly leading to decreased fertility, increased chance of miscarriage and increased risk of some birth defects. Many studies have shown an association between increasing paternal age and adverse birth outcomes, low birth weight and increased incidence of conditions such as Down syndrome and mental disorders.

Semen colour and consistency changes with age, but red or brown coloured semen (haemospermia) is abnormal.

It is also important to note that the ejaculated volume may change due to the effects of drugs and treatment for conditions associated with old age (e.g. alpha blockers for the LUTS causing retrograde ejaculation).

Sexual function in the ageing male

Sexual function in men is complex and comprised of separate stages: the sexual desire (libido), erectile function (arousal), plateau, ejaculation, detumescent (loss of turgidity), ejaculation and refractory phases. All these phases involve a complex interplay of hormones, blood vessels and nerves, which change as part of the normal ageing process. This is compounded by social, emotional and cultural factors; the availability of a partner; and treatment for conditions affecting other organ systems.

Libido

Libido decreases with normal male ageing. To produce arousal, testosterone acts on the brain and these nerve cells become less hormone responsive with age. In contrast, men tend to produce more female hormones (oestradiol and prolactin) as they age. Peripheral stimulation of the genital area, therefore, becomes more important for sexual stimulation in the ageing man. Changes in testosterone and its effects are discussed below.

Erection

An erection is a neurochemically mediated (i.e. release of nitric oxide from the nerve endings of the parasympathetic system in the cavernous tissues) hydraulic event (blood flow into expansile cavernous tissue through sinusoidal relaxation, arterial dilatation, and venous compression) in hormone-primed tissue. With age, penile responsiveness to sensory stimulation slows and there may also be a decrease in penile blood flow as men grow older, even if they stay healthy. Most men experience decreased sexual responsiveness with increasing age. Erections occur more slowly and they become more dependent on physical stimulation than on erotic thoughts. Even when erections develop, most men in their 60s report that they are more difficult to sustain and not as hard or rigid.

Night-time erections

These diminish with age. Between the ages of 45 and 54 years old, men average 3.3 erections per night; between ages 65 and 75, only 2.3 erections. The erections also tend to become briefer and less rigid with age. Morning erections are also reduced. The complexity of expressed sexual function is best captured by population-based epidemiological studies (e.g. Massachusetts Male Aging Study, European Male Aging Study). These studies have shown that ED is closely linked to age: while only 5% of men under 40 years old experience ED, the prevalence increases to 44% in men aged 60–69 years old.

Plateau

This stage usually lasts from 30 seconds to 2 minutes. During this phase, heart rate and blood pressure increase and more blood is pumped to the body's tissues. Blood flow increases not just to the penis; most men also experience facial flushing and the testicles swell by about 50%. During the plateau phase, the prostate and seminal vessels begin to discharge fluid to prepare for ejaculation. There are no reported changes in the plateau phase with ageing.

Ejaculation

During ejaculation, the muscles in the epididymis, vas deferens, seminal vesicles and prostate contract automatically (via the sympathetic system pathways). This propels the semen forwards. At the same time, nerve impulses tighten muscles in the neck of the bladder so that semen is forced out through the urethra instead of flowing back into the bladder. The pleasurable sensation of orgasm usually occurs with ejaculation. In nearly all men, the heart rate reaches its peak during ejaculation.

Ejaculation changes with age. The muscular contractions of orgasm are less intense, ejaculation is slower and less urgent, and the semen volume is smaller. Possibly the most important psychophysiological alteration of sexual pattern to develop in men between 50 and 70 years of age is an increase in ejaculatory control and much less dependence on ejaculation for sexual enjoyment during intercourse.

Refractory phase

The penis cannot respond to sexual stimulation during this phase, which can last from 30 minutes (in younger men) to 3 hours (in older men). However, at any age, worry, stress or depression can interfere with sexual interest, activity and satisfaction, even if a man's physical apparatus remains intact. So, too, can marital issues, poor communication, poor sexual technique and boredom; many of these problems become more common with age.

In summary, while sexual desire and response continue into later life, there are numerous physical alterations that can affect sexual activity. With age, men experience a decrease in the number of spontaneous and morning erections. The rigidity of the erection diminishes, the force and volume of the ejaculate diminishes and there is faster detumescence. The pre-ejaculatory sensation also diminishes. These changes often lead to distress in men unless they can be made aware that they are normal changes associated with ageing.

Testosterone and ageing

The testicles are the main source of testosterone in men. As men age, testosterone levels fall, as has been confirmed in several populations. Cross-sectional and longitudinal studies in men have indicated consistent age-related declines in total and free testosterone levels from the age of 30–40 years onwards

On average, levels of testosterone fall by about 1% per year beyond age 40, but most older men still have enough testosterone to function sexually. In the Massachusetts Male Aging Study, total testosterone levels were estimated to decline at 0.8% per year and free and albumin-bound testosterone levels at 2% per year in a cross-sectional analysis, whereas a longitudinal analysis revealed declines of 1.6% per year and 2%–3% per year for free and albumin-bound testosterone levels, respectively.

Age-related decline in testosterone levels is not only thought to be responsible for changes in various aspects of sexual function but also to affect many other systems, including bone, muscle and cognition. Short-term (3 months) testosterone supplementation to healthy older men who have serum testosterone levels near or below the lower limit of normal for young adult men results in an increase in lean body mass and, possibly, a decline in bone resorption, as assessed by urinary hydroxyproline excretion, with some effect on serum lipoproteins, haematological parameters and PSA. The sustained stimulation of PSA and the increase in haematocrit that occur with physiological testosterone supplementation suggest that older men should be screened carefully and followed up periodically throughout therapy.

THE FEMALE REPRODUCTIVE SYSTEM

In women, the effects of ageing on the reproductive system consist of multiple endocrine and non-endocrine processes. The epithelial and secretary health of genital tissues are dependent on pituitary-ovarian function. Progressive atrophy of the genitalia and reproductive system results from the decreased levels of oestrogens. The ovary is the primary site of hormone change, with decline in the production of oestrogens beginning prior to menopause. Levels of oestrogens (most specifically, that of 17β-oestradiol) drop, whereas hypothalamic and pituitary function appear to be relatively unaffected by ageing, so levels of follicle-stimulating hormone and luteinising hormone rise. Although adipose tissue metabolises androstenedione from the adrenal glands into oestrone, oestrone is biologically less potent than oestradiol.

Most women experience menopause around the age of 50 years old; however, in approximately 8% of women, menopause occurs before the age of 40. Prior to menopause, menstrual cycles often become irregular. As a consequence of the decrease in hormonal levels, changes occur throughout the reproductive system. The vaginal walls become less elastic, thinner and less turgid. The vagina becomes shorter and narrower due to atrophy of the subcutaneous tissues. Secretions become scant and watery. The external genital tissue decreases leading to atrophy of the labia. The changes in the vulva include thinning and greying of pubic hair, thinning and pallor of tissue, diminution of the labia minor and the presence of petechiae in sexually active older women. These vaginal changes, along with skeletal changes (e.g. hip arthritis) may make sexual intercourse and vaginal examination difficult. The cervix atrophies and the external ostium may become stenosed. Basal and immature epithelial cells from the vagina and cervix are a hallmark of oestrogen deficiency (apart from bacterial and fungal overgrowth). Interpretation of a cervical smear test in post-menopausal women can be difficult because of the predominance of basal epithelial cells and the presence of cytological atypia from inflammation. The uterus significantly decreases in size, the endometrium thins and becomes atrophic, and the myometrium is replaced by fibrous tissue. Ovarian size diminishes so that normally ovaries cannot be palpated on bimanual pelvic examination. The breast tissues also become atrophied in response in gonadal-endocrine changes. These changes are summarised in Box 11.1.

BOX 11.1 Changes in the female reproductive system with age

- Shorter, narrower vagina resulting from atrophy of subcutaneous tissues
- Vaginal wall less elastic, thinner, paler and less turgid
- Atrophy of labia
- Atrophy of cervix
- Possible stenosis of external ostium
- Immature epithelial cells in vagina and cervix
- Decrease in size of uterus with replacement of myometrium by fibrous tissue
- Thin atrophic endometrium
- Atrophy of breast tissue
- Atrophy of ovarian size
- Thinning and greying of pubic hair

Sexual function in the ageing female

A British study of ageing women, using *not* having had sexual intercourse in the previous year as a proxy for sexual activity, found that 50% of women aged between 55 and 64, 74% of women aged between 65 and 74, 93% of women aged between 75 and 84 and 99% of women aged over 85 years had limited sexual activity. However, this should not be confused with sexual interest or libido. A woman may experience changes in her sex drive (libido) and her sexual response may change but ageing does not prevent a woman from being able to have or enjoy sexual relationships. Most often, factors such as availability of a partner, vaginal dryness and thinning vaginal walls, and psychological and social factors affect a woman's sexual response more than the changes associated with ageing. An American community-based study of women aged over 60 years found that 55.8% of married women and only 5.3% of unmarried women were sexually active, suggesting the influence of factors other than just age. However, a more recent study concluded that the majority of older adults are engaged in sexual activity and regard sex as an important part of life. The physical and mental health of the individual as well as that of their partner, the availability of a willing partner and the individual's previous level of sexual activity all play important roles in sexuality in ageing.

Sexual dysfunction is common in middle-aged and older women, from the effects of declining oestrogens on genital and sexual structures, mood (post-menopause syndrome), musculoskeletal changes, lack of partner (as women live longer than men) and other physical and mental illnesses. It has been reported that while the proportion of women with low sexual desire increases with age, the proportion of women distressed about their low desire actually decreases with age. Sexuality in older people, in particular, should be seen in the context of a couple. The ability of couples to adapt to the changes of ageing, and to understand them, is essential to maintaining a healthy lifestyle.

FURTHER READING

Coyne KS, Sexton CC, Kopp ZS et al. The impact of overactive bladder on mental health, work productivity and health-related quality of life in the UK and Sweden: results from EpiLUTS. *BJU Int.* 2011; **108**(9): 1459–71.

Kuzmarov IW, Bain J. Sexuality in the aging couple – Part I: the aging woman. *Geriatrics & Aging.* 2009; **11**(10): 589–94.

Llorente C. New concepts in epidemiology of lower urinary tract symptoms in men. *Eur Urol Suppl.* 2010; **9**(4): 477–81.

Siroky MB. The aging bladder. *Rev Urol.* 2004; **6**(Suppl. 1): S3–7.

Yeap BB. Testosterone and ill-health in aging men. *Nat Clin Pract Endocrinol Metab.* 2009; **5**(2): 113–21.

QUESTIONS: THE UROGENITAL SYSTEM

1 Regarding LUTS in older people, all of the following statements are correct, except:

A compliance of the urinary bladder in both sexes decreases with age

B in women, LUTS are most commonly due to problems in voiding function

C judicious use of local oestrogens may improve overactive bladder symptoms in older women

D LUTS are as common in ageing women as they are in men

E other co-morbid conditions and iatrogenic factors contribute significantly to LUTS in both sexes.

Answer: B

2 Regarding sexual function in men, all of the following statements are true, except:

A haemospermia is abnormal in ageing men

B neurological autonomic pathways responsible for erectile function are mostly parasympathetic

C nitrous oxide release is the most important signalling pathway for erectile function in men

D the refractory phase following ejaculation decreases with age

E semen parameters deteriorate with age.

Answer: D

3 With regard to the prostate, which one of the following statements is true?

A as part of the normal ageing process the prostate, like other tissues, gradually atrophies, due to a decrease in the male hormones

B as most semen is produced by the prostate, removing the prostate will result in failure to produce semen

C PSA is normally produced by the prostate

D PSA is a cancer-specific enzyme

E the zonal anatomy of the prostate does not change as part of normal ageing process.

Answer: D

4 Only one of the following is true in relation to the decline in oestrogens in ageing women.

A immature epithelial cells are found in the cervix and vagina, leading to difficulty in the interpretation of a cervical smear test

B is partly responsible for thickened vaginal discharge and leucorrhea in old age

C is often due to subclinical pituitary hypofunction

D leads to decrease in libido

E weakens pelvic floor muscles leading to prolapse.

Answer: A

5 Regarding testosterone, which one of the following statements is true?
   A longitudinal studies have shown that there is no change in testosterone levels as part of normal ageing in men
   B supplemental testosterone can cause anaemia
   C testosterone has a significant effect on non-genital tissues and function
   D testosterone supplementation does not require careful supervision
   E testosterone suppresses PSA production in the prostate.

Answer: C

CHAPTER 12

The skin

TAMARA GRIFFITHS AND RACHEL WATSON

INTRODUCTION

The skin is a large and complex organ whose primary purpose is to provide a mechanical protective barrier. Other critical functions include temperature regulation and immunosurveillance, as well as endocrine and neurosensory roles. Furthermore, the psychosocial impact of skin health should not be underestimated.

Skin function deteriorates with chronological ageing but environmental factors also play an important role. Extrinsic lifestyle choices greatly affect the appearance and function of skin and there is significant evidence that the major environmental factor to influence skin biology is chronic sun exposure or ultraviolet (UV) radiation. There is also increasing evidence that cigarette smoking and hormonal status contribute to the appearance of aged skin. Both intrinsic and extrinsic ageing result in a common endpoint – the decline of skin's physiological function. Recent evidence suggests intrinsic and extrinsic ageing may share fundamental pathways with common mediators (*see* Figure 12.1; Table 12.1).

Deterioration of skin function combined with increased likelihood of co-morbidities can present unique challenges in the dermatological care of older people. Greater understanding of the molecular mechanisms and pathways that regulate processes associated with skin ageing will enable the development of improved strategies to treat and prevent diseases. This will become increasingly relevant with the anticipated expansion of the population of older people over the next decades.

Skin is comprised of two major interrelated, though functionally distinct, layers. The outermost epidermis provides a physical barrier between the individual and the external environment. It is highly cellular (comprised

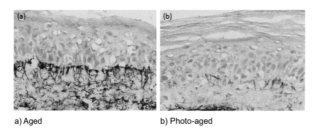

a) Aged   b) Photo-aged

FIGURE 12.1 Images from the skin of the same individual demonstrating the fibrillin-rich microfibril network: (A) aged, sun-protected (buttock) and (B) photo-aged (dorsal forearm) skin. Note the paucity of fibrillin in the photo-aged skin compared with the sun-protected skin. Sections were stained with antibody to identify microfibrils using standard immunohistochemistry techniques and counterstained with methyl green. Magnification ×200

TABLE 12.1 Features of intrinsic and extrinsic skin ageing

	Intrinsic ageing	Extrinsic ageing
Fine wrinkles	Yes	Yes
Coarse wrinkles	Minimal	Yes
Skin laxity	Yes	Yes
Solar lentigines (age/liver spots)	No	Yes
Xerosis (dryness)	Yes	Minimal
Epidermal changes	Atrophic	Hypertrophic then atrophic
Dermal changes	Atrophic	Dystrophic/Elastotic

predominantly of keratinocytes) and avascular, and has the capacity for constant renewal: keratinocytes derived from the basal cell layer cycle through an organised maturation process and are finally shed as anuclear corneocytes. The most superficial epidermal layer, the stratum corneum, acts as a protective barrier from environmental assault and infection. Though its thickness does not appear to alter with age, its moisture content and cohesiveness diminishes.

In comparison, the dermis is relatively cell poor. It is primarily composed of a complex network of fibrillar collagens, microfibrillar proteins and elastic fibres, all embedded in a proteoglycan-rich 'ground substance', and is collectively known as the extracellular matrix (ECM). The ECM provides the skin with strength, resilience and compliance. The dermis also supports the organ by housing intricate vascular, lymphatic and neuronal systems, as well as skin appendages such as the hair follicle, sebaceous glands and eccrine and apocrine sweat glands.

At the dermal–epidermal junction (DEJ), lies an elaborate basement membrane structure that provides an active interface between the epidermis and dermis. Undulating rete pegs, finger-like epidermal projections into the underlying dermis, increase the surface area of the DEJ.

MOLECULAR AND CELLULAR CHANGES

Epidermis

It has long been known that the aged epidermis is atrophic, with reduced capacity for barrier repair and function. Impairment of lipid processing as a result of rising surface pH plays an important role in barrier disruption. Enzymes such as acid and neutral sphingomyelinase, ceramide synthase and acid ceramidase that are required to produce key structural components in epidermal barrier function – ceramides – are diminished in older people. Glycerol acts as a humectant in the stratum corneum and is important in the maintenance of hydration and effective barrier function. The reduction of aquaporin-3, a glycerol and water membrane channel required to maintain adequate glycerol concentration in the stratum corneum, contributes to barrier insufficiency; its gene expression is diminished in those over 60 years of age. Epidermal CD44, the keratinocyte transmembrane glycoprotein thought to play a regulatory role in keratinocyte proliferation and maintain local hyaluronic acid (HA) homeostasis, is decreased in aged and photo-aged skin when compared with young skin. This may contribute to epidermal thinning and reduction of its viscoelastic properties. Furthermore, linearisation of the epidermis with flattening of the rete pegs is an alteration seen in intrinsic ageing and in extrinsically aged skin from younger individuals. The resultant reduction in the active interface between the epidermis and dermis at the DEJ may contribute to the skin fragility associated with increasing age.

Dermal–epidermal junction

The component molecules resident in the basement membrane have been studied extensively, in the context of both health and disease, and ageing. These molecules include bullous pemphigoid antigen 1, type IV collagen and laminin-5, and several other proteins have also been shown to play structural and biochemical roles in the basement membrane. A number of studies have identified an increase in basement membrane thickness in intrinsic ageing, while the amount of type IV collagen decreases with advancing age but is not exaggerated by photo-ageing. There is little published evidence that either intrinsic or extrinsic ageing alters other DEJ components. Flattening of the rete pegs results in a reduced basement membrane area. Transmission electron microscopy has identified duplication of the basement membrane, which may be an attempt at a reparative mechanism to ensure tissue cohesiveness.

Dermis

The dermal ECM exhibits structural and functional changes in both intrinsically and extrinsically aged skin (*see* Figure 12.2). With increasing age, atrophy of the dermal matrix is observed, including reduction in the deposition of type I and type III collagens. Synthesis is also impaired. Sites chronically exposed to UV irradiation, such as the face, anterior chest and forearms, show magnified changes. Degradation of elastic fibres is observed in intrinsically aged skin. However, photo-damaged skin has masses of dystrophic, tangled elastic fibres, which are recognised as the key histological finding of solar elastosis. This accumulation can be explained in part by the increase in tropoelastin expression with UV irradiation. The collagenous and elastic matrices are embedded in a carbohydrate-rich ground substance. There are three distinct forms of oligosaccharides in human skin: glycoproteins, proteoglycans and glycosaminoglycans (GAGs). Collectively, these hydrophilic molecules are distributed throughout the dermis where they perform a key role in maintaining skin hydration. Two primary GAGs in the ECM are dermatan sulphate and HA. Diminution in dermal HA may contribute to skin fragility by reducing the skin's protective mechanical function.

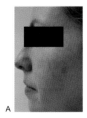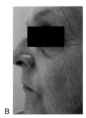

A   B

FIGURE 12.2 Images of facial skin: (A) young and (B) older – extrinsic ageing superimposed on intrinsic ageing. Minor signs of extrinsic ageing, such as hyperpigmentation, are apparent in A, but there is an absence of coarse wrinkles and laxity, which are the predominant features of extrinsic ageing, a marked feature of B

CHANGES IN METABOLIC PROCESSES
Vitamin D synthesis

Skin synthesis of vitamin D_3 and 1,25-dihydroxyvitamin D_3 [1,25$(OH)_2D_3$] is mediated by UVB exposure. There is increasing evidence that vitamin D_3 and its metabolites are important for functions involving immune response and cellular growth and regulation in a wide range of tissues, for example breast, lung and colon. Furthermore, 1,25$(OH)_2D_3$ also protects against UVB-induced skin damage and carcinogenesis, as well as playing a role in preventing opportunistic infection.

The skin's ability to produce vitamin D_3 declines with age. The concentration of 7-dehydrocholesterol, a vitamin D_3 precursor, declines by approximately 50% between ages 20 and 80 years, and the total amount of previtamin D_3 in young individuals is at least twice that in older people. The overall result is reduction in vitamin D_3's protective effects, many of which go beyond the boundaries of the integument (*see also* Chapter 10, 'The kidneys', and Chapter 13, 'The musculoskeletal system: bone').

IMPACT OF CHANGES ON ANATOMY AND PHYSIOLOGICAL FUNCTIONS

Dry skin and irritant dermatitis

Dry skin, or xerosis, is characterised by reduced lipid content and impaired repair of the epidermal barrier after insult. The typical dermatitis associated with old age is asteatotic eczema, or *eczema craquelé*, which is most common in the winter months and associated with diminished ambient humidity. It may be exacerbated by frequent washing with hot water and soap or other detergent-based cleansing products.

Impaired barrier function predisposes to irritant contact dermatitis. Common chemical irritants include detergents, solvents, oil, dusts and fibre, acids and alkalis. Physical irritants are heat, sweat, friction, pressure, vibration, UV irradiation and occlusion. Urine or faecal incontinence with diaper occlusion can result in recalcitrant perineal dermatitis, which can be of particular relevance in the older population.

Immune function

Impairment of the immune system associated with age or immunosenescence may be related to a pro-inflammatory state in combination with abnormal T- and B-cell functions. Age-related changes in the cutaneous immune system result in defective Th1 function and enhanced Th2 function, promoting a pro-inflammatory state predisposed to eczematous dermatitis. The loss of naive T-cells reduces the ability of older persons to respond effectively to infections to which they have had no prior exposure. Age-related reduction in the Langerhans cell population and inhibition of their trafficking to draining lymphatics results in a reduction in immunosurveillance. This disinhibition may promote development of skin cancers, the incidence of which increases with photo-ageing superimposed on intrinsic ageing (*see* Chapter 4, 'The immune system').

Wound healing

Slowed epidermal turnover, epidermal thinning and increased fragility result in greater susceptibility to trauma and poor wound repair in older people. Age-associated reduction in cutaneous vessel size and loss of dermal vessel density also plays a role. Although UV exposure may induce angiogenesis and formation of new blood vessels, these new immature vessels may be hyperpermeable and initiate local inflammation. Furthermore, with time, the number of blood vessels decreases in chronically photo-damaged skin.

Hormonal influences in wound healing are not insignificant. Reduced oestrogen levels in post-menopausal women are linked to abnormalities in tissue regeneration due to altered cytokine pathways and inflammatory response, in particular through macrophage inhibition. In healthy older men and women, topical oestrogens applied to chronic ulcers have induced fibronectin expression with reduction in elastase levels, as a result of diminished neutrophil response, leading to improved wound healing.

Thermoregulation

The ability to effectively thermoregulate oneself diminishes with age and this is linked to reduction in sweat output and ability to respond to peripheral stimuli. Older people have higher core and skin temperatures. Impaired vascular responsiveness may also play a role.

IMPACT ON DISEASE MANAGEMENT

Pruritus

Pruritus is a common complaint among older people and is often multifactorial. Contributing factors include diminished epidermal barrier repair, enhanced Th2 immune function and neurodegenerative impairment, centrally and/or peripherally. Medications can induce pruritus through various mechanisms; for example, by direct interaction with mast cells or by induction of hepatobiliary disease. The increased likelihood of polypharmacy in older people requires careful consideration with regard to the temporal relationships between commencement of the suspicious agent and the onset of itching. However, it should be noted that the implicated medication may have been started some time prior to pruritus and that itching may persist for several months after the offending medication is discontinued. Other causes of pruritus in older people include scabies, mycosis fungoides, dermatitis herpetiformis, lichen planus and bullous pemphigoid. Underlying causes must be considered, including renal or hepatic disease, diabetes mellitus, iron deficiency, lymphoreticular malignancy (e.g. Hodgkin lymphoma) or, rarely, solid tumour. Neuropathic disease can result in dysaesthesia and pruritus, for example brachioradial pruritus and notalgia paresthetica. Avoidance of irritants and allergens in addition to liberal use of bland emollients to promote the skin barrier function may help, after any underlying aetiology has been addressed.

Skin tumours

Skin tumours that arise in older people can range from benign, such as seborrhoeic keratosis, sebaceous hyperplasia and cherry angiomata; pre-cancerous, such as actinic keratosis; to frank malignancies, such as basal cell carcinoma (BCC), squamous cell carcinoma (SCC), melanoma and others. Senescence and oxidative stress together could encourage a tumour-promoting state and the most common types of skin cancer are BCC and SCC. Increased vigilance in the older population is required for early detection, particularly on chronically sun-exposed sites such as the face, neck and dorsal hands. In addition, sensible behaviours for avoiding excess sun exposure are recommended.

Infectious diseases

Age-related cutaneous immunosenescence plays an important role in the older patient's increased susceptibility to infections such as herpes zoster, candidal infection, staphylococcal impetigo and streptococcal cellulitis. Clinicians should lower their threshold for consideration of these diagnoses in older people and be aware that atypical presentations may arise, particularly if the patient is taking immunosuppressive therapies for other disease. Likewise, systemic immunosuppressive agents used to treat skin disease in older people should be prescribed with appropriate care.

Co-morbidities

The presence of co-morbidities in older people, such as metabolic syndrome, hypertension, renal insufficiency, diabetes mellitus, reduced hepatic function, dementia and cancer, complicate the treatment of skin disease. One must also remain vigilant for signs of dermatologic manifestations of systemic disease, such as hypothyroidism and diabetes. Clinicians should be cognisant of drug toxicities when prescribing systemic agents for treatment of dermatologic disease in these complex patients; for example, impaired renal function is a relative contraindication for the use of cyclosporin in the treatment of psoriasis and methotrexate toxicity is a potential risk in the same patient due to reduced renal excretion.

Physical, psychological and logistical limitations must also be considered in the older patient. Mobility, transportation and cognitive ability are all issues that may affect treatment compliance, as are depression and anxiety, which are sometimes related to isolation. Healthcare assistance, nursing and support from family and friends can be invaluable.

CONCLUSION

There are numerous age-associated changes that occur in the skin, resulting in compromised skin function and a varied presentation of disease states. Furthermore, physiological changes are often superimposed on cumulative damage from environmental, particularly UV, exposure. Variations between the healthy older patient and one who is the same age but has multiple medical problems may dilute the effectiveness of chronological age-specific criteria. What is clear is that age-related decline in skin function coupled with extrinsic ageing and co-morbidities present unique challenges for the dermatologist and geriatrician alike. Better understanding of molecular mechanisms and the pathways that regulate processes related to skin ageing may translate ultimately into improved patient care.

FURTHER READING

Berger TG, Steinhoff M. Pruritus in elderly patients: eruptions of senescence. *Semin Cutan Med Surg*. 2011; **30**(2): 113–17.

Kaya G, Saurat JH. Dermatoporosis: a chronic cutaneous insufficiency/fragility syndrome;

clinicopathological features, mechanisms, prevention and potential treatments. *Dermatology.* 2007; **215**(4): 284–94.

Veysey EC, Finlay AY. Aging of the skin. In: Fillit HM, Rockwood K, Woodhouse K, editors. *Brocklehurst's Textbook of Geriatric Medicine and Gerentology.* 7th ed. London: Churchill Livingstone; 2010. pp. 133–7.

Wong JW, Koo JY. Dermatogeriatrics: a case for developing a new dermatology subspecialty. *J Dermatolog Treat.* Epub 2010 Apr 12.

Zouboulis CC, Makrantonaki E. Clinical aspects and molecular diagnostics of skin aging. *Clin Dermatol.* 2011; **29**(1): 3–14.

QUESTIONS: DERMATOLOGY

1 The primary function of the skin is:
   A as a barrier to prevent dehydration and infection
   B as an endocrine organ involved in the production of vitamin D
   C thermoregulation through sweat and vasoactivity
   D to act as a sensory organ
   E to produce dendritic immune-modulating cells.

   Answer: A

2 Compared with the skin of the upper inner arm, the skin of the dorsal forearm of an older person:
   A is less likely to develop BCC
   B is less likely to show solar lentigines
   C is less likely to synthesise vitamin D_3
   D is more likely to demonstrate changes associated with extrinsic skin ageing
   E will show thin, regular elastic fibres.

   Answer: D

3 Changes associated with intrinsic skin ageing include all of the following, except:
   A increased area of the DEJ
   B reduction in ability to produce vitamin D_3
   C reduction in cohesiveness of the stratum corneum
   D reduction in the number of Langerhans cells and a shift to the Th2 cytokine profile
   E stiffening of the dermal extracellular matrix.

   Answer: A

4 Common skin complaints in older people include all of the following, except:
   A asteatotic eczema
   B herpes zoster
   C hyperhidrosis
   D scabies
   E seborrhoeic keratosis.

   Answer: C

5 Factors that complicate dermatological treatment in older people include:
   A all of the following
   B central and/or peripheral neurodegenerative impairment
   C diminished ability to apply topical creams due to mobility issues
   D polypharmacy and drug interaction or allergy
   E poor wound healing and skin fragility.

   Answer: A

CHAPTER 13

The musculoskeletal system: bone

MARK BIRCH AND TERRY ASPRAY

THE STRUCTURE OF BONE

Bone and cartilage are specialised connective tissues that combine extracellular matrix biomolecules and complexes of inorganic ions to give mechanically competent and structurally durable materials that meet functional requirements. The formation, development and maintenance of these tissues throughout life are dependent on the coordinated activity of several different cell types.

The macro-, micro- and nanoscale structures of bone can be considered in the context of their functional roles. The macrostructure of bone consists of a tough outer layer that is termed 'compact' or 'cortical' bone, while the inner marrow cavity is traversed by struts of trabecular (cancellous) bone. This organisation of a reinforced hollow cylinder provides both a structure that resists load with an optimised strength-to-weight ratio and a protective environment for haematopoietic cells. At the microscale, compact bone is built up from arrays of Haversian systems, or osteons, which consist of cylinders of mineralised matrix surrounding a central canal that contains a blood vessel. At the nanoscale, hydroxyapatite $[Ca_{10}(PO_4)_6(OH)_2]$ is deposited on collagen fibrils arranged in parallel bundles, ensuring bone is a mechanically strong biocomposite.

Cells of bone are distributed throughout the skeleton according to their roles in regulating bone mass. Within compact bone, osteocytes are entombed within lacunae, remaining in contact with each other and cells at the surface through tiny canaliculi through which extend intercommunicating cellular processes. On the surface of bone, osteoblast lineage cells are found. They may be flattened and resting or more rounded cells, which, under the microscope, can be seen to stain intensely for the presence of alkaline phosphatase. In addition, at discrete sites on the bone surface, cells of haematopoietic origin may be identified, fusing to form multinucleated osteoclasts that are capable of breaking down and resorbing all of the components of bone. The activities of these cells are controlled by hormones, cytokines and growth factors, together with immobilised signals from the extracellular matrix components.

Cartilage is found principally at the junctions and articulations between bones, helping to provide smooth movement of the joints and resistance to load. In addition, cartilage forms the nasal septum, larynx, trachea and bronchi of the respiratory tract. Cartilage is principally composed of fibrillar type II collagen and the large aggregating proteoglycan aggrecan. Collagen is arranged to provide great tensile strength, while the highly charged glycosaminoglycan side chains of aggrecan attract water into the tissue ensuring its resistance to compressive load. In cartilage, there is a single cell type, the chondrocyte, which can be found embedded within a pericellular matrix isolated from surrounded cells. Cartilage is an avascular tissue, so chondrocytes are dependent on nutrient diffusion from synovial fluid and surrounding tissues.

Cellular mechanisms

Bone remodelling

In adult cartilage, the ability to remodel the extracellular matrix constituting the tissue is restricted to a small pericellular area. As chondrocytes have a limited ability to proliferate, cartilage has poor capacity for repair. However, bone is constantly remodelled throughout adult life in response to metabolic and physical demands. This is achieved by the coordinated activity of the cells of bone working in a sequential chain of events that results in the replacement or repair of bone at discrete foci throughout the skeleton.

OSTEOCLASTS

These are terminally differentiated cells that are easily distinguished *in vivo* by their multinuclearity, apposition to bone and expression of tartrate-resistant acid phosphatase. Osteoclasts are derived from mononuclear haematopoietic precursors that fuse to give the multinucleated cell (*see* Figure 13.1b) at the surface of bone. Osteoclasts interact with the mineralised matrix through cell surface extracellular matrix receptors, integrins, to create a tightly sealed region. Specialist ion transporters, including a V-ATPase H^+ pump and carbonic anhydrase, then acidify this sealed zone, creating a localised environment that solubilises the mineral component of bone. Proteinaceous residue is then liberated by the action of enzymes like cathepsin K and matrix metalloproteinase-9 that can work at a low pH. The action of these enzymes is further enhanced by the migration of osteoclasts along the bone surface with loss of the tightly sealed zone allowing the pH to return towards physiological values in the resorption pit.

OSTEOBLASTS

Osteoblasts are derived from mesenchymal stem cells (MSCs) that can be found within bone marrow and also at several other sites including in adipose tissue, periosteum and muscle. No single marker describes the MSC phenotype and they are characterised based on positive staining for specific surface proteins. MSCs are multi-potent cells that can differentiate to the chondrocyte, adipose and other connective tissue lineages, as well as the osteoblast. Recruitment of MSCs to the osteoblast lineage involves a number of processes including changes in the activity of nuclear transcription factors, including runt-related transcription factor 2, osterix and Sox9, resulting in appropriate gene expression to promote the osteoblast phenotype, which includes the expression of alkaline phosphatase, type I collagen, parathyroid hormone receptor and osteocalcin. The mature osteoblast (*see* Figure 13.1a) is intensely metabolically active and produces a highly organised matrix consisting mostly of type I collagen. Having laid down the protein scaffold, the osteoblast secretes matrix vesicles that contain large amounts of Ca^{2+} and PO_4^{3-} ions as well as lipoproteins that combine to give the hydroxyapatite crystals found in bone. Once bone has been deposited, mature osteoblasts suffer one of three fates: 1. apoptosis (programmed cell death; thought to be greater than 80%); 2. return to a resting state on the surface of bone (so-called bone-lining cells), and; 3. entombment within bone (termed 'osteocytes').

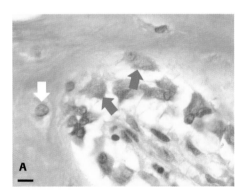 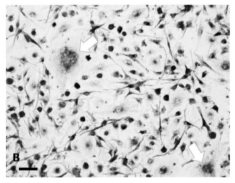

FIGURE 13.1 (A) Osteoblasts: mature osteoblasts are large metabolically active cells directly apposed to the bone surface (blue arrows), while matrix-entombed osteocytes can also be observed (white arrow). Scale bar = 10 μm. (B) Osteoclasts: peripheral blood mononuclear cells can cultured *in vitro* with receptor activator of nuclear factor kappa-B ligand and macrophage colony-stimulating factor to produce multinucleated osteoclasts that are positive for tartrate-resistant acid phosphatase (white arrows). Scale bar = 50 μm

OSTEOCYTES

The most abundant cell in bone is the osteocyte (tens of thousands per cubic millimetre). Thus, osteocytes constitute 90%–95% of all bone cells with osteoblasts making up 4%–6% and osteoclasts, 1%–2% respectively. Osteocytes are fully encased within bone but remain in contact with each other and with cells on the surface of bone through gap junctions at the ends of numerous cyto-plasmic projections that extend through tiny canaliculi. As osteoblasts become osteocytes, their metabolic activity is drastically reduced in preparation for their new environment. Osteocytes express several genes that can also be found in osteoblasts, such as osteocalcin and matrix extracellular phosphoglycoprotein. However, phosphate regulating endopeptidase homolog, X-linked *PHEX* and sclerostin are associated with the osteocyte lineage. It is believed that osteocytes form a mechano-sensory network that gives bone its propensity to remodel in response to physical loading.

COORDINATION OF BONE REMODELLING

At the start of the remodelling process, cells lining the bone surface peel away and osteoclasts then resorb bone matrix at the site. After a short period, often termed 'reversal', the site becomes populated with mature osteoblasts that deposit new mineralised bone. Once complete, the cells at the surface return to a flattened resting phenotype. This programme of events is termed the 'remod-elling cycle' (*see* Figure 13.2); it can easily be envisaged how small changes in the balance of the individual elements can lead to significant alterations in bone mass.

A complex array of molecular mediators ensures that the activities of bone cells are coordinated in the remodelling cycle. Osteocytes are believed to ini-tiate the process, in response to mechanical factors and bone microdamage, by undergoing apoptosis, which leads to the creation of a permissive envir-onment on the surface of bone for osteoclast formation (osteoclastogenesis). Several mechanisms have been proposed to drive osteoclast recruitment, including the loss of osteocyte-expressed transforming growth factor-beta (TGF-beta) and osteoprotegerin (OPG), both of which suppress osteoclas-togenesis. The bone-lining cells are responsive to parathyroid hormone (PTH), 1,25-dihydroxyvitamin D_3 [1,25$(OH)_2D_3$], prostaglandins and numerous cytokines that help to trigger a change in the local biology, including the pro-duction of chemokines (e.g. monocyte chemoattractant protein-1 [MCP-1] and stromal cell-derived factor-1 [SDF-1]), which aid in the recruitment of mononuclear osteoclast precursors to the region. However, the most signific-ant alteration in the local molecular framework is the production of receptor activator of nuclear factor kappa-B ligand (RANKL), which, together with mac-rophage colony-stimulating factor, potently induces osteoclastogenesis.

During bone resorption, proteinaceous components of the matrix are released, including bone morphogenetic protein (BMP)-1, insulin-like growth factor (IGF)-1 and TGF-beta 1, which are believed to recruit osteoprogenitor cells to the remodelling site. BMPs, in particular, are potent regulators of bone formation and are able to drive the process of cell differentiation through to the production of a mineralised matrix. As bone formation nears completion,

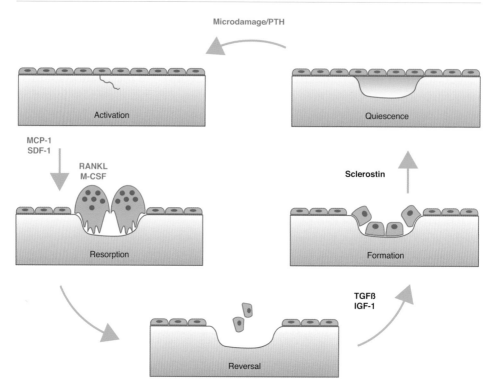

FIGURE 13.2 Bone remodelling cycle: a quiescent bone surface is activated by accumulation of microdamage and/or the action of parathyroid hormone. Recruitment of osteoclasts and their activity is influenced by a number of factors including receptor activator of nuclear factor kappa-B ligand (RANKL). During bone resorption, liberated factors such as transforming growth factor-beta (TGF-beta) are believed to play a role in the recruitment of osteoblasts. Sclerostin produced by osteocytes contributes to the termination of bone formation

the production of sclerostin by osteocytes begins to slow the process of osteogenesis. Sclerostin acts by binding to low-density lipoprotein receptor-related protein (LRP)-5 and inhibiting its role in transducing signals from a lipid-modified signalling protein called 'Wnt'. This pathway is of fundamental importance in the commitment and differentiation of osteoprogenitors, therefore, the production of sclerostin antagonises this process.

Changes in bone with age

The skeleton grows *in utero* and throughout childhood and young adult life, with 90% of adult bone mass achieved by adolescence, although skeletal growth continues into the fourth decade. A number of factors determine the growth and maintenance of skeletal mass, including sex, race and heritable factors (constituting up to 80% of variability). Other factors are also important, such as nutritional status, exercise and adequacy of hormonal status. In adult life, there is a slow decline in bone mass and, for women in particular, a more rapid loss of bone mineral at the menopause, under the influence of a decline in sex hormone levels. At a macrostructural level, these changes are readily assessed using dual-energy X-ray absorptiometry (DXA), commonly used to measure bone mineral density (BMD). However, as DXA measures BMD in only two planes (vertical and horizontal), it does not represent a true *density*; rather, it represents an estimate of the bone mineral content of the area of interest (spine or hip). This is particularly relevant to the growing (and, to some extent, the shrinking) skeleton, as bone size changes but is not measured in the third dimension of depth. In children, total body BMD can be a useful measurement.

During the course of life, the determinants of bone mass (expressed as BMD) vary (*see* Figure 13.3). In childhood and young adult life, bone growth is an important determinant, which appears to have a strong hereditary component with other influences including diet, exercise and, in some cases, chronic illness. From the fourth decade, there is a slow decrease in BMD, which is accelerated, particularly in women at the menopause. In old age, the decrease in bone mass is associated with progressive sarcopenia and decreased physical activity and may be promoted by hyperparathyroidism, associated with vitamin D deficiency.

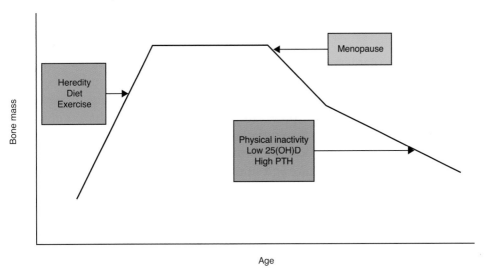

FIGURE 13.3 Schematic diagram (not to scale) showing BMD increasing throughout childhood and young adult life, with peak BMD achieved in the fourth decade. Following this, a slow decline continues until the menopause (in women) around the age of 50 years, when there is an accelerated decrease in BMD and a less rapid decrease thereafter

Ageing bone and cartilage matrix

As the skeleton ages, there is a marked decrease in BMD that correlates with increased fracture risk. However, studies of large patient cohorts have suggested that only 10%–44% of fractures are directly attributable to low BMD. This highlights that bone quantity and bone quality – that is, architectural organisation and physical properties – combine to determine fracture risk.

With age, there is a remarkable reduction in the number of trabecular bone struts and consequent loss of their connectivity. The thickest and longest trabecular elements are oriented parallel to the loading axis with smaller interconnecting trabeculae. The interconnecting struts are lost first in age-associated bone loss and this explains an increased susceptibility to buckling and failure under compression loading. Cortical bone is affected less with ageing. However, periosteal porosity increases, which is believed to contribute approximately 55% of yield stress and 70% of elastic modulus (the bone's tendency to deform elastically, rather than permanently). Porosity increases towards the endosteal surface and result in Haversian (osteonal) canals merging with the medullary space, causing significant architectural changes. This type of bone loss is observed in post-menopausal women with osteoporosis and contributes to their disease severity.

Another type of microstructural change observed in bone is the development of micro-cracks, due to microdamage accumulating in response to loading and part of the mechanism to dissipate energy and resist failure (fracture). Micro-cracks run through the osteocyte canalicular network and can thus influence cell activity; they accumulate with age and are often associated with decreased osteocyte density.

At the molecular level, non-enzymatic cross-link densities increase in bone with age. These are advanced glycation end products (AGEs), such as pentosidine, that form both intra- and interfibrillar links within collagen. Stiffening of the collagen fibres occurs, preventing them from sliding when under load and a loss of plasticity results in more micro-cracks.

Molecular changes also occur in cartilage as an individual gets older, with alterations in the size, structure and sulphation of aggrecan. The reduced levels of charged glycosaminoglycans result in cartilage having a decreased capacity to imbibe water and therefore less structural resilience and durability. Similar to bone, there is also an age-related increase in AGEs causing a stiffening of the collagen scaffold in cartilage, making the tissue more brittle and susceptible to fatigue failure.

Age-related changes in skeletal cell activity

The changes in skeletal mass and architecture already described reflect a shift in the activity of those cells responsible for the continued maintenance and adaptation of bone and cartilage. In perimenopausal women, in particular, there is a rapid decline in skeletal mass, characterised by accelerated bone remodelling with enhanced bone resorption by osteoclasts, which is not matched by bone formation by osteoblasts. As the rate of loss decreases in old age, osteoclast activity is still reduced but recruitment of cells to the osteoblast lineage and their subsequent differentiated function is even poorer, resulting in a continued reduction in bone mass.

In post-menopausal women, there is an overall increase in the number of cells expressing RANKL. Loss of oestrogen seems to increase expression of RANKL by a range of cells, including marrow stromal cells, T- and B-cells, and ageing osteoclast precursors also appear to have an increased sensitivity to RANKL. There is a resultant shift in the RANKL-OPG axis towards osteoclast activity, together with a pro-inflammatory state, increasing the abundance of mediators such as tumour necrosis factor-alpha and interleukin (IL)-1, IL-6 and IL-17, which all lead to increased osteoclastogenesis and bone resorption.

The recruitment, differentiation and activity of osteoblasts are impaired with ageing and an age-related decline in the lifespan of MSCs is also seen. With age, in the bone marrow environment, MSCs appear to differentiate away from the osteoblast lineage to the adipocyte. Increased levels of inflammatory mediators, together with decreased levels of IGF-1 and TGF-alpha contribute to alter signalling in cells of the osteoblast lineage, also reducing bone formation.

Other cellular changes

Underlying mechanisms relevant to ageing are discussed in detail in Chapter 2, 'The concept of ageing: theories and mechanisms', and Chapter 3, 'The ageing cell'. Telomeric shortening, disruption to the cell cycle, hormonal influences and increased levels of reactive oxygen species (ROS) are implicated as underlying mechanisms, acting at a cellular level, to promote ageing in health and disease; the skeletal system provides an excellent model for considering these processes.

There is some evidence supporting telomere shortening as a mechanism in the development of osteoporosis, with a decreased telomere length associated with lower BMD at the spine and forearm. However, evidence is inconsistent and telomere length appears not to relate to change in BMD, bone loss or fracture risk.

Cell cycle, apoptosis and hormones

The intimate relationship between osteoblasts and osteoclasts at the bone surface has already been discussed. The mechanism of bone formation and resorption is controlled by the regulation of the osteoblast and osteoclast cell cycle. Apoptosis of osteoclasts occurs after a cycle of bone resorption and this process is promoted by sex hormones, allowing the bone formation to continue. With ageing (and a decrease in oestrogen levels in women) normal bone resorption and formation are interrupted. Both processes seem to be up-regulated, but with an increase and prolongation in osteoclast activity and a net effect of resorption. However, the balance between bone formation and resorption is complex and influenced by the interactions between a range of hormones, cytokines and stromal cells, osteoblasts and osteoclasts. The relevant hormones include PTH, oestrogen and metabolites of vitamin D and their effects are mediated through cytokines, including receptor activator of nuclear factor kappa-B, RANKL and OPG.

ROS

ROS are believed to contribute to decreases in osteoblast numbers, with oxidative stress inducing forkhead box class O transcription factors to inhibit elements of the Wnt signalling pathway, while oxidised lipids activate peroxisome proliferator-activated receptor signalling, leading to reduced osteoblast activity and increased adipogenesis. In cartilage, replicative senescence is unlikely to be relevant, since these cells rarely divide. However, a senescence secretory phenotype has been identified that is linked to accumulated ROS damage. The elevated production of IL-1, IL-6, IL-8 and metalloproteinases, together with decreased responsiveness to IGF-1, characterise this chondrocyte phenotype and contribute to the altered cartilage physiology with ageing.

Molecular changes with age

Genetics

Evidence from studies in twins suggest that there is a strong genetic influence on bone structure, with between 60% and 80% determined by genetic predisposition, whether evaluated by BMD, bony architecture or rate of bone turnover. For fracture risk there is a weaker association, although a discrete relationship (independent of BMD), particularly with parental fracture, especially at the hip. However, although multiple genetic effects are postulated, a number of candidate genes have been investigated in an attempt to identify specific determinants of osteoporosis and fracture risk, in particular.

Genes responsible for collagen formation may affect bone quality. One extreme example of abnormal collagen formation is due to mutations of loci encoding collagen type I, alpha 1 chains (and some other genes) causes osteogenesis imperfecta, which is associated with a very high fracture risk in childhood, mimicking the effects of osteoporosis with low BMD. Rarely, cases of osteogenesis imperfecta are not seen until adulthood. However, it may be that there are more subtle effects on collagen and its quality that influence the development of osteoporosis and fracture risk in old age of which we are not currently aware. Another potential area of genetic effect is the vitamin D receptor (VDR). Studies have identified phenotypic differences on calcium absorption and BMD relating to VDR genotype.

An exciting example of a disease process relating to a specific genotype has been the discovery that the autosomal-recessive osteoporosis-pseudoglioma syndrome is associated with a specific gene mutation, coding for the LRP-5 gene on chromosome 11. Impairment of LRP-5 production is thus associated with osteoporosis in this very rare condition. However, LRP-5 gene mutation has also been found in subjects with *idiopathic* osteoporosis and in subjects with an effective increase in LRP-5 production, associated with an increase in BMD (a condition termed 'osteopetrosis'). These real-life experiments have identified the importance of LRP-5 in promoting osteoblast activity through a separate mechanism on the Wnt pathway, which is responsible for a wide range of processes in other organs of the body, as well as in bone. Thus, from a rare disease associated with osteoporosis in childhood, insights are gained into the regulation of osteoblast activity, bone formation and potential targets for novel treatments.

Vitamin D

Many of the principles outlined so far are well reflected in the relationship between vitamin D and musculoskeletal health. Vitamin D can be viewed as a nutrient, pro-hormone or biomarker and the term 'vitamin D' applies to a range of species. Dietary vitamin D from animal sources is cholecalciferol (vitamin D_3) and a non-animal source is ergocalciferol (vitamin D_2). However, vitamin D is also synthesised in the skin from the conversion of 7-dehydrocholesterol to vitamin D_3, which is subsequently hydroxylated in the liver to 25-hydroxyvitamin D [25(OH)D]. This pro-hormone is further hydroxylated in the kidney to $1,25(OH)_2D_3$, which is a potent metabolite.

Vitamin D is important for bone health and muscle function. Deficiency is associated with rickets in childhood and osteomalacia in adult life, while myopathy may be associated with insufficiency or deficiency of vitamin D. It is particularly relevant in old age, when a decline is observed in vitamin D status. This decline is hypothesised to be due to a number of reasons:

- decreased conversion of 7-dehydrocholesterol to vitamin D in the skin, which may be related to less sunlight exposure and/or specific age-related impairments in the characteristics of the skin, resulting in decreased vitamin D synthesis (*see* Chapter 12, 'The skin')
- decreased dietary vitamin D intake in old age
- a possible decline in the hormonal effects of vitamin D with age
- potential failure of the hydroxylation of vitamin D to 25(OH) vitamin D in the liver
- decrease in the hydroxylation of 25(OH)D to $1,25(OH)_2D_3$ as renal function declines with age (*see* Chapter 10, 'The kidneys').

To evaluate vitamin D status, we usually measure plasma 25(OH)D levels. There is no universal consensus on a plasma level of 25(OH)D that reflects sufficiency; current guidelines indicate that a plasma 25(OH)D level greater than 50 nmol/L reflects sufficiency and less than 25 nmol/L reflects deficiency (which is associated with a significant risk of osteomalacia). A plasma 25(OH)D level between 25 and 50 nmol/L reflects insufficiency. However, these thresholds for the measurement of plasma vitamin D reflect the lack of a satisfactory biomarker for vitamin D status, since 25(OH)D in the plasma is merely a pro-hormone and a substrate for conversion to $1,25(OH)_2D_3$. Unfortunately, the variation and short half-life of $1,25(OH)_2D_3$ prevent its use as a marker of vitamin D status.

Until recently, plasma $25(OH)D$ level was difficult to measure, so it was necessary to infer the presence of vitamin D deficiency from abnormalities in plasma levels of calcium, phosphate and PTH. Indeed, for patients with probable vitamin D insufficiency, the identification of a raised PTH level (reflecting secondary hyperparathyroidism) is a valuable aid in the identification of a clinically significant abnormality.

Vitamin D deficiency

As already mentioned, the musculoskeletal consequence of vitamin D deficiency is osteomalacia (rickets in the growing skeleton), which results in a mineralisation deficit, causing bone pain, deformity (with rickets) and fractures, which may be micro-fractures. At intermediate levels of plasma $25(OH)D$, there is an increased risk of myopathy, which is typically painful. However, the most contentious area of clinical risk relating to vitamin D concerns the potential for extra-skeletal effects. At a molecular level, vitamin D is believed to have anti-inflammatory and immune-modulatory effects. In some population studies, vitamin D deficiency has been identified as a possible cardiovascular risk factor and to have effects on diabetes and infection risk. However, such epidemiological data are not consistently supported by intervention studies. Similarly, there is epidemiological evidence that the prevalence of multiple sclerosis (MS) is related to northern latitude and an inference that this reflects the effect of worsening vitamin D status on the disease. Vitamin D supplementation has also been shown to decrease the recurrence of episodes of demyelination in MS.

CLINICAL IMPLICATIONS AND IMPACT ON DISEASE MANAGEMENT

Perhaps the most important consequence of age-related change in bone is osteoporosis, which results in bone fragility and an increased fracture risk. At a macrostructural level, it is clear that osteoporotic fractures affect certain sites, particularly the hip, spine and radius, although many other sites can be affected and fractures can result at these after minimal trauma. The predilection for certain fracture sites may be related to anatomical factors, such as the width of the bone (neck of femur and distal radius), the accelerated loss of trabecular bone (vertebra) and co-morbidity/behavioural issues, such as the tendency to fall on an outstretched hand with increasing age (distal radius fracture). When a fracture is unlikely to heal adequately, it is important to replace bone tissue with a functional prosthesis. Often, this will be a metal alloy, particularly if a weight-bearing bone is to be replaced, such as the proximal femur, where it should be strong and light. However, the combination of mechanical and structural durability needed to meet functional requirements cannot be fully met with inorganic material and the fantastic ability of bone to repair itself can never be reproduced.

With regard to microstructure and function, it is fortunate that bone continues to turnover with a balance of osteoblast and osteoclast activity into old age, so that fracture healing is not impaired. Mal-union of fractures can occur and a number of methods have been used to promote bone formation, including ultrasound and impulse waves as well as limb casts and basic surgical options such as autogenous cancellous bone grafting. In such cases where it is hypothesised that osteoblasts do not seem to be recruited locally, BMP has also been used to recruit osteoprogenitor cells to the remodelling site and promote healing. The combination of modified implant material, biological therapeutic agents and/or cell therapy are part of a regenerative medicine approach that orthopaedic surgeons are beginning to explore. Understanding how biomaterials can be fabricated and engineered at the nanometre length scale allows for the fine control of biological molecules interacting with that scaffold and the opportunity to influence biological events at the implant site. It is hoped that these approaches will be able to provide tailored surgical solutions to the often-unique orthopaedic problems facing older patients.

With regard to vitamin D, the clinical implications of a high prevalence of deficiency present a major public health concern. Currently, there is no United Kingdom reference nutritional intake for vitamin D in adults under the age of 65 years. For those aged 65 years and older, a dietary intake of 400 iu per day is recommended. However, it is recognised that such an intake level cannot be achieved in many groups without supplementation, particularly for frail older people and those living in care homes. The more recent recommendations, from the North American Institute of Medicine, that older populations should consume 800 iu per day is an even greater challenge.

We are increasingly aware of the potential contribution of vitamin D to health generally and bone health in particular. Aside from the recognised diseases of vitamin D deficiency (rickets in childhood and osteomalacia in adult life), low 25(OH)D levels promote secondary hyperparathyroidism and low BMD (as already outlined), thus contribute to osteoporosis in old age. Overall, this area is an exciting one and we anticipate continued developments in both basic and clinical science in the future.

FURTHER READING

Rosen CJ, Compston JE, Lian JB, editors. *Primer on the Metabolic Bone Diseases and Disorders of Mineral Metabolism*. 7th ed. Hoboken: John Wiley & Sons; 2008.

Ross AC, Manson JE, Abrams SA *et al*. The 2011 report on dietary reference intakes for calcium and vitamin D from the Institute of Medicine: what clinicians need to know. *J Clin Endocrinol Metab*. 2011; **96**(1): 53–8.

QUESTIONS: BONE

1 A number of cell types are found in bone and cartilage with a range of functional responsibilities.

Which one of the following cells is principally responsible for coordinating skeletal tissue response to physical loading?

A chondrocytes
B mesenchymal stem cells
C osteoblasts
D osteoclasts
E osteocytes.

Answer: E

Comment: *The osteocyte is believed to respond to physical loading by directing bone remodelling.*

2 A new pharmacological agent is being developed that increases the population of cells responsible for bone formation, while decreasing bone resorption.

Under the microscope, one would expect to see increased numbers of cells:

A containing calcium and phosphate ions
B staining for alkaline phosphatase
C staining for tartrate-resistant acid phosphatase
D that are multinuclear
E with reduced metabolic activity.

Answer: B

Comment: *Increased numbers of* osteoblasts*, which stain for alkaline phosphatase. They* secrete *large amounts of calcium and phosphate.*

3 A 19-year-old woman of short stature fractured her distal radius in a fall. As part of her assessment, DXA was performed to evaluate her BMD.

What is the reason for measuring total body BMD in her case?

A it is a better predictor of fracture at this age
B it is not influenced by bone length
C she has not achieved peak bone mass
D she may be hypogonadal
E the fracture will affect regional measurements.

Answer: C

Comment: *There is no clear evidence on fracture risk prediction at this age and, although total body BMD is not influenced by bone length, the skeleton is growing, so total bone mass can be monitored.*

4 A 54-year-old woman fractured her left femoralneck in a fall. Her last menstrual period was 3 years previously. During surgery, a bone biopsy sample was sent for histopathology.

Compared with bone from a 40-year-old, what would one expect evidence of?

A decreased osteoblast activity and decreased osteoclast activity
B decreased osteoblast activity and increased osteoclast activity
C increased osteoblast activity and decreased osteoclast activity
D increased osteoblast activity and increased osteoclast activity
E more osteocytes.

Answer: D

Comment: *This is perimenopausal bone loss. Both bone formation and resorption increase (but resorption more so than formation), as opposed to later stages, when formation starts to decline.*

5 Vitamin D deficiency has been associated with impaired bone health and lower BMD.

The negative effect on bone health is believed to be mediated through:

A decreased conversion of 7-dehydrocholesterol to vitamin D in the skin
B decreased dietary vitamin D intake
C hypocalcaemia
D secondary hyperparathyroidism
E tertiary hyperparathyroidism.

Answer: D

Comment: *Although many of these statements are correct, the best explanation for the underlying process contributing to lower BMD in vitamin D deficiency is mediated through secondary hyperparathyroidism.*

CHAPTER 14

The musculoskeletal system: muscle

DANIEL BAYLIS AND AVAN AIHIE SAYER

INTRODUCTION

Skeletal muscle is the most abundant tissue in the human body and the changes that occur with advancing age constitute a significant part of the general ageing process. The human muscular system includes over 630 separate muscles and these contribute up to 50% of total body weight. Skeletal muscle is essential for posture and movement as well as being central to metabolic processes and thermoregulation.

The two most common causes of age-related muscle loss are sarcopenia and cachexia. Sarcopenia, which occurs universally, is the unintentional loss of muscle mass and function that occurs with age. Cachexia is a complex metabolic syndrome associated with sustained inflammation and characterised by the loss of muscle mass with or without loss of fat mass.

Loss of skeletal muscle mass is directly associated with ageing and individuals who lose muscle mass at greater rates experience increased morbidity and mortality and reduced independence and quality of life. Recent estimates suggest that sarcopenia costs the United States (US) over US$18 billion per year, a sum close to the economic consequences of osteoporosis. Therefore, an understanding of the role and importance of skeletal muscle within the ageing process is essential knowledge for all doctors and health professionals looking after older people.

NORMAL MUSCLE PHYSIOLOGY

Skeletal muscle consists of longitudinally arranged muscle fibres (myofibres). Groups of myofibres are innervated by a single motor neurone forming a motor unit and generation of muscle power is proportional to the number of motor units recruited. Myofibres may be classified into two major groups according to myosin heavy chain content. Type I myofibres have a high capacity for oxidative phosphorylation with high myoglobin levels and mitochondrial density. They are characterised by a slow contraction time and relative resistance to fatigue. Type II myofibres have a greater reliance on glycolytic enzymes and are used for short powerful bursts of movement. Typically, they have a fast contraction time but tend to fatigue rapidly.

Muscle composition depends on anatomical location and functional requirement. For example, in the eye, precision movement is attained by a reduced number of myofibres per motor unit within ocular muscles. Axial muscles involved in the maintenance of posture have a higher ratio of type I myofibres for sustained controlled contractions.

Microscopically, myofibres are multinucleated single cells containing long protein bundles called 'myofibrils' (*see* Figure 14.1). These are the basic contractile units of muscle, incorporating thin and thick filaments – primarily actin

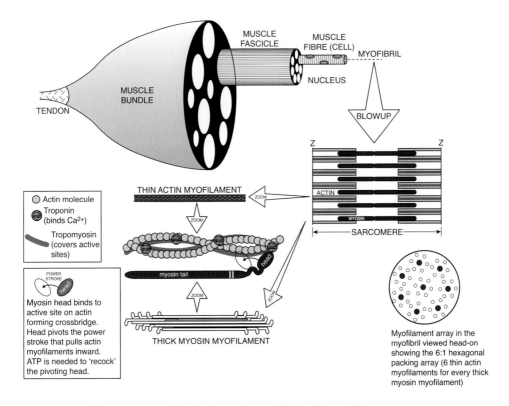

FIGURE 14.1 The structure of skeletal muscle and sliding filament theory

and myosin, respectively – organised longitudinally into repeated subunits called 'sarcomeres', which give skeletal muscle its striated appearance. Pools of satellite cells lie quiescent between the basal lamina and plasma membrane of myofibres. Upon injury or mechanical loading, satellite cells are activated and start to proliferate, adding new myonuclei to myofibres to achieve hypertrophy or replenish the satellite cell pool.

Contraction is initiated by the propagation of an action potential into myocytes via T-tubules. This causes calcium ion influx through voltage-gated ion channels and from the sarcoplasmic reticulum. Calcium binds to troponin C on thin filaments leading to the allosteric modulation of tropomyosin and subsequent unblocking of myosin binding sites, enabling binding of myosin to actin and the release of adenosine diphosphate (ADP) plus a phosphate. The bond is broken via the binding of adenosine triphosphate (ATP) to myosin, which is subsequently 're-primed' through hydrolysation back to ADP. Calcium is actively pumped back into the sarcoplasmic reticulum and the cycle finishes when levels of intracellular calcium fall causing the re-blocking of myosin binding sites.

ANATOMICAL CHANGES WITH AGE

Muscle mass and strength peaks in early adulthood and subsequently declines with age from approximately the fifth decade. In individuals over the age of 50 years, muscle mass is lost at a rate of 1%–2% per year and strength at a rate of 1.5%–3% per year. Determinants of muscle ageing can be considered using a life-course approach (*see* Figure 14.2) and include early life influences that determine maximum muscle mass and strength in addition to mid- and later life influences that affect rate of decline (*see* Table 14.1).

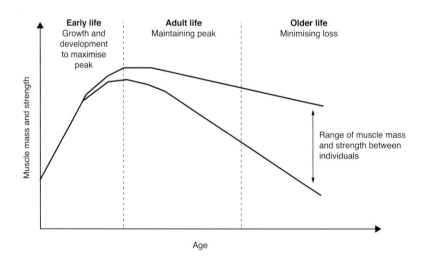

FIGURE 14.2 Muscle ageing: a life-course approach

TABLE 14.1 Life-course influences on muscle ageing

Intrauterine	Maternal influences
	Early size and growth
	Co-morbidity
	Genetic and epigenetic variation
Childhood	Size, growth and body composition
	Nutrition
	Physical activity
	Co-morbidity
Adulthood	Size and body composition
	Nutrition
	Physical activity
	Co-morbidity
	Ageing: intrinsic (skeletal muscle) and extrinsic (e.g. neurodegeneration, immune-endocrine axis changes, anorexia of ageing)

MOLECULAR AND CELLULAR CHANGES

Macroscopically, ageing is associated with a reduction in muscle mass and infiltration of adipose and connective tissues (*see* Figure 14.3). This loss of muscle may be missed by clinicians because *total* body size and leg circumference may not decline but remain constant or even increase due to a corresponding increase in fat mass. This is called 'sarcopenic obesity' and is discussed later in this chapter.

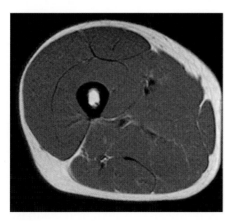 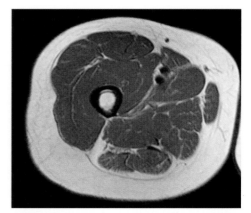

Aged 24   **Aged 62**

FIGURE 14.3 Cross-sectional magnetic resonance images at the thigh

Microscopically, ageing is associated with a global decline in myofibre numbers as well as a reduction in myofibre size, and there is some evidence for a preferential effect on type II myofibres. Skeletal muscle is infiltrated with connective tissue and non-contractile proteins that reduce structural integrity; this is accompanied by a reduction in blood flow. Satellite cells become more resistant to activation and reduce in number, causing less regenerative capacity and impaired myofibre maintenance.

Remodelling occurs, which is partly driven by changes to innervation. Myofibres undergo a continuous denervation and re-innervation due to the loss of motor neurones in the spinal cord; overall there is a 10%–15% decrease in motor neurones with age. This contributes to the loss and atrophy of myofibres, a reduction in the number of motor units and an increase in motor unit size. Furthermore, regeneration by surviving axons is often incomplete, causing uncoordinated muscle contraction. Overall, these microscopic changes cause reduced mass and strength and also reduced speed and precision.

CHANGES IN METABOLIC PROCESSES

Muscle protein synthesis declines with age by approximately 28%, particularly affecting the myosin heavy chain and contributing to reduced contractile function. Although there are few age-related changes to the enzymes of the glycolytic pathway, there is a reduction in mitochondrial volume and activity, which causes a reduced muscle respiratory capacity, partly explaining the reduction in aerobic endurance that is noted with ageing.

Within the sarcoplasmic reticulum, there is reduced expression of the faster calcium ATPase proteins and increased expression of slower calcium-channel release proteins. This results in a slower flux of calcium into the myofibre following depolarisation from an action potential and contributes to the slowing of muscle contraction that is seen with age. Table 14.2 summarises the changes that occur in skeletal muscle with ageing.

Muscle is a dynamic organ that is consistently under both anabolic (hypertrophic) and catabolic (atrophic) influences (*see* Figure 14.4); this balance determines myofibre size and, as a consequence, total muscle mass and strength.

Anabolic effectors include insulin, amino acids and muscle contraction. The principal anabolic pathway is via the polypeptide hormone IGF-1, which is predominantly secreted by the liver in response to growth hormone. When activated, IGF-1 receptors on skeletal muscle trigger intracellular signalling cascades (phosphoinositol 3-kinase/Akt and Ras/mitogen-activated protein kinase pathways) causing protein synthesis and hypertrophy. IGF-1 levels decline with age, resulting in a balance shift away from anabolism and towards catabolism. This is compounded by anabolic blunting with an observed decline in response to anabolic effectors and a down-regulation of anabolic intracellular signalling molecules.

TABLE 14.2 Age-associated changes to skeletal muscle

Decreased muscle mass and cross-sectional area

Reduced contractile function

Infiltration of adipose and connective tissue; reduced structural integrity

Decreased number of type II myofibres and reduction in their size

Decreased number of type I myofibres and possible reduction in their size

Decreased motor units

Decreased blood flow

Reduced number of satellite cells and increased resistance to their activation

Decreased protein synthesis, especially myosin heavy chain

Decreased mitochondrial volume and activity; reduced anaerobic endurance

Slower calcium flux; slowing of muscle contraction

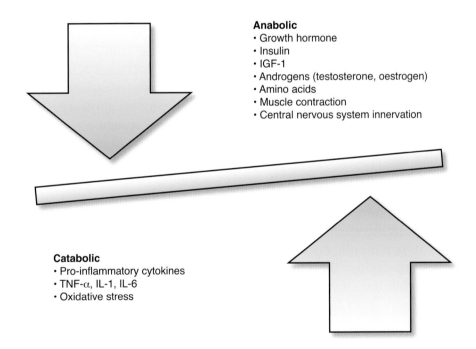

Anabolic
- Growth hormone
- Insulin
- IGF-1
- Androgens (testosterone, oestrogen)
- Amino acids
- Muscle contraction
- Central nervous system innervation

Catabolic
- Pro-inflammatory cytokines
- TNF-α, IL-1, IL-6
- Oxidative stress

FIGURE 14.4 Anabolic and catabolic influences on skeletal muscle

Forkhead box class O (FoxO) transcription factors play a central catabolic role in skeletal muscle myocytes. In its normal state, FoxO is phosphorylated and inactivated by anabolic factors (including IGF-1) via intracellular protein kinases. However, as the balance shifts towards catabolism and away from anabolism, FoxO translocates into the nucleus and causes the transcription of skeletal muscle-specific E3 ubiquitin ligases. These label skeletal muscle proteins for degradation and this is believed to be the major pathway in skeletal muscle atrophy in muscle-wasting conditions. However, evidence in sarcopenia is conflicting, with several studies demonstrating up-regulation of ubiquitin pathway components in sarcopenia and others finding that it is down regulated or unchanged. The relative contributions of the other major proteolytic pathways in sarcopenia (lysosomal, Ca^{2+}-dependent, caspase-dependent) currently lack evidence.

The immune and endocrine systems are closely related, forming an immune-endocrine axis. This generates a 'metabolic milieu' within the human body that influences the majority of cellular biological processes via interaction with cellular receptors and the activation of signalling cascades that affect protein expression. The immune-endocrine axis is affected by a number of intrinsic and extrinsic influences, including genetic variation, adiposity and environmental antigens/pathogens. Age-related change in the immune-endocrine axis is characterised by an expansion of mature T-cell clones and a chronic rise in pro-inflammatory cytokines, termed 'inflammaging'.

These changes are increasingly implicated in the pathogenesis of many age-related diseases, including ischaemic heart disease, stroke, osteoporosis and Alzheimer's dementia. Indeed, the extent of these changes is believed to influence the rate and likelihood of these conditions progressing and has been independently associated with mortality and quality of life measures. This is discussed in a greater detail in Chapter 4, 'The immune system'.

Therefore, it is unsurprising that the age-related changes in the immune-endocrine axis also affect the anabolic–catabolic balance within myocytes, causing a shift towards catabolism, atrophy and progression of sarcopenia. As with other age-related disease processes, it is believed that the degree of shift towards catabolism affects the rate of sarcopenic decline. Pro-inflammatory cytokines, in particular tumour necrosis factor (TNF)-α, appear to play a particularly important role through inhibition of mRNA for myosin heavy chain synthesis, activation of the ubiquitin system and nuclear factor-kappa B, which in turn inhibits muscle cell differentiation. A number of epidemiological studies have shown both cross-sectional and longitudinal associations between sarcopenia and the immune-endocrine axis.

IMPACT OF CHANGES ON PHYSIOLOGICAL FUNCTIONS
Sarcopenia
Epidemiology and diagnosis
As already mentioned, sarcopenia is the loss of muscle mass and function with age. It is common, with prevalence estimates ranging from 9% to 18% in those aged over 65 years, to 30% in men over 80 years and even higher in hospitalised patients. Sarcopenia has recently been reviewed by the European Working Group on Sarcopenia in Older People (EWGSOP). This group defines

sarcopenia as 'a syndrome characterised by progressive and generalised loss of skeletal muscle mass and strength with a risk of adverse outcomes such as physical disability, poor quality of life and death'. Diagnosis depends on demonstrating both low muscle mass and low muscle function (*see* Figure 14.5).

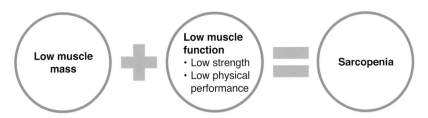

FIGURE 14.5 Criteria for the diagnosis of sarcopenia

Assessment techniques

MUSCLE MASS

A wide range of techniques can be used to characterise muscle mass in both clinical and research environments (*see* Table 14.4). Whole-body and peripheral computed tomography as well as magnetic resonance imaging scans are very precise and can accurately differentiate muscle from other soft tissues of the body, thus these methods are the gold standards. For clinical purposes, dual-energy X-ray absorptiometry (DXA) is a suitable alternative technique to determine lean mass that is readily available. It is less expensive than the gold standards and involves minimal radiation.

Bioimpedance analysis can be used to estimate the volume of fat and lean body mass. It utilises portable equipment, so can be used in a range of settings, including in hospitalised patients confined to bed and within people's homes. Under standardised conditions, it is reproducible and correlates reasonably well with the gold standards. However, standardised conditions can be difficult to reproduce in older populations with co-morbidities and polypharmacy.

MUSCLE STRENGTH

Muscle strength is often characterised using isometric hand-grip strength measurement. This correlates with lower-limb muscle strength and is independently associated with poor clinical outcome as well as incident disability for activities of daily living. Measurement is by handheld dynamometry. The Jamar® dynamometer (*see* Figure 14.6) is most widely used and a standardised (Southampton) protocol has been described (*see* Box 14.1).

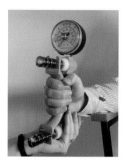

FIGURE 14.6 Measurement of grip strength by Jamar® dynamometer

BOX 14.1 **Southampton Protocol**

1 Sit the participant comfortably in a standard chair with legs, back support and fixed arms.
2 Ask them to rest their forearms on the arms of the chair with their wrist just over the end of the arm of the chair, in a neutral position, thumb facing upwards.
3 Demonstrate how to use the dynamometer to show that gripping very tightly registers the best score.
4 Start with the right hand.
5 Position the hand so that the thumb is round one side of the handle and the four fingers are around the other side. The instrument should feel comfortable in the hand. Alter the position of the handle if necessary.
6 The observer should rest the base of the dynamometer on the palm of their hand as the subject holds the dynamometer. The aim of this is to support the weight of the dynamometer (to negate the effect of gravity on peak strength), but care should be taken not to restrict its movement.
7 Encourage the participant to squeeze as long and as tightly as possible or until the needle stops rising. Once the needle stops rising the participant can be instructed to stop squeezing.
8 Read grip strength in kilograms from the outside dial and record the result to the nearest 1 kg on the data entry form.
9 Repeat measurement in the left hand.
10 Do two further measurements for each hand alternating sides to give three readings in total for each side.
11 The highest value of the six grip strength measurements is recorded.
12 Also record hand dominance.

Roberts HC, Denison HJ, Martin HJ *et al.* A review of the measurement of grip strength in clinical and epidemiological studies: towards a standardised approach. *Age Ageing.* 2011; **40**(4): 423–9.

PHYSICAL PERFORMANCE

There are a number of well-validated measures of physical performance in older people. Perhaps the most comprehensive is the Short Physical Performance Battery, which measures gait speed, balance, strength and endurance, as summarised in Table 14.3. Other simple measures include the usual gait speed and the Timed Up and Go tests.

TABLE 14.3 Short Physical Performance Battery

Three-metre walk	Time taken to walk 3 m at usual pace
One-legged (flamingo) stand	Time standing on one leg (eyes open or closed)
Five chair rises	Time taken to rise to a fully standing position from sitting

CUT-OFF POINTS

Age-related loss of muscle mass and function is a continuous variable. However, identifying individuals with sarcopenia requires defining cut-off points and a number of alternative approaches have been proposed. The EWGSOP recommends that skeletal muscle mass is adjusted for height and compared against a healthy younger population with cut-off points at two standard deviations below the mean reference value as used to identify osteoporosis from continuous bone mass data. With muscle mass measured by DXA, this equates to a cut-off point of $7.26 \, kg/m^2$ for men and $5.5 \, kg/m^2$ for women. Suggested cut-off points when measuring hand-grip strength are less than 30 kg in men and less than 20 kg in women. It is noteworthy that when using these definitions in older hospitalised populations the majority of patients will have sarcopenia.

TABLE 14.4 Tools for diagnosing sarcopenia

Variable	Research environment	Clinical environment
Muscle mass	Computed tomography	Bioimpendance analysis
	Magnetic resonance imaging	DXA
	DXA	Anthropometry
	Bioimpendance analysis	
Muscle strength	Hand-grip strength	Hand-grip strength
	Quadriceps strength	
	Peak expiratory flow	
Physical performance	Short Physical Performance Battery	Short Physical Performance Battery
	Usual gait speed	Usual gait speed
	Timed Up and Go test	Timed Up and Go test

The EWGSOP have suggested an algorithm for the identification of sarcopenia in older people (*see* Figure 14.7).

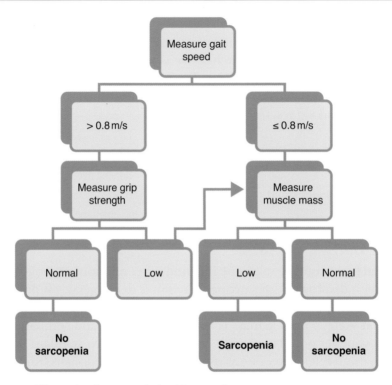

FIGURE 14.7 Diagnosis of sarcopenia in older people

Associations with disease and clinical outcomes

Loss of skeletal mass and function with age occurs universally and is associated with a range of adverse health outcomes including increased all-cause mortality and increased morbidity from osteoporosis, type 2 diabetes, ischaemic heart disease and chronic lung disease as well as frailty (*see* Chapter 18, 'Frailty and ageing'). It is also a major risk factor for physical disability, admission to supported accommodation and hospitalisation, where it is associated with increased length and cost of hospital stay and increased hospital-acquired complications.

FALLS, BONE HEALTH AND FRACTURE

There is a clear relationship between muscle and bone mass throughout the life course and a number of studies have demonstrated the association between sarcopenia and increased fracture risk. Hip fracture may also be a precipitant for development or worsening of sarcopenia and recurrent falling. The Sarcopenia and Hip Fracture Study reported that 75% of participants with hip fracture were also sarcopenic. Over 1-year follow-up, 56% fell at least once, 28% had recurrent falls and 5% sustained a new hip fracture. Sarcopenia is also significantly associated with falling in non-hip fracture patients. Findings from the Hertfordshire Cohort Study demonstrated an inverse relationship between grip strength and falls in the last year in both men and women. Joint American and British Geriatric Society Guidelines for the prevention of falls in older people describe muscle weakness as the single greatest intrinsic risk factor for falling, with an estimated relative risk of 4.4.

Obesity and sarcopenic obesity

Rising levels of obesity in the context of an ageing population are resulting in an increasing prevalence of the body composition-phenotype sarcopenic obesity. Identifying individuals with sarcopenic obesity depends on first defining obesity in older populations. Although this varies by study, the most common definitions use either percentage body fat greater than the median or body fat in the highest two quintiles. In 2000, the prevalence of sarcopenic obesity was estimated to increase from approximately 3% to 10% from 65 to 80 years of age, with other studies in older people reporting a range from 4% to 12%.

The associations between sarcopenia and obesity are far from independent; in fact, there are many biological and behavioural reasons why the conditions are connected and reinforce each other. Sarcopenia causes an increased mismatch between energy expenditure and intake, resulting in positive energy balance, mostly stored as fat. Sarcopenia also causes a reduction in basal metabolic rate that is further exacerbated by reduction in physical activity and active metabolic rate. Adipocytes are far more than simple fat storage vessels; they secrete signalling molecules called 'adipokines' including pro-inflammatory cytokines, oestrogen and leptin. Consequences include a raised inflammatory milieu and an increased shift towards catabolic effects on myocytes in addition to central effects on energy homeostasis and appetite.

The clinical consequences of sarcopenic obesity are significant. It is more strongly associated with disability than either reduced muscle mass or increased fat mass alone. Recent studies have demonstrated a 2.5- to 3.0-fold increased risk for disability and a mortality risk that is 1.39 times higher than in people of normal weight.

Cachexia

Epidemiology and diagnosis

Cachexia (Greek, *kakos* 'bad', *hexia* 'condition') was recognised by Hippocrates, who noted 'the shoulders, clavicles, chest and thighs melt away. This illness is fatal'. It has since been described by consensus definition (Evans 2008) as 'a complex metabolic syndrome associated with underlying illness and characterised by loss of muscle with or without loss of fat mass. The prominent clinical feature of cachexia is weight loss in adults'. It must be distinguished from starvation, age-related loss of muscle mass, primary depression, malabsorption and hyperthyroidism. Diagnostic criteria have been defined (*see* Box 14.2).

Cachexia is a systemic process mediated by the body's immune system. Chronic administration of pro-inflammatory cytokines such as TNF-α, interleukin (IL)-6 and interferon-γ, either alone or in combination, is capable of reducing food intake and reproducing the distinct features of cachexia, a mechanism with strong evolutionary roots. Specific proteins within skeletal muscle are targeted to yield amino acids that are subsequently consumed in the liver for the synthesis of acute-phase proteins such as C-reactive protein (CRP).

This highly conserved system is beneficial during acute inflammation for repair and provision of energy but has severe implications during chronic catabolic states. In addition to effects on skeletal muscle, cytokines also lower serum albumin concentrations, enhance lipolysis and are responsible for the anorexia associated with cachexia. Pro-inflammatory cytokines cause decreased activity of the hypothalamic orexigenic signal neuropeptide Y, which stimulates hunger and reduces energy expenditure. Cytokines also delay gastric emptying and increase feelings of fullness.

BOX 14.2 Diagnostic criteria for cachexia

Unintentional weight loss of at least 5% in 12 months (or body mass index less than 20 kg/m^2)

    Plus at least three of:

1 decreased muscle strength*
2 fatigue
3 anorexia
4 low fat-free mass[†]
5 abnormal biochemistry
    a increased inflammatory markers[‡]
    b anaemia (haemoglobin <12 g/dL)
    c low serum albumin (<32 g/L)

* Lowest tertile grip strength.
[†] Lean tissue depletion, i.e. mid-arm circumference less than tenth percentile for age and sex.
[‡] Defined as any inflammatory marker above two standard deviations of the age and sex matched means, e.g. CRP >5.0 mg/L and IL-6 >4.0 pg/mL.

Cachexia is an underestimated and under-diagnosed consequence of any chronic or severe inflammatory process including infection, chronic obstructive pulmonary disease (COPD), congestive cardiac failure (CCF), chronic kidney disease, inflammatory arthritis and human immunodeficiency virus/acquired immune deficiency syndrome. Twelve-month mortality rates range from 15% in COPD and 30% in CCF to 80% in certain cancers. It is also of great relevance to clinicians involved with the care of older people, where it is the second most common cause of muscle loss. A recent study in the US found a prevalence of

28% among nursing home residents. Little is known about the prevalence in the United Kingdom. Older people are particularly vulnerable to becoming cachexic as a consequence of chronic illness, background sarcopenia, reduced physical activity, dysgeusia, dysosmia, orogingival disease, depression, dementia and social isolation. Furthermore, ageing is associated with a physiologic anorexia that results in reduced energy intake and puts older people at risk of developing cachexia even during minor illnesses.

Previously, cachexia was believed to be associated with the end stages of a disease process. However, it has recently been reported that cachexia occurs far earlier in the course of a disease. Indeed, there is now good evidence that cachexia is an early phenomenon, emphasising the importance of recognition and treatment. The diagnostic criteria for cachexia have been further modified to facilitate timely early recognition and intervention. Therefore, cachexia can be classified as mild, moderate or severe depending on the degree of weight loss in the preceding 12 months: greater than 5%, greater than 10% or greater than 15%, respectively. Furthermore, for the recognition of individuals at high risk of developing cachexia and facilitation of preventative interventions, *pre-cachexia* has also been defined (*see* Box 14.3).

BOX 14.3 Criteria for the diagnosis of pre-cachexia

All of:
1 underlying chronic disease
2 unintentional weight loss ≤5% of usual body weight during the last 6 months
3 chronic or recurrent systemic inflammatory response
4 anorexia.

The relationship between sarcopenia and cachexia is subject to much debate. The current rationale is that cachexia is a component of sarcopenia, but the two disease processes are not the same. Sarcopenia occurs universally whereas cachexia occurs in the presence of severe or accumulative disease processes. Thus, most cachexic individuals are also sarcopenic, but few people with sarcopenia are also cachexic. The hallmark of cachexia is a sustained, measurable systemic inflammatory response with associated weight loss whereas sarcopenia is a multifactorial age-associated condition of skeletal muscle.

PREVENTION AND TREATMENT
Exercise

It is now well established that exercise can slow the loss of skeletal muscle mass and function and that inactivity accelerates loss. However, a recent 3-year longitudinal study of body composition reported that physical activity in older people caused body weight to remain stable, while lean body mass *decreased* and fat mass *increased*. This study reinforces the principle that total body weight and body mass index are not useful techniques to assess loss of skeletal muscle; it also emphasises the importance of the *mode of activity* in the preservation of lean body mass.

Resistance exercise (strength training) is the most effective mode of activity to combat age-related changes in muscle especially at high velocity. This includes the very old and those admitted to nursing homes; benefits can still be demonstrated more than 30 weeks after stopping an exercise programme. A recent Cochrane review of 121 trials that included 6700 participants found that high-intensity resistance training performed two to three times per week had a positive effect on muscle strength and that this was associated with a modest improvement in gait speed and getting out of a chair. The authors concluded that progressive resistance training is an effective intervention for improving strength and physical functioning in older people including functional performance of some simple and complex tasks.

Nutrition

Nutrition is also important in maintaining muscle mass and strength in later life, although the findings from studies have not been as consistent as those from exercise interventions and a recent Cochrane review found no definite functional benefit of nutritional supplementation. For example, increasing daily protein intake to 1.2–1.5 g/kg has been reported in some studies to be beneficial. However, this needs to be consumed as a small amount of high-quality protein with each meal and with a reduction in carbohydrate intake. Such a diet is very difficult to achieve, especially as 40% of people aged over 70 years do not consume the recommended minimum dietary allowance of 0.8 g/kg/day.

Other examples include the essential amino acid leucine, which is found in leguminous products, fish and beef, and is believed to increase protein anabolism while reducing muscle breakdown. Vitamin D was recently the subject of a meta-analysis that concluded the evidence for supplementation was strong, although questions still remain about dosing, efficacy and long-term safety. A number of current trials combine nutritional supplementation with resistance exercise, which remains the most effective treatment to date in combating age-related loss of skeletal muscle.

Drugs

There is considerable interest in drug development to combat the age-related loss of skeletal muscle. The commonest pharmacological target is the immune-endocrine axis, but results of randomised controlled trials to date have been disappointing. Currently, there is no recommended drug treatment; examples of candidate targets/drugs are summarised in Table 14.5.

TABLE 14.5 Example candidate targets/drugs for use in sarcopenia

Intervention	Effect	Pros/Cons
Testosterone	Varying evidence of increased muscle mass and strength	Masculinisation of women, risk of prostate cancer in men
Oestrogen	Some evidence for increased muscle mass, nil for function	Risk of breast cancer
Growth hormone	Some evidence for increased muscle mass, varying for strength	Extensive side-effect profile
Vitamin D	Varying evidence for increasing muscle strength, reduced falls in nursing home residents	Fracture reduction, possible cardiovascular benefits
Angiotensin-converting-enzyme inhibitors	Some evidence for increased exercise capacity	Other cardiovascular benefits, already well used
Creatine	Variable evidence for increased muscle strength and endurance, especially when combined with exercise	Risk of nephritis
Myostatin antagonists	No trials in older people	
Peroxisome proliferator-activated receptor-γ agonist	No human trials	
AICAR enzyme*	No human trials	

* 5-aminoimidazole-4-carboxamide-1-β-D-ribofuranoside.

Modified from Burton LA, Sumukadas D. Optimal management of sarcopenia. *Clin Interv Aging.* 2010; **5**: 217–28.

CONCLUSION

Ageing of the muscular system is a central part of the ageing process and is associated with mortality, morbidity, frailty and disability. The two most common causes of age-related muscle loss are sarcopenia, which is multifactorial and occurs universally, and cachexia, which is caused by underlying sustained inflammation. New consensus definitions have recently been developed for both conditions that will underpin both clinical recognition and research. At present, the only established beneficial intervention is resistance exercise, although there is growing interest in nutritional approaches as well as drug development. A life-course perspective to skeletal muscle ageing includes consideration of the determinants of peak muscle mass and function in early adulthood as well as those factors influencing the subsequent rate of decline.

FURTHER READING

Baylis D, Bartlett DB, Sayer AA *et al.* Immune-endocrine biomarkers as predictors of frailty and mortality: a 10-year longitudinal study in community dwelling older people. *Age (Dordr).* Epub 2012 Mar 3.

Cruz-Jentoft AJ, Baeyens JM, Bauer JM *et al.* Sarcopenia: European consensus on definition and diagnosis; report of the European Working Group on Sarcopenia in Older People. *Age Ageing.* 2010; **39**(4): 412–23.

Evans WJ, Morley JE, Argilés J *et al.* Cachexia: a new definition. *Clin Nutr.* 2008; **27**(6): 793–9.

Liu CJ, Latham NK. Progressive resistance strength training for improving physical functioning in older adults. *Cochrane Database Syst Rev.* 2009; (3): CD002459.

Sayer AA. Sarcopenia. *BMJ.* 2010; **341**: c4097.

Sayer AA, Cooper C. Aging, sarcopenia and the life course. *Rev Clin Gerontol.* 2006; **16**(4): 265–74.

ACKNOWLEDGEMENTS

Mark Meyer, Figure 14.1.
Helen Roberts, Figure 14.6.

QUESTIONS: MUSCLE

1 Which one of the following is incorrect regarding type I myofibres?
A they are principally used for aerobic activity
B they have a low endurance
C they produce a lower force relative to type II myofibres
D their ratio with type II myofibres varies depending on anatomical location
E they reduce in number with age.

Answer: B

2 After the age of 50 years old, muscle strength is lost at an average rate of:
A loss of muscle strength with age is not a universal process
B less than 0.5% per year
C 0.5%–1.5% per year
D 1.5%–3.0% per year
E 3.0%–4.5% per year.

Answer: D

3 Which one of the following is correct regarding the diagnosis of sarcopenia?
A bioimpedance has no role in the characterisation of muscle mass
B clear cut-off points have been defined and are widely accepted
C hand-grip dynamometry is a useful technique to characterise muscle strength
D ultrasound scanning is normally used to characterise muscle mass
E the measurement of gait speed is rarely required.

Answer: C

4 Trials have suggested that the most effective intervention for the treatment of sarcopenia is:
A androgen replacement therapy
B high protein diet
C immune-modulating drugs
D nutritional supplements
E resistance exercise.

Answer: E

5 Which one of the following statements regarding cachexia is incorrect?
A up-regulation of IGF-1 is strongly implicated
B cachexia is a cause of sarcopenia, but the two disease processes are not the same
C cachexia is an immune-mediated disease process
D early recognition and timely intervention are important
E cachexia in older people is commonly multifactorial.

Answer: A

CHAPTER 15

The brain

ROXANNE STERNICZUK, SULTAN DARVESH
AND KENNETH ROCKWOOD

INTRODUCTION

Virtually every major neurodegenerative illness becomes more common with age, with most seen chiefly in old age. Therefore, understanding how the brain ages is a critical part of understanding how this immense burden of illness eventuates. Of great interest, too, is that most of these late-onset neurodegenerative disorders have long prodromes that can span decades in their preclinical stages. During this period, knowing whether given symptom constellations represent disease or 'just ageing' can be impossible to discern without the passage of time, which is hardly a satisfactory diagnostic approach.

Understanding brain ageing is a daunting task, as it combines two formally complex problems: how the brain works and how this changes with age. Perspective is everything; thus, several themes will be emphasised in this chapter. The first is to view ageing as a stochastic process of deficit accumulation, in which, on average, things gradually function less effectively. This on-average decline is mitigated by the fact that change typically happens slowly and that some improvement (although, like the decline, usually only modest) is also possible at any time. Second, we note that brain ageing results from changes to the metabolic triad of altered mitochondrial functioning, reactive oxygen species (ROS) formation and altered intracellular calcium homeostasis; together, these ultimately impair homeostatic responses. Brain homeostasis is of particular interest because post-mitotic neurons depend on intracellular repair processes (not cellular replacement) in response to injury. This repertoire can be limited or ultimately injurious, which is the subject of the third theme: although age-related decline is small, in the face of what we call disease, it typically accelerates. In part, this reflects long prodromes of subclinical decline and that responses, which initially help in adaptation, may themselves become maladaptive, giving rise to vicious cycles at sub-cellular and then higher levels, again impairing homeostasis. Finally, we note that methodological aspects are key, with the consequence that significant parts of our understanding are technology dependent. With this, it is necessary only once to point out just how tentative our conclusions about brain ageing are.

Brain ageing in context

Almost all organisms experience ageing. Ageing (compared with the simple passage of time) can be understood as an increase in the risk of death. Even considering only brain changes, there is no shortage of theories of ageing (*see* Chapter 2, 'The concept of ageing: theories and mechanisms') or of how it might be controlled. Between the idea of ageing as genetically programmed cell death and the idea of ageing as susceptibility to entirely random processes, a broad middle ground exists in the notion of ageing as the accumulation of unrepaired deficits. Damage slowly builds to impair the organism's ability to respond to stress. Theories differ as to what gives rise to the damage, how that affects the ability to repair and how energy used in repair is traded off against energy that could be used for reproductive success. Different theories can reflect differences in methodology as much as in concepts: it is possible to consider only data that are visible and 'visibility' is typically technology dependent.

The most obvious impact of methodology comes from advances in molecular biology. For example, techniques to visualise green fluorescent protein-LC3 have allowed identification of autophagosomes *in vivo*. With this, the concept of 'mitophagy' offered a means of understanding how damaged mitochondria could be removed. For clinicians, the dramatic advances in neuroimaging now allow detailed visualisation of brain anatomy *in vivo*.

Any account of how biological processes change over longer time intervals must consider how factors associated with ageing interact. The brain itself appears to influence the rate of ageing. Major depression has been linked not just to physical disease but also to cellular markers of so-called accelerated ageing. In women, time since menopause, itself related to life stress events, has been related to an array of age-related disorders, with older age at menopause being protective. Even so, caution about attributing too much of brain ageing, especially in relation to dementia-like changes, to the experience of stress is warranted. As we shall see next, sometimes stress can serve as much to unmask age-related change as to cause it. This occurs not just at the clinical level where, for example, physical illness can give rise to delirium in people whose cognition never recovers, but also at cellular and sub-cellular levels.

MOLECULAR AND CELLULAR CHANGES

Sub-cellular and cellular deficit accumulation

Ageing represents the accumulation of unrepaired sub-cellular damage, which eventually compromises the functioning of cells, tissues and organs, that becomes at some stage clinically evident. Clinical manifestations of ageing are often subtle and only seen under stress, in which the ability to respond becomes compromised. Ageing characteristically affects cell membrane lipids and proteins involved in metabolism and structural roles, in addition to causing well-recognised damage to the DNA present in cell nuclei and mitochondria (*see* Chapter 3, 'The ageing cell').

Mitochondrial activity

The brain's huge energy consumption makes it an ongoing site of damage to mitochondria (*see* Figure 15.1). ROS are also by-products of fatty acid metabolism in organelles known as 'peroxisomes', wherein hydrogen peroxide is generated. When ROS are not balanced by antioxidant activity, damage ensues, which accumulates if it cannot be repaired.

Essential to understanding neuronal ageing is that these cells are substantially post-mitotic, having little cell division in adult life. The brain is rarely capable of diluting and repairing the accumulation of biochemically altered harmful macromolecules (e.g. DNA and proteins) and organelles (e.g. mitochondria) as stem and progenitor cells can by cellular replacement. In consequence, it must rely on repair and clearance mechanisms. The brain also responds to its environment via so-called neuronal plasticity. 'Neuroplasticity' can refer both to cellular mechanisms of change and to the ability for new synaptic formation to carry out functions performed by circuitry that has become damaged. The recognition of neuroplasticity has proved to be one of the most influential changes in thinking about how brains age.

Neuroplasticity

Long-term potentiation (LTP) is the most studied form of neuroplasticity and is a strong neural correlate for learning and memory. LTP links neurons by facilitating transmission between them. Usually *N*-methyl-D-aspartate (NMDA)-type glutamate receptor activation gives rise to Ca^{2+} influx. This activates additional intracellular pathways, such as Ca^{2+}/calmodulin-dependent protein kinase II and other kinases. These enzymes can then act either pre- or post-synaptically to modify neuronal synaptic efficacy (e.g. regulate processes such as ion channel conductance, gene expression and protein synthesis).

Age-dependent cognitive impairment is increasingly linked to problems in synaptic plasticity. In the aged brain, LTP takes significantly longer to develop and decays more rapidly than in younger controls; these changes parallel impaired new learning capability. In rats, older animals require stronger stimulation to achieve the same signal induction than that observed in their younger

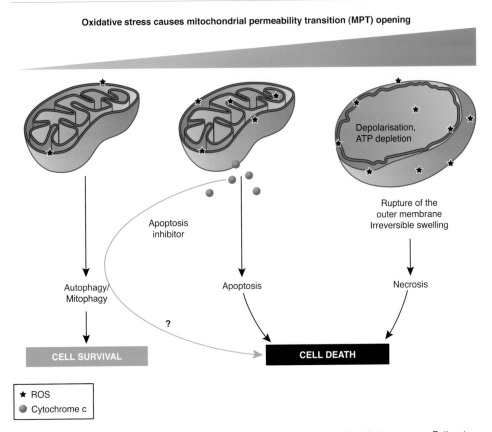

FIGURE 15.1 Mitochondrial activation following varying degrees of oxidative stress. Following low oxidative stress, or the initial encounter of ROS, as seen in the leftmost pathway, autophagy and mitophagy may be induced to ensure survival of the neuron. Here, mitophagy is a means of countering ROS damage. As the number of ROS increases, cellular damage accumulates and causes cytochrome c to be triggered and apoptosis to be activated. Following extreme mitochondrial damage from high levels of oxidative stress, mitochondria become swollen and the membrane may rupture, inducing necrosis. Reproduced from Yen WL, Klionsky DJ. How to live long and prosper: autophagy, mitochondria, and aging. *Physiology (Bethesda).* 2008; 23: 248–62; used with permission[1]

counterparts. Likewise, older synapses appear to be less capable of sustaining the depolarisation required to activate downstream cascades involved in LTP. For example, there is a shift from the primary NMDA-type glutamate receptor Ca^{2+} influx to voltage-gated Ca^{2+} channel activation during ageing; if this does not sufficiently increase intracellular Ca^{2+}, it will not trigger vital Ca^{2+}-dependent kinases. Without the LTP-dependent changes in proteins required by neuronal axons and dendrites to grow and form new connections, learning and memory consolidation is impaired.

The accumulation of biological waste products

As noted, with oxidative stress, mitochondria produce ROS. Intracellular damage, neuronal dysfunction and death can also arise from nitrosative stress. Determining the role of nitrosative stress has required an understanding of intricacies of the NMDA-type glutamate receptor, which can increase intraneuronal calcium, in turn activating neuronal nitric oxide synthase and ultimately producing peroxynitrite-associated free radicals. A key challenge to understanding the biological role of nitric oxide has been that its effect depends on its concentration: it can participate in neuronal signalling, being either protective or harmful.

Although aerobic cells have developed antioxidant defence systems, they are not fully capable of defending against the accumulation of macromolecular waste products that results from sub-cellular deficits. Aged cells are often larger than younger ones; in the former, this reflects accumulation of intracellular debris and compensatory enlargement of functionally degenerating structures. This represents another example of the theme that initially compensatory mechanisms come at a later cost. These larger cells are less bio-energetically efficient than their smaller and younger counterparts. Intracellular lipofuscin also accumulates with age, mainly in long-lived post-mitotic cells. This yellowish-brown non-degradable pigment is formed from compounds of ageing lysosomes, specifically complexes of aldehydes and free protein fragments. Lipofuscin arises from macromolecular cross-linking, which prevents lysosomal degradation. Increased formation of intracellular hydrogen peroxide or minimal cytosolic degradation of hydrogen peroxide contributes to increased lipofuscin formation. Only mitotic activity is known to dilute the pigment and remove this form of waste product from the intracellular space.

Despite these evident age-related changes, the brain has various mechanisms to defend itself against ongoing insults; just as some features mean that the brain participates in and can ultimately accelerate its own ageing, it also has the means through which it can fight back. An analogy to quality control is sometimes made in describing what are known as 'housekeeping' and 'chaperone' proteins and their protective functions. As noted, for their viability to be maintained, post-mitotic neurons need intracellular debris (abnormal proteins, damaged organelles) to be removed. Autophagy itself is also susceptible to age-related compromise; this is felt to be an important step in how neurodegenerative disorders develop. Likewise, the triggering of apoptosis as a defence against the accumulation of misfolded proteins, which arise in the setting of cell stress and can elude repair when such mechanisms fail, is an example of how damage can accelerate.

Taken together, cellular ageing can be viewed as the accumulation of deficits that override neuronal repair mechanisms. Tellingly, this build-up can occur with positive feedback loops, so that, for example, ROS production causes an increase in mitochondrial damage and a decrease in mitochondrial autophagy, which propagates ROS production and lipofuscin accumulation; ultimately, this decreases adenosine triphosphate (ATP) production and causes cellular apoptosis.

Synaptic dysfunction

Deleterious alterations to the metabolic triad ultimately lead to dysfunctional synaptic activity and the decline in cognition that is observed in old age. Changes to the number and size of synapses and various components of synaptic signalling may be altered during ageing. These include shrinkage of the soma, loss or regression of dendrites and dendritic spines, myelin dystrophy, and altered neurotransmitter release and reception. These structural changes ultimately affect the neurons' electrophysiological properties. Although an increase in action-potential rates is visible with ageing, there is an overall decrease in excitatory synaptic transmission; most probably due to increased gamma-aminobutyric acid (GABA) release from presynaptic interneurons.

The blood–brain barrier (BBB)

The protective BBB network of the cerebral vascular system regulates the passage of substances between the central nervous system (CNS) and external systemic circulation. The BBB is composed of a neurovascular unit, which consists of vascular endothelial cells, pericytes, neurons and astrocytes. In response to trauma or injury, this unit regulates the proliferation, migration and branching of brain microvascular endothelial cells. Age-related compromise of the BBB can alter the transport of crucial nutrients and metabolites to and from the brain and/or permit the entry of toxins; either can lead to CNS dysfunction and diminished behavioural and physiological functioning. Many factors contribute to microvascular injury and subsequent cognitive impairment, particularly hypertension, hyperlipidaemia, diabetes mellitus and various medications. Impairment in the BBB has been linked to age-associated neurological and cognitive decline and to geriatric syndromes such as executive dysfunction, delirium, impaired mobility and incontinence.

The ageing BBB exhibits less cortical and white matter microvascular density, smaller capillary lumen size, fewer endothelial cells, fewer mitochondria per endothelial cell, less enzymatic activity and greater basement membrane thickness. Compared with that of younger brains, the BBB of healthy older adults exhibits significantly greater permeability, which is further increased in disease (e.g. vascular dementia or Alzheimer's disease [AD]). Transport of glucose, amino acids and hormones across the BBB is diminished in old age, contributing to brain hypoglycaemia and cognitive decline.

CHANGES IN METABOLIC PROCESSES

In addition to glucose (and, to a much lesser extent, free fatty acid) metabolism, a large number of other metabolic processes change with age.

Calcium homeostasis in the brain

Maintaining intracellular Ca^{2+} homeostasis is crucial to both synaptic neurotransmission and the genetic regulation of structural protein production. Synaptic neurotransmission critically depends on the maintenance of a charge differential across the neuronal membrane. This membrane potential is maintained chiefly by a 50-fold difference in the intracellular versus extracellular concentration of Ca^{2+}. Within the neuron, calcium is sequestered within the endoplasmic reticulum. A theme of many types of neuronal death is leakage from the endoplasmic reticulum into the intracellular space, giving rise to Ca^{2+} overload.

Calcium handling is altered in other ways. Age-dependent changes to voltage-gated Ca^{2+} channels within pyramidal neurons of the CA1 region of the hippocampus and neurons of the basal forebrain are well described. These regions exhibit either an increase in Ca^{2+} after hyperpolarisations or a drop below resting membrane potential due to increased L-type Ca^{2+} channels. Another robust effect of age is a decrease in the effectiveness and number of NMDA subtypes of glutamatergic receptors, which permits Ca^{2+} entry during neuronal activation. The NMDA receptor 2B subunit appears to be chiefly affected, with decreased mRNA expression detected in old age. The number of Ca^{2+}-binding proteins decreases, specifically, calbindin and calretinin in the cerebral cortex. A decrease in calbindin is also found in the basal forebrain, but an increase is observed in the temporal cortex, suggesting that changes to Ca^{2+}-binding proteins are region specific.

Another instance of initial changes in ageing being associated with potentially compensatory changes in cell function is how ageing affects intracellular compartments that regulate Ca^{2+} signalling. Inhibition of Ca^{2+} release from intracellular stores appears to activate, rather than inhibit, LTP. Furthermore, a significant decline in LTP in hippocampal neurons (and memory decline) is observed following an increase in Ca^{2+} release, possibly due to the activation of slow after hyperpolarisations.

Chronic mitochondrial depolarisation is the most robust age-related change. This causes an increase in the threshold required to activate mitochondrial Ca^{2+} uptake. With it comes a delay in recovery of resting Ca^{2+} channels, or a decrease in Ca^{2+} clearance, following stimulation. Proton leakage within the respiratory chain is increased and causes a decrease in ATP synthesis; this leakage may be a cause or the effect of mitochondrial depolarisation. In general, altered Ca^{2+} handling can arise in many circumstances (e.g. damage by ROS, dysfunction of Ca^{2+} channels or loss of intracellular Ca^{2+}-binding proteins).

Excitotoxicity

The toxic effect of excessive receptor activation by excitatory amino acids (e.g. glutamate) appears to underlie excitotoxicity. Excitotoxicity is a major mechanism in cell death and may mediate the neuronal damage seen in both ischaemic and neurodegenerative diseases (e.g. AD). Overstimulation of glutamate receptors produces several negative effects intracellularly, including altered Ca^+ homeostasis and organelle functioning, increased production of nitric oxide and other free radicals, activation of proteases and kinases, and an increase in transcription factors and immediate early genes that promote cellular death. NMDA-receptor activation also depolarises mitochondrial membranes, which may lead to an increase in ROS. Non-NMDA receptors, such as those that respond to 2-amino-3-(5-methyl-3-oxo-1,2-oxazol-4-yl)propanoic acid (AMPA) and kainite, may also play a role in cell death, as their activation causes neuronal depolarisation.

In addition to the effects that glutamatergic transmission have on neuronal excitation, several other mechanisms play a role in mediating excessive intracellular activation, especially changes in intracellular organelles. Neurons undergoing excitotoxic death exhibit several dysfunctional organelles, including swelling of endoplasmic reticulum, vesiculation of Golgi apparatus, mitochondrial disruption and an increased number of secondary lysosomes. For example, the endoplasmic reticulum contributes to the excitotoxic process by releasing Ca^+ from its intracellular stores via ryanodine receptors. At the same time, other processes (e.g. necrosis, autophagy) contribute to neuronal injury and death.

As the brain ages, neuronal energy supplies primarily generated in the mitochondria (e.g. ATP, nicotinamide adenine dinucleotide [NAD^+]) decrease. This prevents requisite restoration of ion gradients across the neuronal membrane after generation of activation and action potentials. This reduction in energy supply is associated with the increased intracellular Ca^+ levels that are observed in ageing. Both the sustained influx of Ca^{2+} through glutamatergic channels as well as impaired ion-motive ATPase activities – which are enzymes that regulate the exchange of ions, particularly Ca^{2+}, across the membrane – contribute to this effect. Decreased levels of ATP and NAD^+ are also associated with age-related cognitive impairments.

IMPACT OF AGEING ON NEUROANATOMY AND NEUROPHYSIOLOGICAL FUNCTIONS

Neuroanatomy

The ageing brain undergoes structural and functional changes that manifest clinically as alterations in everyday performance but that are typically more visible with formal testing. With age, the brain's complex interconnected networks of anatomically and physiologically distinct regions become even more heterogeneous between and within individuals. Systematic study in humans is challenged by the limited control for the effects of disease, which significantly contribute to neurodegeneration and cause both anatomical and neurochemical alterations. For example, examination of the brain at autopsy makes it seem that the most striking feature of ageing is age-related atrophy (*see* Figure 15.2). How this is confounded with disease can be difficult to determine. Comparisons of cross-sectional and longitudinal analyses reveal that longitudinal measures of neuronal atrophy exceed cross-sectional reports. That said, both cross-sectional and longitudinal designs have demonstrated that healthy brain ageing occurs in a spatially specific manner. Generally, brain volumes shrink with age, by approximately 5% per decade after about the age of 50 years. A more rapid decline in volume is visible after 70 years, especially in the hippocampus and temporal regions, although it has been suggested that this effect can be reversed by aerobic exercise.[2] The decrease in size is relatively uniform throughout the cerebral white matter. In contrast, the extent of grey matter loss varies between different brain regions. Grey matter appears to be lost more at a younger age (i.e. 20–50 years) than white matter, which deteriorates more at an older age (i.e. 70–90 years). The brainstem nuclei appear to be well preserved into old age.

No Dementia Female 60 year old	No Dementia Female 90 year old	Alzheimer's Disease Female 91 year old
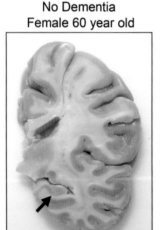	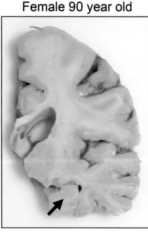	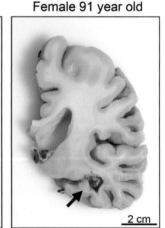

FIGURE 15.2 Coronal slices demonstrating the gross neuroanatomical changes during ageing and disease. (A) A healthy younger-old female without dementia and minimal atrophy within the hippocampal region (as indicated by the arrow). (B) An older-old female without dementia and mild atrophy within the hippocampal region, as well as ventricular enlargement. (C) An older-old female with advanced AD and significant atrophy within the hippocampal and cortical regions, as well as severe enlargement of the ventricles. While not untrue on average, in recent years, this picture of visible atrophy with age, and markedly worse atrophy with dementia, has become considerably more nuanced

Volumetric changes appear to be due less to loss in the number of neurons (which appears not to change in normal ageing) rather than to loss of synaptic spines and synapses and shorter myelinated axons. As the brain shrinks, the ventricles and subarachnoid space expand to fill in the space created by the loss of volume. The production of cerebrospinal fluid also decreases with age. In this regard, anatomy appears to give rise to metabolic change, rather than just the opposite, as sclerosed arachnoid villi increase outflow resistance, thereby maintaining higher levels of cerebrospinal fluid and consequently hindering the normal exchange of nutrients and oxygen.

These changes in structure and function manifest themselves in clinically detectable ways. Acknowledging at the outset that what we call 'cognition' and its components represent semantic categories for the functioning of complex neuronal networks that are not sensibly reduced to cellular events, convention allows us to talk about purposeful directed activities that can be understood as cognitive functions such as executive memory, language and visuospatial functions. It is impossible to give a brief account that has any claim to comprehensiveness, thus, in describing each brain area, just a few important points will be highlighted. In keeping with the theme of technology dependence noted in the introduction to this chapter, communication about the impact of ageing on cognitive functioning can be challenging when various disciplines describe essentially similar phenomena in different ways, reflecting the varied approaches and technologies of their disciplines. This is especially important when talking about memory and attention, which are commonly affected in ageing, that can be described in multiple ways.

REGIONAL BRAIN CHANGES WITH AGEING

The frontal lobes

The most prominent neuroanatomical alterations during ageing occur in the frontal lobes (*see* Table 15.1). There is reduction in volume and preferential synaptic density decline in this region. Atrophy is greatest within the prefrontal cortex, which comprises the majority of the frontal lobes and exhibits the largest reduction in white matter. This region is associated with cognitive operations such as working memory, episodic memory, sequencing, organisation, abstraction and planning. Other forebrain structures, namely the basal ganglia thalamo-cortical circuits, are consistently affected by ageing as well.

Compared with younger individuals, older individuals who exhibit greater frontal lobe activation tend to perform better on cognitive tasks; that is, the greater activation appears to be compensatory. Because memory impairment is a hallmark of ageing, many neuroimaging studies focus on working and episodic memory tasks. Region-specific differences in activation are associated with age-related changes in performance, with primary deficits occurring in the right anterior, right dorsal and bilateral ventral regions of the prefrontal cortex. Both increases (interpreted as compensation) and decreases (interpreted as loss) to prefrontal cortical activity have been reported in older individuals. Most increases, or compensations, tend to occur within the left dorsal and anterior prefrontal cortex. The functional compensation view states that increases in activation reflect either successful compensation, and in turn no visible age-related differences, or attempted compensation and subsequent deficit in old age. Others have suggested that the apparent reduction in hemispheric specialisation seen with neurocompensation may simply reflect deficits in neurotransmission causing diminished cortical activation. In other words, increased activity is not always compensatory, since reduced regionally specific processing may cause aberrant neural activity; behaviourally, this can lead to better or worse performance. Prefrontal atrophy strongly correlates with impaired performance on working memory tasks in aged non-human primates. There appears to be an optimal level of neuronal activity that is necessary when processing such tasks. For example, single and multi-unit recordings of pyramidal cells within the prefrontal cortex of alert monkeys show increased action-potential frequencies during working memory tasks. Changes to these firing patterns may underlie age-related alterations to cognition. During peak performance, aged animals appear to require higher rates of firing than the lower rates exhibited by their younger counterparts when so challenged. The frequency of action-potential occurrence is U-shaped: very low and very high firing rates are observed following poor performance, but higher firing rates are seen during accurate performance of working memory tasks.

Although selective attention remains relatively well preserved, decrements in executive functioning contribute to impaired attention on demanding tasks. For instance, age-related declines are observed in divided attention tasks, inhibiting automatic response and ignoring irrelevant information. Functional neuroimaging demonstrates that age-related impairments during working memory and attention tasks are associated with less activity within the prefrontal cortex. Supporting the idea of neurocompensation, studies examining perceptual and episodic memory tasks have reported increased activity in the prefrontal cortex. This compensatory recruitment is speculated to be due to age-related white matter deterioration between the frontal and posterior regions, and subsequent loss of functional connectivity. Even so, such conclusions must be tentative, as this over-recruitment only appears to be visible in cross-sectional analyses, not longitudinal estimates, and is task dependent. For example, older subjects engaged in a visual attention task exhibit greater frontal activation when compared with younger subjects, who exhibit increased posterior activity.

Deficits in motor performance can be attributed to impairments in both the central and peripheral nervous systems. Older individuals often exhibit difficulty in coordinating movements, maintaining balance and gait as well as an overall slowing of movement. However, there is contradictory evidence regarding the extent to which the motor cortex (posterior frontal lobe) is affected by age. Some studies have shown no effect, whereas others have found significant decreases in volume and cortical thickness, as well as increased sensorimotor activation during motor tasks. It is possible that atrophy in this region contributes to the slowing of movement, since older subjects tend to have smaller sensorimotor regions, which has been linked to shorter steps and longer support times while walking. Other structures related to gait, such as the cerebellum, also play a vital role in the coordination of movement; they, too, show decreases in volume with age. In addition, the basal ganglia exhibit age-related decline, especially the caudate nucleus, which is important for skill acquisition during motor learning.

The temporal lobes

The temporal cortex is affected by ageing to a lesser extent than the frontal lobes. Even so, it is most susceptible to the early degenerative effects of disease and is often implicated in the memory impairments that characterise unhealthy ageing. A reduction in temporal lobe size, and of the underlying hippocampus, is associated with increased ventricular volume. Age-related decrease in hippocampal volume is associated with impaired learning, whereas a decrease in the volume of the surrounding entorhinal cortex is associated with impaired recognition. The impact of ageing on atrophy of the frontal and temporal cortices appears to be greater in men.

The medial temporal lobe, which is important for memory encoding and retrieval, exhibits a significant reduction in activation during old age. The hippocampus is critical for learning and memory, especially spatial and episodic memory, so that any impairment in this region causes significant memory deficits. Although a reduction in neuronal expression might be expected to underlie these deficits, hippocampal neurons mostly remain preserved. Synapses appear to be preserved within the CA1 region and no changes are apparent in the presynaptic fibre potentials from Schaffer collaterals to CA1 cells. Despite some cell loss in the subiculum and hilus of the dentate gyrus, the granule cells of the dentate gyrus and pyramidal cells of the hippocampus appear to be largely unaffected by ageing. Several other changes that underlie behavioural deficits are decreased excitatory post-synaptic potentials within the perforant pathway or input to the hippocampus, decreased amplitude of presynaptic fibres from the perforant pathway to the dentate gyrus, and reduced excitatory post-synaptic potentials to the CA1 sector of the hippocampus. It has been proposed that brain-derived neurotrophic factor (BDNF) is critical to the maintenance of hippocampal functions with age, given that disruption is associated with dysfunction, whereas exercise – which induces reversal of age-related hippocampal atrophy in older adults – is also associated with increased BDNF levels. There is also a significant reduction to neurogenesis in the dentate gyrus, one of the only regions to acquire new neurons throughout life; however, this does not appear to be associated with deficits in memory. Hippocampal place cells, responsible for selectively firing to, and encoding of, a novel location in space, do not appear to be consistently affected by ageing. Finally, in contrast to the frontal and other aspects of the temporal lobes, the hippocampus and parietal cortex, discussed following, appear to be more affected by ageing in women.

The parietal lobes

Compared with the temporal and occipital lobes, cortical grey matter decreases largely in the parietal region. The parietal lobes contain the primary somato-sensory cortex, which is associated with somatic sensations, and the secondary cortices that are closely connected to the visual, auditory, gustatory and olfactory networks. Atrophy of the somatosensory cortex may contribute to poorer balance and increased falls, or even increased reliance on visual feedback during a motor task. Specifically, older individuals exhibit impairments in sensation, strength, reaction time and vestibular function that are attributable to a loss of distal myelinated sensory fibres and receptors.

The occipital lobes

Both cross-sectional and longitudinal analyses demonstrate age-related declines in occipital activation. Even so, the occipital cortex appears to be the least affected part of the brain. The primary visual cortex stays relatively stable through old age, even given decreases in dendritic spine density and dendritic thickness, as well as changes to the electrophysiological properties of visual cortical cells (e.g. prolonged firing latency). During visual processing tasks, such as encoding faces and houses, older individuals tend to exhibit bilateral activation of the prefrontal region in response to decreased activity in visual areas, as opposed to right-hemispheric activation in younger subjects, suggesting a greater need for compensation. Ageing results in slower visual processing speed, as is demonstrated by fewer cells being recruited to encode rapidly moving bars or flickers of light; even so, no changes are observed in cortical receptive fields. Another explanation for visual deficits could be altered processing speed at the neuronal level, as previous work has demonstrated diminished myelin sheaths of axons in the fibres passing through deep layers of the visual cortex.

The hypothalamus

The hypothalamus participates in the regulation of various behavioural and physiological functions, including circadian rhythms, feeding, body temperature, blood pressure and sexual activity. The preoptic area exhibits one of the most prominent reductions, especially in males aged between 50 and 60 years old; however, cell death is more prominent in women over the age of 70, in whom only 10%–15% of cells from childhood remain. The suprachiasmatic nucleus (SCN) decreases to 59% of its original size by age 80 years. Although total cell density does not significantly change, the total number of SCN cells drops to 55% over the age of 80. Decreases in the number of neuropeptides involved in SCN regulation, such as vasoactive intestinal polypeptide and vasopressin, are also prominent in ageing, as is an overall decrease in neuronal firing. Nocturnal melatonin levels decrease during ageing, whereas daytime levels tend to increase, which may result in virtually no distinct day–night rhythm. These alterations appear to contribute to the earlier onset of sleep and wakefulness in older individuals. Other hypothalamic systems, such as oxytocin neurons in the paraventricular nucleus, vasopressin in the supraoptic nucleus, as well as the dorsomedial and ventrolateral nuclei, appear to remain intact in old age. Despite preservation of these functions, a significant increase in corticotrophin-releasing hormone in the paraventricular nucleus is seen with ageing; in turn, this is associated with age-related increases in cortisol. Finally, because of decline in the noradrenergic system, secretion of luteinising, growth and thyroid-stimulating hormones may also be altered (*see* Chapter 17, 'The endocrine system').

TABLE 15.1 Summary of the major neuroanatomical changes that occur during ageing

Lobe	Region	Deficit(s) observed during ageing
Frontal lobe	Prefrontal cortex	Working and episodic memory Sequencing, planning and organisation Abstract thinking Attention
	Primary motor cortex	Motor execution
	Basal ganglia (caudate nucleus)	Motor control and learning
Temporal	Hippocampus	Spatial and episodic memory
Parietal	Primary somatosensory cortex	Sensation Strength Reaction time Vestibular function (balance)
Occipital	Primary visual cortex	Visual processing
Hypothalamus	Preoptic area	Reproductive and sexual activity Thermoregulation
	Suprachiasmatic nucleus	Circadian rhythms

IMPACT OF AGEING ON NEUROTRANSMITTER SYSTEMS

Neuronal alterations that occur during ageing have profound effects on the transmission of various neurotransmitter systems in the brain (*see* Table 15.2). The cholinergic, serotonergic, dopaminergic and glutamatergic systems exhibit significant declines in signalling, which can impair chemical transmission within various corticocortical pathways, such as those connecting the prefrontal and superior temporal cortices.

Acetylcholine

Cholinergic neurotransmission in the human brain is regulated by the neurotransmitter acetylcholine and its synthesising enzyme choline acetyltransferase, muscarinic acetylcholine receptors (mAChRs) and nicotinic receptors, and by the catabolic enzymes acetylcholinesterase and butyrylcholinesterase. The cholinergic basal forebrain innervates several regions of the cerebral cortex, including the amygdala and the hippocampal formation, which are involved in cognition and behaviour. The basal forebrain is parcellated into four regions. The medial septal nucleus provides a cholinergic innervation to the hippocampal formation. The nucleus of the vertical limb of the diagonal band of Broca also provides the innervation to the hippocampal formation. The nucleus of the horizontal limb of the diagonal band of Broca provides innervation to the olfactory bulb. The nucleus basalis of Meynert provides the cholinergic innervation to the amygdala and the entire cortical mantle.

All cholinergic muscarinic receptor subtypes are found in the brain, albeit to different extents. M1, M2, M4 predominate in the brain. M3 and M5 also are expressed but in low abundance. M1 and M4 are important in striatal dopaminergic transmission. M1 is a post-synaptic mAChR located on the surface of cell soma and dendrites. It predominates in the cerebral cortex (mainly layers II and III, somata in layer V and VI, lightest in layer IV). It is more abundant in frontoparietal regions than the retrosplenial cingulate cortex; in the amygdala (especially in basolateral nucleus); hippocampus, where it is particularly intense in the molecular layer of dentate gyrus, striatum oriens and radiatum; stratum pyramidale (CA1 and CA2 but not CA3); striatum (diffuse); globus pallidus (transversing fibre bundles); habenula of the thalamus (medial edge); magnocellular basal forebrain; olfactory tubercle; locus coeruleus; dorsal raphe; and, to a lesser extent, in the thalamus and brainstem. M2 is an autoreceptor located pre- and post-synaptically, mainly within neuropil with little neuronal staining. It predominates in basal forebrain, certain thalamic nuclei, striatum and the brainstem, hippocampus, and, to a lesser extent, in the cerebral cortex. M4 is found in neuropil and cell soma, predominates in striatum, globus pallidus, basal forebrain, thalamus, hippocampus, and, to a lesser extent, in the cortex. M3 and M5 are expressed in the brain but at consistently low levels.

Nicotinic receptors are much more diverse and widespread throughout the brain. Even so, they appear to play an important role in the regulation of calcium. In addition to being permeable to Na^+ and K^+, nicotinic receptors are also permeable to Ca^{2+} ions, thereby altering intracellular Ca^{2+} levels by activating various downstream signalling pathways.

Cholinergic innervation of the human brain is important for attention, memory and a number of cognitive functions. For example, pharmacological blockade of mAChRs temporarily produces impairment in learning and memory that is seen in normal ageing. Loss of cholinergic neurons in the basal forebrain is observed in the ageing brain, but such loss appears to be chiefly related to disease. In normal ageing, there is a loss of cholinergic functioning caused by dendritic, synaptic and axonal degeneration. In addition, impaired intracellular signalling, neurotrophic signalling and cytoskeletal transport, as well as altered gene expression, contribute to age-associated dysfunction of the cholinergic system. Nerve growth factor (NGF) appears to be particularly important for the maintenance and protection of cholinergic neurons in the basal forebrain; furthermore, a decrease in NGF signalling, but not a reduction in NGF levels, may result in atrophied cholinergic cells. During ageing, there is a marked reduction in presynaptic cholinergic cortical boutons, specifically in large layer-V pyramidal neurons of the forebrain, which contain a dense projection of cholinergic terminals. These findings demonstrate that alterations to signalling and innervation within the cholinergic basal forebrain system appear to primarily underlie the learning and memory impairments that are observed in ageing. It has also been observed that those neurons within the basal forebrain that are deficient in calbindin are particularly vulnerable to AD pathology.

Serotonin

Declines in serotonergic levels are variable throughout the brain, however, total brain levels significantly decrease with age. Reductions to serotonin receptors $5\text{-}HT_{1A}$, $5\text{-}HT_{1B/D}$ and $5\text{-}HT_{2A}$ are found in aged frontal and occipital lobes, as well as the hippocampus; $5\text{-}HT_2$ cortical binding also declines. Changes to the integrity of the serotonergic system have implications in altered cognition, mood, circadian sleep–wake rhythms and aggression levels. In particular, deficiencies in serotonin are strongly associated with depression. An increase in monoamine oxidase, the enzyme that breaks down serotonin, may be an underlying causative factor in the development of depression later in life. The circadian clock, or SCN, has one of the densest serotonergic plexus in the brain. Impairments to this system in aged animals result in inappropriate adaptations to changing temporal environmental cues. Alterations to daily serotonin rhythms may underlie the disturbed sleep and circadian rhythms that are commonly observed in old age.

Serotonin has long been known to play a role in psychiatric diseases, such as schizophrenia, and mood disorders, such as depression, but there is also evidence demonstrating a strong association between serotonergic signalling and AD. In particular, $5\text{-}HT_{2A}$ and $5\text{-}HT_6$ receptor subtypes appear to be important in how AD arises. Not only is there a reduction in serotonin reuptake transporters but also the binding and expression of both receptor subtypes is significantly decreased in cortical pyramidal cells of AD patients. In addition, $5\text{-}HT_{2A}$ receptors have been shown to activate the secretion of amyloid precursor protein, the break down of which generates the primary component of amyloid plaques. Interestingly, the raphe nucleus, which contains a dense cluster of serotonergic neurons, is highly susceptible to the formation of neurofibrillary tangles and exhibits significant neuronal loss in patients with AD. These findings suggest that serotonin and its receptors have the potential to serve as drug targets for the therapeutic treatment of AD.

Dopamine

Dopaminergic cells steadily decline within the nigrostriatal pathway. By 60 years of age, approximately half of the neurons that are present at birth are lost within the basal ganglia, specifically in the substantia nigra, which plays an important role in movement, reward seeking and addictive behaviours. The pattern of striatal loss observed during ageing is substantially different from that seen in Parkinson's disease. Dopamine receptor D2 exhibits that greatest decrease in the substantia nigra, caudate nucleus, putamen and globus pallidus; D1 receptor levels have been shown to increase or remain the same. Significant decreases in dopamine are also visible in the hypothalamic tuberoinfundibular system, where the most marked changes are found in the medial basal hypothalamus and median eminence. Here dopamine acts as a hormone to stimulate the secretion of prolactin from the anterior pituitary gland, which begins to decrease around menopause in women.

Amino acids

The concentration of GABA in the cortex declines significantly with age. Glutamic acid decarboxylase, the enzyme that breaks down GABA, likewise declines in the primary auditory and visual cortices. Interestingly, the number of GABA binding sites appears to increase with age (or to not change at all), suggesting a significant alteration to $GABA_A$ receptors and binding affinity. Cortical GABAergic projections and interneurons are remarkably diverse in their functional role. Functional degradation to cortical neurons may result from increased GABA-mediated cortical inhibition and higher resting motor threshold. Age-related alterations to this system are associated with various sleep and psychiatric disorders.

Changes in the glutamatergic system are more complex. As with GABA, glutamate is involved in functionally diverse cortical projections, and age-related changes vary according to region. Altered glutamatergic signalling in the aged brain has been linked to changes in learning and memory, emotion and motivation, motor function, and neurodegenerative diseases. Decreased glutamate concentrations appear to be the greatest within the prefrontal cortex and hippocampus, which may be due to age-related alterations in the regulation of glutaminase, the enzyme required for the hydrolysis of glutamine to form glutamate. To a lesser extent, diminished glutamate expression has also been described in the striatum, nucleus accumbens and substantia nigra. However, contradictory findings have been demonstrated in all regions examined (e.g. increased glutamate concentrations or no change). There is also no change to the level of cortical or striatal glutamate released during ageing, but these regions have been found to exhibit reduced presynaptic glutamate uptake and affinity for glutamate transporters. Most consistently noted is the decrease in NMDA and AMPA receptor density (i.e. up to 50%) within the cortex and hippocampus.

TABLE 15.2 Summary of the effects of ageing on the major neurotransmitter systems

Neurotransmitter	Regions affected the greatest	Deficit(s) observed during ageing
Acetylcholine	Basal forebrain	Learning and memory
Serotonin	Frontal and occipital cortices	Depression and mood
	Suprachiasmatic nucleus	Circadian rhythms
	Raphe nucleus	Sleep–wake cycles
Dopamine	Basal ganglia	Movement
	Medial basal hypothalamus and Median eminence	Prolactin secretion
GABA	Primary auditory cortex	Auditory processing
	Primary visual cortex	Visual processing
Glutamate	Prefrontal cortex	Emotion, motivation, motor function
	Hippocampus	Learning and memory
	Basal ganglia	Motor control and learning

IMPACT OF CELLULAR AGE-RELATED CHANGES ON COGNITIVE FUNCTION

Ageing is marked by the accumulation of not just intracellular waste, as already described, but also intracellular amyloid plaques and extracellular neurofibrillary tangles. The standard account is that the pathology of AD is characteristically described by widespread cerebral atrophy (preferentially involving frontal and temporal – especially medial temporal and parietal – regions) with microscopically visible amyloid plaques, dystrophic neurites and neurofibrillar tangles, which have characteristic distributions; this is true, but lacks the negative control: people with such features who do not have the disease. Here, we briefly mention one of the more dramatic shifts to be made in our understanding of the relationship between normal brain ageing and dementia.

Surprisingly, it has been found that cognitive function is not affected in everyone who has evidence of enough changes in their brains (e.g. amyloid plaques and neurofibrillary tangles) to be clinically diagnosed with various types of dementia. A series of studies, especially those from community-based or special samples (e.g. the Cognitive Function and Ageing Study[3] in the United Kingdom and the Religious Orders Study[4] in the United States), is causing a major shift in the way we understand how age-related changes and disease are linked with cognition. Briefly, the question is now less about why 90% of older people with clinical dementia have amyloid plaques and neurofibrillary tangles and more about why the one-third of older adults who are cognitively normal can maintain their function in the face of many plaques and tangles. Ironically, much of this change has occurred only after a massive investment, chiefly by the pharmaceutical industry and manufacturers of imaging devices, in so-called dementia biomarkers, based largely on the more traditional understanding of an inevitable progression to dementia by the build-up of plaques, tangles and related pathologic features. Even so, the essential question that remains is why some people accumulate plaques and tangles while others do not, and, perhaps even more promisingly in the near term, why some people resist the deleterious effects of such features, while in others they are associated with dementia. This last question is commonly addressed under the rubric of understanding cognitive reserve and the related construct of brain reserve – a rich area for inquiry and debate.

Heterogeneity of human brain ageing

As we have noted, understanding about how brain ageing gives way to dementia is now thought to be considerably more complicated than simply an accumulation of plaques and tangles account. With the new understanding (or newly rediscovered – recent reviews note that autopsy studies from decades ago showed much the same thing) that not everyone with plaques and tangles has dementia, there is a need to understand why this is so. An early suggestion was that co-morbidity was critical – for example, that even a single lacunar infarct could precipitate dementia in someone with a brain at risk from plaques and tangles. Even so, as noted, several community-based autopsy series have shown that this is not viable; as one states, there was no cut-point of plaques, tangles or ischaemic changes, alone or in combination, which would satisfactorily distinguish between those with and those without dementia.

Against this background, it is worth considering again how age-related cognitive decline proceeds. Heterogeneity of disease expression in relation to neuropathological evidence of dementia-associated lesions is likely a subset of overall heterogeneity of age-related changes in cognition. It is irrefutable that cognition declines with age, but this average decline is not uniform. In some people, cognition declines a great deal whereas in others it declines just a little. There is more variability yet: it is not just a matter of rates of decline. Catastrophic change – and detectable improvement – can also occur. Displays of individual test scores over time can look every bit as chaotic as the daily stock market indices did in 2011; however, unlike in stock market fluctuation, there is a high degree of uniformity in how cognitive test scores change. Figure 15.3 shows how cognition changes across nine grades of baseline cognitive function. Cognitive function here is defined in relation to errors on the 100-point Modified Mini-Mental State (3MS) examination. Cognitive states are grouped by three errors, that is, the one in the upper left-hand corner shows the outcomes at two successive 5-year intervals for people who made no errors, one

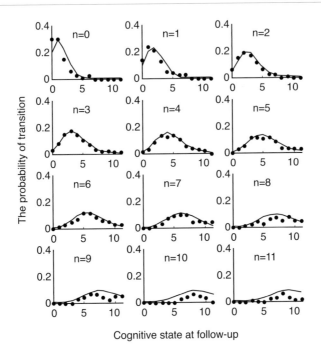

Cognitive state at follow-up

FIGURE 15.3 A novel T-Poisson model for estimating the probability of transition in cognitive status. The figure shows the probabilities of transition over a 5-year period for various baseline states, *n* from 0 to 11. The area under the curve diminishes with baseline state indicating an increase of mortality with baseline state. Mitnitski AB, Fallah N, Dean CB *et al*. A multi-state model for the analysis of changes in cognitive scores over a fixed time interval. *Stat Methods Med Res.* Epub 2011 Sep 20[5]

error or two errors at baseline. As in each panel, it shows the distribution of cognitive scores at follow-up. Consider the uppermost right-hand panel ('n = 2'), which shows cognitive test scores for people who made six to eight errors at the relevant baseline – that is, a 3MS score of 94, 93 or 92. At each of the two follow-ups, the modal score for people in the '2 state' is 3, that is, to have made 9–11 errors (a 3MS score of 91, 90 or 89). A few people improve to the 1 state and very few to the 0 state – in fact, this is the highest error level in which improvement to the 0 state (returning to a perfect or near-perfect test score) is possible. Notice also that the area under the curve decreases as the error state increases: this reflects progressive mortality as cognitive decrements increase. Finally, note that there is no sharp discontinuity between panels, even though these cognitive states cross clinical-diagnostic categories from no cognitive impairment, to mild cognitive impairment, through to mild dementia. This orderly behaviour is captured in a parsimonious model that has high fit across different time periods, in different settings and using different cognitive tests.[5] In general, these outcomes are conditional on two factors: for any individual, the chance of moving from one cognitive state at baseline to another cognitive

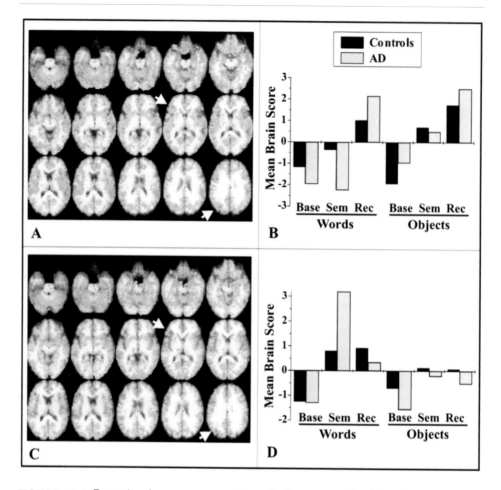

FIGURE 15.4 Example of neurocompensation. Performance of healthy older adults and patients with probable AD, on the first two latent variables (B, D) of a semantic and recognition word task. Positive scores indicate increased brain activity in regions coloured red and yellow (A, C), whereas negative scores indicate increased brain activity in regions coloured blue (A, C). Additional recruitment (bilaterally) of prefrontal areas by AD patients is associated with increased performance in semantic and episodic memory tasks. One of the reasons that progressive atrophy has become considerably more nuanced is because compensatory changes in brain function result in clinical attenuation of disease expression. However, this understanding depends on the development of new technology allowing this to be detected. Reproduced from Grady CL, McIntosh AR, Beig S *et al.* Evidence from functional neuroimaging of a compensatory prefrontal network in Alzheimer's disease. *J Neurosci.* 2003; **23**(3): 986–93[6]

state at follow-up depends on not only their own cognitive state (and the factors associated with that state) but also on their environment.

The fact that some people's cognitive function can change more slowly than does others, has excited a lot of interest in ways to manipulate factors to promote healthy brain ageing. At present, control of vascular risk factors seems reasonable and a long list of potential manoeuvres (i.e. fish oils, resveratrol, rapamycin) needs to be evaluated. The best evidence supports an important role for physical activity.

Overall, there appears to be a great deal of cognitive heterogeneity between individuals. It probably reflects the dynamic changes that occur in brain function, of which cognition is a high-order manifestation. The dynamic nature of cognitive change with age appears to point towards underlying processes in which deficits arise from insults that are initially repaired but accumulate as repair mechanisms fail. Even as deficits accumulate, they can be resisted, either by a large reserve or compensatory mechanisms (*see* Figure 15.4). The ability to first resist insults and then deficits seems highest in certain people with as yet not well-defined genetic profiles; in those who are more highly educated, have favourable early life circumstances, exercise, engage in cognitively stimulating occupations and/or leisure activities; and who lead lives with a high level of social engagement and have an otherwise high satisfaction with life.

CONCLUSION

Understanding brain ageing is challenging and here approached only at a necessarily incomplete level. We have emphasised that, despite its privileged status, the brain ages much like other organs, being especially susceptible to a metabolic triad: the accumulation of ROS, the effect of this on mitochondrial function and the apparent essential role of calcium homeostasis in neuron dysfunction and death. Just as damage is ubiquitous, so too are clearance and repair processes. Post-mitotic neurons depend on repair processes and not on cellular regeneration, so dysfunction of clearance and repair processes is associated with accelerated damage; likewise, many repair processes induce compensatory effects, which themselves can eventually cause damage.

We close by considering that despite the picture of average decline, the picture of brain ageing is not one of doom and gloom, not only because some people show only very slow changes. Consider that as neurocognitive speed robustly declines with ageing, the functional magnetic resonance imaging correlate of this is that more brain areas are recruited into standard tasks. While this may be viewed simply as inefficiency (according to calculation of number of voxels per task), there is another view. The traditional view of wisdom is not one of raw 'cleverness' and speed of processing; instead, we expect a wise person to take more factors into account. If the price of judiciousness is one of speed, it is a price many older adults would be willing to pay.

REFERENCES

1   Yen WL, Klionsky DJ. How to live long and prosper: autophagy, mitochondria, and aging. *Physiology (Bethesda)*. 2008; **23**: 248–62.

2   Erickson KI, Voss MW, Prakash RS *et al.* Exercise training increases size of hippocampus and improves memory. *Proc Natl Acad Sci U S A.* 2011; **108**(7): 3017–22.

3   Neuropathology Group. Medical Research Council Cognitive Function and Aging Study. Pathological correlates of late-onset dementia in a multicentre, community-based population in England and Wales. Neuropathology Group of the Medical Research Council Cognitive Function and Ageing Study (MRC CFAS). *Lancet.* 2001; **357**(9251): 169–75.

4   Negash S, Bennett DA, Wilson RS *et al.* Cognition and neuropathology in aging: multidimensional perspectives from the Rush Religious Orders Study and Rush Memory and Aging Project. *Curr Alzheimer Res.* 2011; **8**(4): 336–40.

5   Mitnitski AB, Fallah N, Dean CB *et al.* A multi-state model for the analysis of changes in cognitive scores over a fixed time interval. *Stat Methods Med Res.* Epub 2011 Sep 20.

6   Grady CL, McIntosh AR, Beig S *et al.* Evidence from functional neuroimaging of a compensatory prefrontal network in Alzheimer's disease. *J Neurosci.* 2003; **23**(3): 986–93.

FURTHER READING

Darvesh S, Hopkins DA, Geula C. Neurobiology of butyrylcholinesterase. *Nat Rev Neurosci.* 2003; **4**(2): 131–8.

Gottlieb RA, Carreira RS. Autophagy in health and disease. 5. Mitophagy as a way of life. *Am J Physiol Cell Physiol.* 2010; **299**(2): C203–10.

Schliebs R, Arendt T. The cholinergic system in aging and neuronal degeneration. *Behav Brain Res.* 2011; **221**(2): 555–63.

White L. Brain lesions at autopsy in older Japanese-American men as related to cognitive impairment and dementia in the final years of life: a summary report from the Honolulu-Asia Aging Study. *J Alzheimers Dis.* 2009; **18**(3): 713–25.

Wolkowitz OM, Reus VI, Mellon SH. Of sound mind and body: depression, disease, and accelerated aging. *Dialogues Clin Neurosci.* 2011; **13**(1): 25–39.

Zeevi N, Pachter J, McCullough LD *et al.* The blood-brain barrier: geriatric relevance of a critical brain-body interface. *J Am Geriatr Soc.* 2010; **58**(9): 1749–57.

Acknowledgements

RS is sponsored by the Canadian Institutes of Health Research (CIHR) and Sir Izaak Walton Killam Postdoctoral Fellowships (Dept. Psychiatry).

KR is supported by the Dalhousie Medical Research Foundation as the Kathryn Allen Weldon Professor of Alzheimer Research.

All authors gratefully acknowledge the support of the CIHR, the Alzheimer's Society of Canada, the Dalhousie Medical Research Foundation and the Fountain Innovation Fund of the QEII Health Sciences Foundation.

They further appreciate the assistance of Andrew Reid, Technician of the Maritime Brain Tissue Bank in the Department Anatomy and Neurobiology, for the creation of the neuroanatomical and histochemical figures.

QUESTIONS: BRAIN

1 Each of the following is observed in usual human ageing, except:
   A cognitive processing speed slows
   B gait speed slows
   C more errors are made in divided attention tasks
   D more time is spent sleeping, especially during the day
   E motor skill acquisition takes longer.

Answer: D

Comment: *Sleep decreases and daytime drowsiness is associated with an increased mortality risk.*

2 Regarding LTP, which one of the following statements is false?
   A compared with younger controls, in the aged brain, LTP decays more rapidly
   B compared with younger controls, in the aged brain, LTP takes significantly longer to develop
   C it is a form of neuroplasticity
   D older synapses appear to be less capable of sustaining the depolarisation required to activate downstream cascades involved in LTP
   E with ageing, there is a shift from voltage-gated Ca^{2+}-channel activation to NMDA-receptor Ca^{2+} influx.

Answer: E

Comment: *With ageing, the shift is from primary NMDA-receptor activation to voltage-gated Ca^{2+} channel. This parallels impaired new learning capability.*

3 Characteristic features of neuroanatomical changes with normal ageing include all of the following, except:
   A decrease in hippocampal volume
   B drop-out of brainstem nuclei
   C increase in ventricular volume
   D loss of synaptic spines, synapses and myelinated axons, compared with preservation of the number of neurons
   E relative sparing of the volume of the occipital cortex.

Answer: B

Comment: *Brainstem nuclei appear to be well preserved in old age.*

4 Limitations in studying normal brain ageing changes include all of the following, except:

  A cohort effects may mimic age-related changes
  B limited control for the effects of disease in clinic-based studies
  C more studies reporting cross-sectional data than longitudinal data
  D no prospective community-based autopsy studies
  E the average decline in cognitive function is non-linear and accelerates with age.

Answer: D

Comment: *Prospective community-based autopsy studies have changed views originally generated by clinic-based studies.*

5 Age-related reductions in serotonin levels are associated with decrements in each of the following, except:

  A circadian sleep–wake rhythms
  B cognition
  C initiative
  D mood
  E neuron numbers.

Answer: E

Comment: *Neuron numbers do not decline with age.*

CHAPTER 16

Balance and ageing

DAINA L STURNIEKS, JASMINE MENANT
AND STEPHEN R LORD

INTRODUCTION

Good balance is an imperative skill for daily life. It requires the complex integration of sensory information regarding the position of the body relative to the surroundings and the ability to generate appropriate motor responses to control body movement. Vision, vestibular sense, proprioception, muscular strength and neuromuscular coordination are involved in balance control, in addition to central processes, such as visual-spatial processing and attention. With increased age, there is a progressive loss of function of these systems, which can contribute to balance deficits. For example, in women, the amount of postural sway while standing has been shown to almost double from young (age 20–39 years) to older adulthood (age 80–84 years). Poor performance in balance and other sensorimotor measures are associated with impairments in tasks of mobility, including walking, stair climbing and standing from a seated position. Consequently, older adults with poorer balance performance have reduced mobility and independence compared with those with better balance. Importantly, balance disorders represent a growing public health concern, due to their association with falls and fall-related injuries, particularly in regions of the world with growing ageing or aged populations.

To plan and coordinate movement to maintain balance, postural control relies on internal sensory representation of the body in space. Continuous information from multiple sensory systems allows a moment-to-moment update of the postural state and the environment for effective navigation. A degree of redundancy exists in the sensory information necessary to control balance, particularly in unchallenging circumstances. However, with increased age, that redundancy is lost and balance disorders or instability can result from sensory, motor or central processing system impairments. Such impairments may be the result of a specific pathology, accelerated loss of function due to inactivity or the general progressive loss of function due to normal ageing impinging on one or more of these systems. This combination of factors leads to increased variability in functioning across all sensorimotor and balance systems in older people, such that some older people perform no worse than younger adults in balance and mobility tests whereas others display marked impairment. This chapter will examine the physiological systems associated with balance and discuss typical age-related changes in each of these and the impact of these on stability.

PERIPHERAL SENSATION

Sensations regarding touch, position and movement come from the skin, muscles and joints of the body. These signals provide a potent source of information that is used to control balance. In fact, input from the lower limbs is arguably the most important contributor to standing balance, as the proprioceptive threshold is lower than visual and vestibular thresholds controlling postural sway. Furthermore, during walking, joint and muscle mechanoreceptors provide information to help coordinate each step and achieve optimal foot placement. As such, age-related loss of peripheral sensation is an important contributor to reduced balance performance in older people. Loss of peripheral sensation can also result from a wide range of age-related conditions such as diabetes mellitus and arthritis. The role of peripheral sensation in balance control is indicated by the significant association between increased postural sway and poor tactile sensitivity, vibration sense and proprioception. Quantitatively assessed impairments in tactile sensitivity at the ankle, vibration sense at the knee and knee joint position sense, have also been identified as significant and independent risk factors for falls in older people.

Proprioception

Receptors in muscles, tendons and joints provide information on the position, movements and the sense of effort of moving the body and its segments. These senses are collectively known as 'proprioception'. Cutaneous receptors, discussed in the next section, are also likely to contribute to movement sense.

The contraction and relaxation of muscle triggers muscles spindles. These receptors sit within muscle fibres and respond to changes in length. Reduced muscle spindle sensitivity has been noted with increased age. Age-related morphological changes such as increased capsular thickness, decreased number of intrafusal fibres, reduced spindle diameter and altered (less spiral) shape of the primary endings of muscle spindles may contribute to reduced sensitivity. It is unclear what level and region of anatomical loss in muscle spindles is associated with impaired proprioception and balance dysfunction.

Located at the muscle–tendon interface are receptors known as 'Golgi tendon organs', which respond to changes in muscle tension. These receptors are extremely sensitive to movement and their signals are used to adjust the level of contraction in a muscle. Mechanoreceptors existing in and around joints respond to distortion of the joint capsule and ligaments also contribute proprioceptive information. However, it is believed that these receptors contribute mostly to end-of-range position and movement detection. Little information exists regarding age-related changes in Golgi tendon organs and joint mechanoreceptors.

Several studies have shown proprioceptive acuity to be significantly poorer in older populations, across different joints of the body, than in younger populations. For static position sense at the ankle, age-related decreases of about 3 degrees have been reported. However, less prominent age-related insensitivity has been found for dynamic position or movement sense, indicating that the use of velocity information is less affected by ageing. There is some suggestion that spindle function is preserved, relative to other receptors that contribute to proprioception. Furthermore, the age-related difference in proprioceptive acuity is reduced in tests that involve weight bearing, when proprioception is generally more accurate.

Poorer proprioception has been shown to be significantly associated with increased postural sway in older people and is a risk factor for falls in this group. For example, performance in tests of joint position sense have been found to be 30%–60% poorer in older people who experienced multiple future falls than in older non-fallers.

Touch sense

Tactile information from body parts in contact with an external surface (particularly the soles of the feet on the ground) provides additional sensory information to assist in standing balance control. Mechanoreceptors in the skin that are sensitive to vibration and pressure provide us with our sense of touch. These receptors include the fast-adapting Meissner's and Pacinian corpuscles and the slowly adapting Merkel discs and Ruffini cylinders. These receptors, together with free nerve endings and hair cells, provide feedback about the environment and can supplement joint position sense and movement detection. Of the fast-adapting receptors, Meissner's corpuscles are located close to the skin surface and respond to physical deformation upon touch and reformation following the removal of the stimulus. Compared with Meissner's corpuscles, Pacinian corpuscles are located deeper, are larger and fewer in number, they provide feelings of deep pressure and are particularly sensitive to vibratory stimuli. Meissner's and Pacinian corpuscles, in particular, show considerable age-related reductions in number and morphological changes. For example, by age 60 years, the average number of Meissner's corpuscles under the skin of the fingertips reduces by half and this is reflected by a loss of touch sensitivity. It has also been found that tactile sensitivity is reduced to a greater extent in the lower limbs than in the upper limbs. Loss of Pacinian corpuscles with age corresponds with reduced vibration sense, which is poorer in the lower limbs than in the upper limbs at all ages and shows a greater age-related decline. Reduced vibration sense at the ankle has been estimated to affect 30%–50% of older people who are free of neurologic disease. Morphological changes in mechanoreceptors are also likely to contribute to loss of touch acuity. Furthermore, the function of these cutaneous receptors is affected by age-related changes in skin, such as thinning of the epidermis and reduced levels of collagen and elastin. The consequences of reduced touch sensation are important for balance in old age. Light touch (for example, resting a finger on a table without utilising mechanical support) can reduce postural sway by about 20%, with greater reductions in conditions that deprive other sensory information, suggesting that the loss of skin receptor acuity can greatly affect balance control, particularly in older people.

VISION

Visual information allows the central nervous system to create a spatial map to detect hazards, judge speed and direction of moving objects and assess spatial relationships to assist in efficient navigation through the environment. Vision also makes an important contribution to balance by continually updating the nervous system on the position of the body segments in relation to each other and the environment, demonstrated by a recorded 20% to 70% increase in postural sway when people stand with their eyes closed. Older adults, particularly those at risk of falls, tend to sway more in response to large-field oscillating visual-motion stimuli than younger or healthy older adults. In addition, older adults, particularly those who are fall-prone, generally take longer to adapt to the conflict between (moving) visual and (static) proprioceptive, somatosensory and vestibular sensory cues during 'moving room' experimental paradigms, than younger or healthy older adults. Such postural responses reflect a preferential weighting of visual information for the control of posture in older adults, particularly those who are prone to falling.

Aside from visual changes resulting from ocular diseases, increased crystalline lens thickness (estimated to be 28% thicker at 70 years than it is at 20) and senile miosis (when the pupil becomes smaller at all levels of illumination) cause an estimated 67% reduction in the amount of light reaching the retina between the ages of 20 and 60 years. Additional age-related physiological changes in the eye include, but are not limited to: reduced flexibility of the lens within the lens capsule, resulting in a decrease in accommodation amplitude, down to zero by the time people are in their 60s; corneal changes, whereby the horizontal meridian of the cornea becomes steeper leading to an increase in against-the-rule astigmatism; decreased depth of the anterior chamber of the eye; and vitreous humour liquefaction and shrinkage. Retinal and neural connection changes occurring with increasing age, such as disorientation and reduction in the number of photoreceptors in the macular zone (central retina) from age 40 years and over, are reflected in a decline in visual functions.

Visual acuity is a common clinical assessment of vision that measures the ability to see fine detail. While uncorrected distance visual acuity has been shown to decline linearly from age 30 to 80 years, near visual acuity appears to decline sharply around the fourth and fifth decades and more slowly in latter years. Contrast sensitivity, the ability to detect edges under low contrast conditions, and depth perception, the ability to judge distances accurately and perceive spatial relationships, both decline in old age. Poor edge-contrast sensitivity may predispose older people to tripping over obstacles within the home and outdoor hazards such as steps, kerbs and pavement cracks, while poor depth perception can impair one's ability to negotiate and avoid obstacles and hazards in the environment. Other visual deficits associated with age and age-related ocular diseases relevant to balance control and navigation include reduction in the size of the visual field, reduced absolute level of dark adaptation, increased difficulty recovering from glare, changes in the refractive error from increased against-the-rule astigmatism and decreased dynamic visual acuity (e.g. visual acuity with head movement while walking).

Several studies involving large samples of participants have shown that poor performances in tests of distance contrast sensitivity and depth perception are independent predictors of increased postural sway in older people. This suggests that the accurate perception of visual stimuli and depth play important roles in providing a visual reference frame for the stabilisation of the body relative to its surroundings. In addition, more so than visual acuity, poor edge-contrast sensitivity, depth perception and visual field loss appear to be important visual risk factors for falls, as determined by prospective fall risk-factor studies in older people.

Finally, longitudinal studies have shown that cataracts – an increased opacity of the lens, leading to cloudy vision – is the most common visual pathology in old age (in 16% of people aged over 65 years), followed by retinal pathologies including macular degeneration (in 9% of older people aged over 65 years), and glaucoma, characterised by pathological changes in the optic disc from raised intraocular pressure (in 3% of older people aged over 65 years). The prevalence of these visual pathologies increases with older age. Furthermore, evidence from prospective and retrospective fall studies indicates that older people suffering from these ocular diseases are at higher risk of falling than their healthy counterparts.

VESTIBULAR FUNCTION

The three orthogonal semicircular canals of the vestibular system detect head angular acceleration, while its two otolith organs, the utricle and the saccule, are sensitive to changes in head linear acceleration and gravity-related tilt. The CNS uses this head position and motion information to generate corrective responses to maintain balance via a range of reflexes. The vestibulospinal reflexes help maintain upright stance and a stable head by triggering muscle activity in the neck, trunk and extremities. The vestibulocollic and cervicocollic reflexes stabilise the head in the vertical position by triggering neck muscle activity. The vestibulo-ocular reflex (VOR) helps to maintain visual fixation during head movements by generating compensatory short latency eye rotations.

Animal and human studies have reported anatomical and morphological changes with age in the vestibular apparatus, including deterioration of calcium carbonate crystals (otoconia) located in the otolith organs, and a decrease in hair cell numbers and vestibular neuron ganglions. Together with age-related loss of neurons and dendritic synapses in the CNS, modifications in neurotransmitter systems and regional changes in cerebral blood flow are likely to contribute to vestibular impairment. Furthermore, common direct trauma, infection, calcium carbonate deposition in the semicircular canals, drug toxicity, migraine, cerebellar ataxia and autoimmune disease can significantly add to the mentioned age-related declines in vestibular function.

A diminution of the VOR with increasing age has been well documented in both cross-sectional and longitudinal studies, with reported reductions in VOR gain, decreased ability to enhance and suppress the VOR and shorter VOR time constants. Vestibulospinal reflexes also show age-related changes. A cross-sectional investigation of responses to galvanic vestibular stimulation in 70 adults aged 24–85 years old showed decreased amplitude and delayed onset of short latency soleus muscle responses with increasing age. Moreover, there was an absence of short latency reflexes in more than a third of participants aged over 60 years.

Vestibular dysfunction in older adults might also be reflected in a decreased ability to cope with sensory conflicts. For example, some research has shown that, despite availability of visual information, increasing galvanic vestibular stimulation intensity applied during goal-directed walking resulted in a significantly greater deviation in path trajectory in older participants than in younger ones. This suggests that older adults have a reduced ability to discount vestibular input compared with younger adults.

Research studies have examined the relationship between specific vestibular function tests and balance and gait assessments in older people with varied conclusions. In one study, small but significant longitudinal changes in VOR, visual-VOR and optokinetic VOR function were not associated with symptoms or signs of poor balance in 57 healthy older adults aged over 75 years over a 5-year period. In contrast, another study showed significant correlations between reduced ocular counter-roll in response to head tilt with age and increased postural sway on firm and unstable support surfaces in a cross-sectional analysis of 151 adults aged 21–93 years. Similarly, in a longitudinal investigation of 53 adults aged 75 years and older, decrements in optokinetic nystagmus, visual-VOR and VOR were associated with poorer performance on a clinical assessment of gait and balance (Tinetti score). The ability to maintain objects in focus while undertaking active head movements also appears compromised in older people with vestibular hypofunction; poorer scores in a gaze stability test were found to be associated with impaired gait in 12 older people with unilateral and bilateral vestibular impairment, compared with 20 healthy older adults.

The evidence for vestibular impairment as an important cause of falls remains weak. The findings of most studies to date should be interpreted with caution given the small sample sizes used and the retrospective nature of the study designs. The lack of a clear relationship between vestibular function loss and falls may be due to sensory reweighting, whereby proprioceptive and visual information is used to compensate for vestibular deficits. It could also be that older people with vestibular impairments take appropriate precautions so as to lessen their fall risk exposure. Finally, it is possible that many of the tests used to assess vestibular function are not sufficiently sensitive to identify subtle to moderate vestibular function loss, hence fail to identify people at increased fall risk.

MUSCULAR STRENGTH

Muscle mass begins to diminish from early adulthood, although relatively slowly until the sixth decade. One study has found an average 40% loss of the number of fibres in a quadriceps group muscle from the second to the eighth decade. There appears to be a preferential atrophy of fast-twitch fibres with age and reduced re-innervation capacity of fast-twitch fibres in older muscle.

Muscular strength is maintained reasonably well until about the fifth decade, after which accelerated losses occur. Compared with adults aged in their 20s, hand-grip strength is reduced by 16% in men and 20% in women aged in their 60s, while leg strength is reduced by 28% in men and 38% in women. Muscle strength losses are even more dramatic after the age of 70 years. The ability to coordinate and produce muscle force quickly (muscle power) is particularly impaired in older people. Leg power has been shown to deteriorate twice as fast (3.5% per year) as leg strength (1%–2% per year) in people aged over 65 years.

Reduced lower-limb strength and power has serious balance and mobility implications for older people. Lower-limb muscle weakness contributes to poor balance, abnormal gait patterns and reduced general mobility. Muscle weakness can restrict physical functioning, limiting activities of daily living and independence. For example, reduced strength is reflected in a difficulty in rising from a chair, and the inability to undertake this task is associated with disability, falls and fractures in older people. Furthermore, a reduced capacity for rapid force generation limits the ability to respond quickly to a loss of balance and increases the risk of falling. Indeed, reduced hip, knee and ankle strength have all been found to correlate with an increased risk of falls. Improvements in lower-limb strength, following exercise, correspond with improvements in balance performance and reduced fall risk.

REACTION TIME

'Reaction time' refers to the speed at which a person can respond when presented with a given stimulus. For movement, reaction time involves the receiving and processing of sensory information and planning and execution of motor tasks. The speed and accuracy of movement are important for maintaining balance, particularly when exposed to an unexpected postural challenge.

Simple reaction time slows 25% from the second to the sixth decade, with progressive marked slowing beyond age 60. Older adults have been shown to be slower in both the decision and movement time components of reaction time tasks than younger people, and these age-related differences are more substantial for more complicated tasks (requiring greater cognitive processing) and movements of the whole body.

Slower reaction times in older adults may be due a range of age-related changes across multiple organs and systems. Within the nervous system, age-related loss of neurons and neuronal function can slow and/or reduce the frequency of signals to and from effector organs. Impaired sensory acuity and poor integration of sensory information can contribute to slower reaction time in older adults. Slowed muscle latencies and increased difficulty in producing and coordinating muscle force may also contribute to slowed response. Furthermore, older adults prefer to use more conservative strategies in moving, preferring to sacrifice speed for accuracy.

Increased simple reaction time is an independent risk factor for falls in populations of older people. Multiple fallers have approximately 40% slower simple reaction times compared with non-fallers. Epidemiological studies have shown reaction time to be an independent risk factor for falls and one of five physiological measures (the others being balance, strength, proprioception and vision) that together predict future multiple fallers with good accuracy.

CENTRAL PROCESSING AND COGNITION

In addition to changes in the individual sensory systems already described, general peripheral neuronal changes and CNS changes may affect sensory acuity and motor responses required for balance control. Changes in central processing mechanisms may impair the ability to integrate sensory information and reduce the ability to compensate for unreliable or discordant sensory input.

There is considerable evidence that balance control requires attentional resources, and an individual's balance may be influenced by his or her information-processing ability when performing two or more tasks simultaneously. Dual-task experiments involving simultaneous balance and cognitive tasks have shown a greater cost of dual tasks in older persons than in younger, suggesting that there is an increase in the cognitive resources required for postural control with age. Table 16.1 summarises the changes in balance control associated with ageing.

TABLE 16.1 Summary of age-related changes in the physiological systems associated with balance control

System/Sense	Physiological changes	Functional changes
Peripheral sensation	Muscle spindles show increased capsular thickness, decreased number of intrafusal fibres, reduced spindle diameter and change in shape of primary endings	Poorer proprioception: reduced sensitivity to static joint position sense and movement detection sense
	Unknown changes to Golgi tendon organs and joint mechanoreceptors	Loss of touch sensitivity, especially in lower limbs
	Reduced number of and morphological changes to skin mechanoreceptors (Meissner's and Pacinian corpuscles)	Reduced vibration sense, especially in lower limbs
	Additional effect of epidermis thinning and reduced levels of collagen and elastin in the skin	
Vision	Increased lens thickness	Reduction in:
	Decreased pupil size	• static and dynamic visual acuity
	Reduced flexibility of the lens	• contrast sensitivity
	Corneal changes	• depth perception
	Decreased depth of the anterior chamber of the eye	• visual field size
	Liquefaction and shrinkage of the vitreous humour	Poor dark and glare adaptation
	Disorientation and reduction in number of photoreceptors in the macular zone	Changes in refractive error
Vestibular function	Deterioration of calcium carbonate crystals of otolith organs	Poorer VOR (loss of gaze stability)
	Reduced number of hair cells and vestibular neuron ganglions	Altered vestibulospinal reflexes
Muscular strength	Reduced number of muscle fibres	Reduced muscle strength
	Preferential loss and reduced re-innervation capacity of fast-twitch fibres	Reduced muscle power (rapid force generation)

(continued)

System/Sense	Physiological changes	Functional changes
Central processing	Loss of neurons Poorer signals to and from the CNS	Decline in sensory integration Increased reaction time Increase in the cognitive load of balance control

EXERCISE IMPROVES BALANCE IN OLDER PEOPLE

It appears that older individuals adapt to resistive and endurance exercise training in a similar fashion to younger people. Cross-sectional studies have found that older people who actively engaged in exercise performed better in a range of sensorimotor function tests, including in terms of reaction time, strength, flexibility and balance, than matched groups of older non-exercisers. Furthermore, randomised controlled trials have now shown conclusively that exercise can improve performance in these sensorimotor parameters and prevent falls.

CONCLUSION

Balance disorders are common in older people and contribute to increased risk of falls. Age-related changes in neurological and muscular systems can lead to balance disorders via deficits in proprioception, vision, vestibular sense and motor control. Functionally, balance disorders affect activities of standing, leaning, stepping, walking, external perturbation responses and general mobility. However, there is good evidence that appropriate exercise can reverse age-related changes to improve balance and reduce falls in older people.

FURTHER READING

Halmagyi GM, Baloh R. Overview of common syndromes of vestibular disease. In: Baloh R, Halmagyi GM, editors. *Disorders of the Vestibular System*. New York: Oxford University Press; 1996. pp. 291–9.

Lord SR, Smith ST, Menant JC. Vision and falls in older people: risk factors and intervention strategies. *Clin Geriatr Med*. 2010; **26**(4): 569–81.

Lord SR, Ward JA. Age-associated differences in sensori-motor function and balance in community dwelling women. *Age Ageing*. 1994; **23**(6): 452–60.

Lord SR, Sherrington C, Menz H *et al*. *Falls in Older People: risk factors and strategies for prevention*. 2nd ed. Cambridge: Cambridge University Press; 2007.

Welford AT. Motor performance. In: Birren JE, Schiae KW, editors. *Handbook of the Psychology of Aging*. New York: Van Nostrand Reinhold Company; 1977.

QUESTIONS: BALANCE

1 Impairment in which five sensorimotor and balance systems are independent risk factors for falls in older people?

A vestibular function, lower-limb proprioception, muscle power, reaction time and postural sway

B vision, hearing, vestibular function, muscle strength and postural sway

C vision, lower-limb proprioception, nerve conduction time, lower-limb muscle strength and postural sway

D vision, lower-limb proprioception, reaction time, lower-limb muscle strength and postural sway

E vision, tactile sensitivity, vestibular function, reaction time and postural sway.

Answer: D

2 Which one of the following statements is incorrect?

A compared with younger people, variability in sensorimotor function is decreased in older people

B sensorimotor function declines with age, even in the absence of documented disease

C the effects of disease processes such as stroke and arthritis on sensorimotor function can be greater than the effects of ageing

D underlying medical conditions cannot fully account for age-related deficits in sensorimotor function

E with increased age, sensorimotor function declines in a non-linear (exponential) manner, accompanied by an increase in variability.

Answer: A

3 By the age of 60 years, hand-grip and lower-limb muscular strength decreases by:

A <5%

B ~10% and ~15%, respectively

C ~20% and ~30%, respectively

D ~50% and ~60%, respectively

E ~70% and ~80%, respectively.

Answer: C

4 Peripheral sensation contributes to balance control via signals from:

A baroreceptors, mechanoreceptors and nociceptors

B cutaneous receptors, muscle spindles and the vestibular system

C Golgi tendon organs, retina, Merkel discs and Ruffini cylinders

D otolith organs and semicircular canals

E receptors in the skin, muscles and joints of the body.

Answer: E

5 When the eyes are closed, compared with open, the amount of postural sway during standing changes in the following way:

A there is a 10% to 15% increase

B there is a 20% to 70% increase

C there is a 20% to 70% reduction

D there is a 50% reduction

E the amount of postural sway remains similar.

Answer: B

CHAPTER 17

The endocrine system

KO LEE

INTRODUCTION

The ageing process has been described as the gradual degenerative changes that occur in the body in the absence of disease. With ageing, the endocrine system is not spared and there is a decline in function of many of the endocrine glands. Thus, the prevalence of endocrine system disorders increases during normal ageing. However, the endocrine system is highly regulated, with precise feedback loops at multiple levels and, with ageing, there is a decline in the degree and speed of responsiveness in these feedback systems. Therefore, the gradual decline with ageing in the specific mechanisms of regulation and feedback of hormonal secretion may be more important in their effects. The endocrine system can also be affected by any dysregulation or decline in function in the brain or the autonomic nervous system, as this disrupts the close coordination of function between these two systems. As ageing is normally accompanied by an increase in disease and medications (which are sometimes given to prevent disease), the study of the changes in the endocrine system relating to 'normal ageing' is difficult.

This chapter will concentrate on some of the main changes associated with ageing that affect clinical disease of the classical endocrine system, and discuss some of the recent debates on whether therapy with endocrine hormones will prevent, retard, reduce or reverse the degenerative changes associated with the ageing process.

Osteoporosis is discussed in Chapter 13, 'The musculoskeletal system: bone'.

GENERAL OVERVIEW: THE COMPLEX INTERACTION BETWEEN THE AGEING OF OTHER BODY SYSTEMS AND ENDOCRINE FUNCTION

The regulation of the internal milieu of the body and its response to internal and external changes is largely mediated by the endocrine and nervous systems. These two major systems work together, with the endocrine system primarily involved in the changes and responses that are less rapid, more sustained and more persistent. An example of the coordination between the nervous and endocrine systems is the adrenal medullary secretion of catecholamines in response to stress. The hypothalamus-pituitary axis, the other main neurological endocrine interphase, regulates many of the better-known endocrine glands. In contrast, the many changes in behaviour and body composition that occur at puberty, and in pregnancy and the menopause in women, are examples of the complex sustained alterations that are regulated primarily by the endocrine system. The secretion of hormones by the endocrine cells or glands is tightly regulated by multiple interacting factors and there is usually feedback from the end-effect achieved to decrease or stop the secretion. There is often a circadian rhythm, and other rhythms (monthly, as in the menstrual cycle, and annual seasonal rhythms) may be present. Recent studies have demonstrated that there may also be important localised paracrine and autocrine regulatory effects within the endocrine glands. An example is the complex group of diverse cells within the pancreatic islets where the regulation of glucagon secretion is thought to be through a localised paracrine somatostatin effect. These have been more difficult to study experimentally but are increasingly thought to be of importance in interactions with the nervous system and other major body systems. Therefore, when disorders or disease occur in this beautifully coordinated and interactive system, the effects are widespread and complicated.

Most endocrine tissues are located in the classical endocrine glands and Table 17.1 summarises the different endocrine hormones and some of the effects of ageing. The unique feature of ageing in the endocrine system is the 'timed' changes during the female menopause in which involution and degeneration of the ovaries occur with normal ageing in the absence of disease.

TABLE 17.1 Major endocrine hormones and changes with ageing

Hormone	Cell or tissue	Endocrine gland/ organ	Change with ageing
Adrenocorticotrophic hormone	Corticotrophs	Anterior pituitary gland	Gradual increase
Growth hormone	Somatotrophs		Gradual decrease
Prolactin	Lactotrophs		Unchanged or slight increase

Hormone	Cell or tissue	Endocrine gland/ organ	Change with ageing
Thyroid-stimulating hormone	Thyrotrophs		Decrease
Follicle-stimulating hormone/Luteinising hormone	Gonadotrophs		Abrupt menopause in women
			Gradual decrease in men
Arginine vasopressin	Hypothalamic neurones	Posterior pituitary gland	Decline in responsiveness
Oxytocin	Hypothalamic neurones		Unknown
Thyroxine, triiodothyronine	Thyroid follicle cells	Thyroid gland	Decrease
Calcitonin	Parafollicular (C) cells		Unknown
Parathyroid hormone	Parathyroid chief cells	Parathyroid glands	Increase
Insulin	Beta-cells	Pancreatic islets	Decrease
Glucagon	Alpha-cells		Uncertain
Somatostatin	Delta-cells		Uncertain
IGF-1	Hepatocytes	Liver	Gradual decrease
Gastrin	G cells	Stomach (and duodenum)	Decrease
Ghrelin	Ghrelin cells (P/D1 granules)	Stomach	Uncertain, possible decrease
Glucagon-like peptide-1	L cells	Ileum	Uncertain, possible decrease
Cortisol (hydrocortisone)	Zona fasciculata cells	Adrenal cortex	Increase
Aldosterone	Zona glomerulosa cells		Increase
Dehydroepiandrosterone, androstenedione	Zona reticularis cells		Decrease
Epinephrine, norepinephrine	Chromaffin cells	Adrenal medulla	Increase
Testosterone	Leydig cells	Testes	Gradual decrease
Oestrogens	Theca and granulosa cells	Ovaries	Abrupt, 'timed' decrease
Progesterone	Corpus luteum		Abrupt, 'timed' decrease

MOLECULAR AND CELLULAR CHANGES

Cellular function has been observed to decline in most cells throughout the body with increasing age. While the potential in cell replacement with circulating stem cells and locally regenerating progenitor cells has been observed even in the very old (regenerating beta-cells in the pancreas have been demonstrated at an age of 95 years), the process of wound healing and cellular damage repair is significantly slower with increasing age. As in other organs, the number of normally functioning cells within each endocrine organ decreases, and there is a decline in function of the entire gland. This has been observed in postmortem studies where several endocrine glands decrease in weight and develop a fibrotic appearance with amyloid-like deposits within the gland accompanied by vascular changes (this is apart from the obvious atrophic changes in the ovaries that occur after the menopause).

At the individual cell level, there is telomere shortening at the chromosomal ends and increase in DNA mutations at each mitotic division. In addition, there is also a decline in the capacity for protein synthesis and secretion, and in the capacity of the cellular response to various signals. This has been attributed in part to a decline in cell receptor numbers and function, of both the membrane-bound receptors and the intracellular nuclear receptors. The decline in the number of storage granules containing the hormones and in the secretion rate of the hormones has also been thought to be responsible for the decrease in some hormone secretions with normal ageing. In addition, this affects the paracrine regulatory functions of hormone secretion.

Normal cellular function in non-endocrine cells is dependent on or significantly influenced by the presence or ambient levels of several hormones. The effects of thyroid hormone are well known in the regulation of 'normal' cellular metabolism. Other hormones that also have important general metabolic regulatory effects include the hormones in the growth hormone (GH)–IGF-1 axis, the glucocorticoid hormones and the sex steroid hormones. All of these hormones have important effects on many tissues at the cellular level, and may also interact to have synergistic or other effects. Deficiency in the thyroid, growth or sex hormones causes many changes in cell metabolism that overlap with the changes that occur with normal ageing.

The presence of increasing somatic mutations with ageing, when accompanied by a failure in apoptosis, may also lead to an increase in the growth of abnormally functioning, poorly functioning or non-functioning endocrine cells. When this is joined by immune system ageing (*see* Chapter 4, 'The immune system') and decreased immune surveillance, there is an increase in clonal clusters of these abnormal cells. It is already well known that there is a general increase in tumours of the endocrine glands (as in the other tissues and organs) with increasing age. However, the increase in these clusters of abnormal cells within the endocrine system, together with a rise in the use of computed tomography scans and magnetic resonance imaging in medical practice, has led to an increase in the detection of small tumours within the endocrine glands (that have not become fully transformed into malignant and metastasising cancer cells), which appear as 'incidentalomas'. This has become clinically important for the endocrinologist and has led to discussion about how extensively these incidentalomas, usually in the pituitary and the adrenal glands, need to be investigated.

CHANGES IN BODY COMPOSITION

There is a general decrease in muscle mass and increase in fat mass with normal ageing. These changes may begin in early or middle adulthood (*see* Chapter 14, 'The musculoskeletal system: muscle'). In the endocrine system, the decrease in muscle mass and the increase in fat mass leads to a rise in resistance to the action of insulin. Insulin resistance has major consequences, as the predominant sites of insulin action in the body are in the adipose tissues, skeletal muscle and liver.

With ageing, there is an increase in both subcutaneous and visceral fat. There has been a greater appreciation recently of the cellular and secretory activity of adipose tissues and several adipokines have been described, including adiponectin, leptin, resistin and visfatin. The increase in adipose tissue with ageing, especially visceral adipose tissue, may lead to changes in the circulation of many of these adipokines, which – with the exception of adiponectin – are associated with further insulin resistance. Therefore, there is a general decrease in glucose tolerance with ageing. However, as obesity is associated with increased bone mineral density, this might mean a reduction in osteoporotic fractures in obese older people.

CHANGES IN THE NEUROLOGICAL SYSTEM

With the age-related decline in function of the central and peripheral nervous systems, the interaction and coordination between the nervous system and the endocrine system is disrupted. The changes in some of these higher brain functions with ageing (for example, decrease in activity, changes in food preferences and appetite) may also affect glucose regulation and insulin resistance. The water–electrolyte balance becomes more difficult to maintain as the posterior pituitary secretion of antidiuretic hormone becomes less responsive, particularly when under stressful conditions. Anterior pituitary secretion of GH may often decline in the absence of any obvious cause and this may reflect a decline in hypothalamic regulatory signalling. Disturbances in sleep patterns with ageing can disrupt the circadian and other rhythmic patterns of hormonal secretion. Deterioration of autonomic nervous system function may also affect and be aggravated by changes in the adrenal aldosterone response to renin. In contrast, serum levels of adrenal catecholamines increase with increasing age, and it has been suggested that this occurs in response to the increase in 'stress' with ageing. Many of these changes are still not well understood. The increasing use of psychotropic medications in older people has revealed many interesting insights into the interaction between the central nervous system and endocrinology, as many of these newer drugs affect appetite and increase prolactin secretion.

INTERACTION WITH THE AGEING IMMUNE SYSTEM

There is an increase in autoimmune disease with ageing, which may be the consequence of the decline in the immune autoregulatory functions that also occurs with ageing, leading to a loss of autoantigen tolerance (*see* Chapter 4, 'The immune system'). For this and yet unknown reasons, the prevalence of autoantibodies to many of the endocrine glands may increase with ageing. Although there is some uncertainty regarding the significance of these autoantibodies, there is often an association with decline in function of the affected endocrine gland. Thyroid autoimmunity has been well studied and the prevalence of thyroid autoantibodies rises with increasing age; similarly, the prevalence of hypothyroidism is higher in older people. The prevalence of gastric parietal cells autoantibodies as well as the prevalence and severity of polyglandular autoimmune disease also increase with ageing. This may lead to a decline in function and secretion of these glands, accentuating the more gradual age-related decline in function. However, the clinical symptoms and signs of such a gradual decline may overlap with many of the changes seen in 'normal ageing', and thus be subtle and not very obvious.

OTHER CHANGES

With ageing, there is a well-described decline in kidney function (*see* Chapter 10, 'The kidneys'), with a significant decline in the glomerular filtration rate. Together with ageing of the heart and decline in the regulation of the natriuretic peptides, maintenance of water–electrolyte and acid–base balance becomes less efficient, thus electrolyte disturbances are more common and persistent with ageing. There may also be an associated decline in the direct endocrine function of the kidneys leading to a decrease in the secretion of erythropoietin and in the conversion of vitamin D to its active form, 1,25-dihydroxyvitamin D_3 [$1,25(OH)_2D_3$]. This decline in vitamin D activation with ageing will also be made worse by the decrease in exposure to sunshine, and decrease in intestinal absorption of dietary vitamin D and calcium that occurs with ageing. Some studies have suggested that low vitamin D is associated with an increase in falls as well as in fragility fractures in older people.

The gastrointestinal tract also changes gradually but significantly with ageing (*see* Chapter 8, 'The gastrointestinal system'). There is a decrease in liver mass, slowing in gastric emptying, decrease in gastric secretions, and decline in gastrointestinal transit time. Some preliminary studies have suggested that with ageing there is a decrease and delay in the secretion of incretins, including of glucagon-like peptide-1 (GLP-1) by the L cells in the ileum, in response to food. This will lead to a decrease in the secretion of insulin in response to food intake and aggravate glucose intolerance.

The combined decline in kidney and liver/gastrointestinal function leads to a decline in metabolic clearance of many hormones, the steroid hormones in particular. All steroid hormones are highly protein bound in the circulation, either to their own specific high-affinity low-capacity binding protein (as in the sex hormone-binding globulins, thyroxine-binding globulins and cortisol-binding globulins) or to albumin, which acts as a low-affinity high-capacity binding globulin for many steroid hormones. Any decrease in albumin synthesis by the liver, or increase in loss of albumin in the kidney, will lower the serum measurement significantly. This complex situation becomes even more complicated in that synthesis of many of the steroid hormone-binding proteins by the liver decreases with age but clearance is usually decreased. This is especially relevant in the measurement of blood hormone concentrations of the highly protein-bound hormones. Most of the commercially available assays of 'free' (unbound) steroid hormones, with the exception of free thyroxine (fT4), have not been validated in older people, in whom the levels of binding proteins and real free hormones differ significantly from those of younger people. Thus, the advocacy of hormonal treatment based on such measurements of free hormones in older people is unwise.

SPECIFIC ENDOCRINE DISORDERS

Disorders and disease of the endocrine system may occur in isolation in a single gland or hormone, but the close coordination and interaction that occur within the endocrine system may often lead to complex changes in multiple hormones at the same time. This is well known in pituitary disease. Excess prolactin secretion from a microprolactinoma may inhibit the secretion of the gonadotrophins luteinising hormone (LH) and follicle-stimulating hormone (FSH), thus lead to deficiency in the sex hormones. If there is a large pituitary tumour, the mass effect may cause a deficiency in the secretion of any or all of the other pituitary hormones. Despite this, it is still useful to consider specific clinical endocrine disorders and the changes with ageing.

DIABETES MELLITUS AND AGEING

Most of the digestible carbohydrate in our food is converted into glucose in the gut and transported in the bloodstream to different organs for metabolism or storage. The blood glucose level rises after food and is brought down rapidly by insulin secreted by the beta-cells in the pancreatic islets. The process is tightly and rapidly controlled and also involves the nervous system (vagus nerve). Dysregulation of this tight control leads to elevated blood glucose levels, which, if higher than the threshold of reabsorption in the kidney, leads to the abnormal state glycosuria, the origin of the term 'diabetes mellitus' (sweet urine). The hyperglycaemia in diabetes is caused by a relative or absolute deficiency of insulin. However, disorders in the regulation of glucagon, normally secreted acutely by alpha-cells in the pancreatic islets to raise the blood glucose, have recently been thought to be important in diabetes, particularly in older people. Several studies have reported that serum glucagon remained at high levels in patients with diabetes even though blood glucose was high, suggesting a disorder in the normal suppression of glucagon secretion via autocrine somatostatin. This leads to a persistence of hyperglycaemia after meals.

The changes that occur with ageing in the secretion of insulin from beta-cells are manifold. They include a decrease in the rate of response to a glucose load, perhaps from the decrease in cell membrane glucose transporter 2 and a decrease in the incretin hormones GLP-1 and glucose-dependent insulinotropic polypeptide (GIP) from the ileum. There is also an increase in autoimmune antibodies to the islet beta-cells with normal ageing. Together with the accompanying increase in fat mass in most normal ageing men and women, and the resulting increase in insulin resistance, this decline in insulin response leads to a higher prevalence in impaired glucose tolerance and diabetes in older people. This has been confirmed by the many studies from different ageing populations that have consistently described an increase in the prevalence of impaired fasting glucose, impaired glucose tolerance and type 2 diabetes mellitus with increasing age. Some studies have reported that the prevalence of diabetes has reached over 40% in those aged over 75 years old.

Diabetes mellitus is the most common endocrine disease in adults. In addition to the relative deficiency of insulin in type 2 diabetes, there is often an increase in insulin resistance as well, especially in the early stages of the disease in obese patients. In addition, lipid metabolism is also deranged in patients with diabetes. This combination leads to an increase in macrovascular disease of the coronary arteries and other arteries, which is similar in pathophysiology to the increase in cardiovascular disease found in normal ageing. There is also a diabetes-specific increase in microvascular disease, which gives rise to microvascular retinopathy, nephropathy and neuropathy. The health burden of diabetes and its complications is a major concern in most developed countries.

Diagnosis of diabetes in the ageing population

The symptoms of hyperglycaemia, namely polydipsia and polyuria, in older people are much less prominent than in the younger people. They may be completely absent, or develop very gradually and overlap with some of the symptoms of 'normal ageing'. On occasion, these symptoms may also be mistakenly attributed to medications for other diseases (e.g. diuretics, antihistamines). Many surveys have shown that a significant number of older people (over 10% of the population over 65 years) may have undiagnosed diabetes. It has therefore been recommended that older people undergo annual screening for the disease.

Fasting blood glucose is still the laboratory investigation of choice for the diagnosis of diabetes in older people. While elevated glycosylated haemoglobin (HbA1c) is increasingly regarded as an acceptable alternative with which to diagnose diabetes, in older people HbA1c may be low due to anaemia, which is more common with age, and give a false-negative result. The oral glucose tolerance test is carried out very infrequently now and is necessary for the diagnosis of diabetes only in rare circumstances in older people; for example, when very discrepant results have been obtained on different days.

Treatment goals in the ageing population

In managing this very lifestyle-related and lifestyle-dependent disease in older people, it is especially important that the goal of treatment should be individualised according to the patient's state of health, pre-existing illness(es), mobility and expectations. Recent clinical studies have shown that it takes about 6–8 years or longer before the benefits of tight blood glucose control are seen in the reduction of vascular complications. In contrast, the benefits of good blood pressure control and lowering of low-density lipoprotein (LDL) cholesterol become significant within 2–3 years. Recent clinical trials have also indicated that the risk, and associated morbidity and mortality, of hypoglycaemia is much more severe in older patients, especially if there is pre-existing cardiovascular disease. The autonomic symptoms of hypoglycaemia become less prominent with ageing, and there is also a less effective counter-regulatory response to hypoglycaemia. (The acute glucagon and GH responses to hypoglycaemia significantly decrease with age, leading to a more severe and prolonged serious hypoglycaemia.) Therefore, in some older patients in whom life expectancy may need to be balanced with quality of life, a moderate level of blood glucose control may be more appropriate. In such patients, it would be reasonable to set the goal of treatment to avoidance of symptoms and complications from hyperglycaemia (e.g. infections), without causing a significant risk of hypoglycaemia. Less rigorous and frequent self-monitoring of blood glucose and an HbA1c target of 7.5% (or higher) may therefore be acceptable.

In older patients without other concomitant disease or significant frailty, a more rigorous pursuit of tighter blood glucose control may be appropriate but would still need to be tempered with the known higher risk of hypoglycaemia. Good education on the risks of hypoglycaemia and careful, deliberate selection of anti-diabetes drugs with a lower risk of hypoglycaemia would be important. Treatment goals may need to be reviewed with the development of other diseases.

In ageing patients, including patients with type 1 diabetes who are now older, their long-standing treatment goal of tight blood glucose control with regular glucose monitoring at home should be maintained, but the situation needs to be reassessed at regular intervals to modify their treatment and goals when necessary.

In all of these groups, good control of blood pressure and LDL cholesterol, which is less dependent on lifestyle changes than glucose control, should be maintained. There is good evidence of a relatively rapid significant and persistent benefit in morbidity and mortality reduction from control of these diabetes-associated disorders.

Therapeutic drugs for diabetes in the ageing population

All patients, young and old, should of course be encouraged to eat in moderation and exercise regularly. The ability to exercise often declines with ageing, primarily because of the development of arthritis or cardiovascular disease. Thus, drug treatment is a necessity in the vast majority of patients with diabetes. There has been an increase in the variety of therapeutic drugs available in the last few years, some of which have been subsequently withdrawn because of their side effects. There is increased awareness that these drugs have to be given for a very long number of years in most patients, thus longer-term studies on cardiovascular and other endpoints are now mandated by regulatory authorities for the newer anti-diabetic drugs. The effect of diabetes and anti-diabetes drugs on cancer is now being very actively studied. A detailed discussion of the use of diabetes medication is beyond the scope of this chapter, but some important precautions in prescribing for older people should be noted.

The biguanide metformin is commonly used in diabetes patients. Patients who have been on metformin for many years should have their blood levels of folate and vitamin B_{12} measured, as there is an association with deficiency of these easily replaced vitamins. The alpha-1 glucosidase inhibitor acarbose is widely used in East Asia, but the increase in flatulence has limited its use in most other populations. In older people, where constipation is a common complaint, the use of acarbose may be helpful in lowering blood glucose and also in increasing intestinal gas, as the benefits may outweigh the social side effects. Both metformin and acarbose have almost no risk of hypoglycaemia and are thus useful in the older diabetes patient.

The sulphonylureas carry with them a high risk of hypoglycaemia, especially glibenclamide. While the other long-acting sulphonylureas, for example glimeparide and gliclazide modified release, have not been associated to the same degree with serious hypoglycaemia, the shorter-acting sulphonylureas are preferable. The glinides, for example repaglinide and nateglinide, also act on the sulphonylurea receptor, but the action is much more rapid and of a shorter duration, thus allowing an important flexibility when there is irregularity and skipping of meals.

Two new classes of oral drugs for diabetes have been introduced in more recent years: the thiazolidinediones, or peroxisome proliferator-activated receptor-γ (PPAR-γ) agonists, and the dipeptidyl peptidase-4 (DPP-IV) inhibitors. Of the three PPAR-γ agonists (troglitazone, rosiglitazone and pioglitazone) marketed, only pioglitazone is still available. Although the mechanism of action is still not fully understood, these drugs reduce peripheral insulin resistance and carry a very low risk of hypoglycaemia. The side effects include weight gain, water retention and an increase in fractures. Most clinicians would use pioglitazone for a limited time period (perhaps 6 months) in patients who are already on maximum oral hypoglycaemic drugs and are reluctant or unable to start on insulin. DPP-IV inhibitors restrict the rapid enzymatic deactivation of the incretin GLP-1, which inhibits glucagon secretion and enhances hyperglycaemia-induced insulin secretion. There is minimal risk of hypoglycaemia. There is some concern about possible long-term side effects, but these are uncertain at the moment. Both of these new classes of anti-diabetic drugs may be helpful in older patients because of the lower risk of hypoglycaemia, but the doses may need to be reduced if kidney disease is present.

If oral medication is unable to control blood glucose, the addition of injected insulin and/or a GLP-1 mimetic is usually recommended. However, good eyesight and dexterity are essential once regular injections become the norm. Although some newer devices have become more older-person friendly in recent years, they still use small disposable needles. In addition, home capillary glucose monitoring is recommended once insulin has been started, also requiring dexterity.

Insulin is extremely effective in lowering blood glucose, but the risk of hypoglycaemia is high. Large swings in glucose levels can also be a significant risk, especially with the newer quick-onset of action insulin analogues. Therefore, starting with low doses and small dose changes should be the rules in older people and a goal of 7.0 mmol/L or higher for a fasting glucose level may be adequate. The choice of insulin should be individualised and tailored according to the expectations and capabilities of the patient, and the additional resources available (caregiver assistance, etc.). GLP-1 mimetics are a useful adjunct for suppression of appetite and weight loss, and have a much lower risk of hypoglycaemia.

THE AGEING THYROID GLAND

The thyroid hormones regulate the metabolic rate of all the cells and tissues in the body. Therefore, blood levels are tightly regulated by the hypothalamus (via the thyrotropin-releasing hormone) and the pituitary (via the thyroid-stimulating hormone [TSH]) with a rapid feedback loop. With ageing, the function of the thyroid gland begins to decline; thus, the second most prevalent endocrine disorder in older people is hypothyroidism. The histological changes in the thyroid gland in normal ageing have been well studied. There is a decrease in the size of the thyroid follicles accompanied by peri-follicular fibrosis. The intrafollicular volume of colloid becomes scant and more basophilic, and follicular cells are flattened. These changes would suggest a decline in thyroid function. However, in many older people, microscopic colloid nodules (on histology) and macroscopic (on ultrasound) nodules increase in number significantly, together with focal lymphocytic infiltration. These changes would be consistent with the observed increase in functioning and non-functioning nodules and toxic multi-nodular goitre with ageing. The effects of these histological changes with ageing are thus varied. So, while the prevalence of hypothyroidism increases steadily with ageing, there is also an increase in the frequency of autonomous functioning nodules and toxic multi-nodular goitre (while Graves' disease decreases with ageing). Non-functioning thyroid nodules and thyroid cancers also increase with ageing. Figure 17.1 describes some of the tumours found in the thyroid gland with ageing.

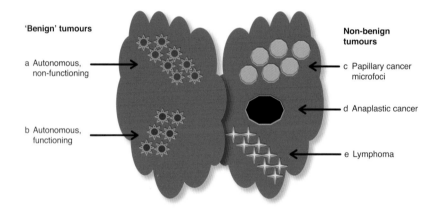

FIGURE 17.1 Thyroid tumours and ageing: there is an increase in benign and non-benign thyroid tumours with ageing; most are benign or slow growing (papillary cancers)

Subclinical hypothyroidism (where the fT4 is normal and TSH is elevated) and subclinical hyperthyroidism (where the fT4 is normal and TSH is suppressed) are increasingly diagnosed in older people. The presenting clinical symptoms and signs of thyroid disease overlap with many features of 'normal' ageing, and are often misinterpreted by the patient as 'normal'. Some have recommended that in older people, there should be routine screening for thyroid disease every few years.

Hypothyroidism
Clinical features and diagnosis
Hypothyroidism causes an increase in body weight with lethargy, depression, constipation and cold intolerance – all of which are present in many normal

older euthyroid men and women. Some of the increasing prevalence is due to the rise in use of radioiodine ablative treatment in younger hyperthyroid patients, medications that trigger autoimmune thyroid disease (e.g. interferons and monoclonal antibodies) and iodine-containing medications (e.g. amiodarone) and radiographic contrast dyes. The diagnosis of hypothyroidism is easily made once there is the awareness of such a possibility (the TSH is elevated and fT4 low). Hypothyroidism secondary to pituitary insufficiency (where both the TSH and fT4 are low) is rare and should be suspected in the increasing number of patients who have received radiation therapy to the head and neck. These patients, if they have concomitant adrenocorticotrophic hormone (ACTH) deficiency, do not gain weight and do not have many of the usual signs of hypothyroidism.

Investigation and treatment

Older patients who have previously received radioiodine therapy or radiation therapy to the head and neck should be screened regularly for hypothyroidism. Treatment with oral thyroxine should be started at a low dose and increased very gradually to reduce cardiovascular stress. If there is an accompanying cortisol deficiency, thyroxine treatment should only be started after cortisol treatment. If the patient has significant coronary artery disease, the recommendation is that intervention of the coronary artery disease be undertaken before treatment with thyroxine is commenced. Studies have shown that cardiac morbidity and mortality is significantly higher in these patients if there is an attempt to restore euthyroidism before cardiac surgery.

Although there is still some disagreement, the benefits of treatment in subclinical hypothyroidism to bring the TSH level to normal outweigh the risks, especially if care is taken to start with low doses of thyroxine and the dose is increased very gradually. Although symptoms are non-specific and difficult to assess, well-monitored treatment of subclinical hypothyroidism has been shown to improve serum lipids, cardiac function, appetite, constipation and various psychometric measurements. If the decision is made not to start treatment, there should certainly be regular monitoring of the fT4.

Hyperthyroidism

Clinical features and diagnosis

Although the prevalence of Graves' disease decreases with ageing, hyperthyroidism is still significant, and there should be awareness of the differences between the clinical features in older and younger age groups. Unlike younger patients, older hyperthyroid patients have very few of the usual symptoms, such as palpitations, heat intolerance and tremors, and may even be completely asymptomatic. The clinical signs are primarily in the cardiovascular system. Thus, atrial fibrillation and congestive heart failure are relatively common as presenting features. The features of Graves' disease resulting from the thyroid-receptor antibody – ophthalmopathy, pre-tibial myxoedema and acropachy – are not common, as Graves' disease is not a common cause of the thyrotoxicosis in older people. Therefore, in any older patient with new onset atrial fibrillation, heart failure or unusual symptoms of weight loss, thyroid function tests would be a very reasonable investigation.

Investigation and treatment

The fT4 is elevated and TSH suppressed in hyperthyroidism. However, in any acute non-thyroidal illness, the results of thyroid function tests may be similarly deranged and the tests may need to be repeated after the patient has recovered. Treatment can be with the anti-thyroid hormone synthesis drugs carbimazole or propylthiouracil; however, in older people, ablative radioiodine is now increasingly the treatment of choice. The oral medications may have serious side effects and require more regular dose adjustment.

There is increased awareness that subclinical hyperthyroidism (low TSH and normal fT4, and distinguished from non-thyroidal illness by measurement on more than one occasion) may be more common than previously thought. Untreated subclinical hyperthyroidism is associated with an increase in subsequent atrial fibrillation and bone turnover and osteoporosis. There are different views concerning the treatment modality, with some physicians preferring to trial low-dose anti-thyroid drugs for a year, and others preferring ablative radioiodine.

Thyroid nodules and thyroid cancer

Investigation and treatment

Thyroid nodules and thyroid cancer increase with ageing. With the increasing use of ultrasound scans, there is a huge increase in investigation of these nodules. Some studies have detected thyroid nodules in over 50% of the older-aged population using high-resolution ultrasound scans. The vast majority of these thyroid nodules are benign, but the prognosis for older patients with malignant nodules is worse than for younger patients. Ultrasound criteria have low sensitivity in identifying malignancy in these nodules and ultrasound-guided fine-needle biopsy of every nodule is neither practical nor definitive in distinguishing malignancy in most patients. There is ongoing discussion as to the follow-up of these nodules. Some consensus is emerging on the criteria for ultrasound and further investigation, so hopefully there will soon be sensible guidelines regarding the investigation and follow-up of nodules detected by ultrasound of the thyroid.

Well-differentiated papillary cancer microfoci have been very frequently observed in autopsy studies of the thyroid, but such microfoci are likely to be insignificant. Thyroid cancer in older people is more likely to be of the anaplastic cell type, and presents in euthyroid patients as a hard neck mass that is locally invasive. The prognosis is poor.

PARATHYROID DISORDERS AND AGEING

Serum calcium is regulated by several interdependent factors, including parathyroid hormone (PTH) secreted by the parathyroid glands. The prevalence of hypercalcaemia from hyperparathyroidism with ageing has increased, partly because of the increase in biochemical screening. Hypoparathyroidism is much less common and is associated with the increase in autoimmune disease with ageing. Both may be mild, asymptomatic or have their symptoms wrongly attributed to 'normal ageing'.

Hyperparathyroidism, if symptomatic and with relatively high serum calcium levels, should be treated as in the younger age groups. After accurate localisation, parathyroidectomy by an experienced surgeon is the treatment of choice. Intraoperative serum PTH measurements give a good and reliable indication of successful treatment. In frail patients with asymptomatic elevation of serum calcium, individualised treatment guided by the most recent consensus is the best option. The recommended guidelines for the treatment of asymptomatic mild hyperparathyroidism have all used an arbitrary age cut-off of 50 years. Surgery is only recommended in people over 50 years if serum calcium is very elevated, there is significant osteoporosis and/or chronic kidney disease. Otherwise, a watch and wait approach is recommended, together with medical treatment with a bisphosphonate. The recently introduced oral calcium mimetic cinacalcet has increased the options available for patients who are not fit or suitable for surgery.

Autoimmune hypoparathyroidism in older people may occur in isolation or together with the other hormone deficiencies in the autoimmune polyglandular syndromes. The established treatment is with oral calcium and vitamin D. The shorter-acting preparations of vitamin D are preferable: calcitriol or alpha-calcidol. Physiological replacement of hypoparathyroid hormone deficiency with recombinant PTH has not become widespread because of the necessity of daily subcutaneous injections and the unproven cost-to-benefit ratio.

PITUITARY, GONADAL AND ADRENAL HORMONES

Normal ageing is associated with a gradual slow decline in function of the pituitary. However, there is also a decline in the autoregulatory feedback mechanisms. This forms the basis of our present understanding of the changes in pituitary hormones with ageing. There is a decline in GH secretion and, in men, of the gonadotrophins LH and FSH. However, the increase in cortisol with ageing is thought to be caused by hyper-responsiveness to chronic stress resulting from dysfunction of the rapid feedback loop. This has been clearly demonstrated in animal studies but difficult to prove in men. In addition, these changes in pituitary hormones have been seen predominantly in frail older people. Studies of healthy older people have shown that in many older-old individuals, there can be completely normal GH-IGF-1, testosterone and ACTH-cortisol levels.

The ill effects of excessive glucocorticoids are well known. The effects of the hypercortisolic state in many older patients may contribute to the increase in glucose intolerance, hypertension, skin fragility and infections. There is no consensus as to the assessment or treatment of this condition in older people. In clearly proven non-suppressible endogenous Cushing syndrome, investigation and treatment should be the same as that in younger people.

Serum levels of androgens, testosterone from the testes and dehydroepiandrosterone/dehydroepiandrosterone sulphate from the adrenals decrease with ageing in most, but not all, men. This decrease is associated with impaired sexual function and also with reduced muscle mass and osteoporosis. Male hormone replacement is strongly advocated in some quarters, but the results from studies on long-term androgen replacement have not been sufficiently convincing for most health authorities to make it a recommendation in older people. Prostate cancer is still an important risk of androgen treatment. Phosphodiesterase type-5 inhibitors may be used for the treatment of male sexual function.

The fall in female hormones at the menopause, with a clear increase in pituitary LH and FSH, is associated with many effects on the female body and psyche. The present consensus is that hormonal treatment with oestrogens and progestogens should be for a limited period only, of 6 months or so, at a low dose, and primarily for symptomatic relief. Testosterone implants are reported to improve libido in post-menopausal women and may be considered for some women requiring this.

AGEING AND HORMONES

Brown-Séquard's publication in *The Lancet* in 1889 was the first modern report of an attempt to use hormones for rejuvenation. It is reported that within 1 year of his publication, 12 000 physicians had similarly injected aqueous extracts of animal testes into patients, probably with similarly strong placebo effects. The search in more recent times has continued. Early studies with female hormone replacement had very positive conclusions, but these have not been supported by further longer-term controlled studies. The effects of oestrogens are still very clearly positive for many women, but the risks of cancer and vascular complications are considered too high. This has been the dilemma for all attempts in endocrine rejuvenation therapy. There is an increase in atherosclerosis and in many cancers with ageing. Most hormones enhance cell growth and stimulate cell mitosis, thus will stimulate and enhance early cancer growth. Oestrogen-dependent cancers will be enhanced by oestrogens and androgen-dependent cancers will be enhanced by androgens. GH will enhance colonic cancer growth and possibly, to a lesser extent, prostate and breast cancer.

GH has many effects on metabolism and tissue maintenance in the adult, long after cessation of height gain. Many of these effects are seen in younger adults with GH deficiency from pituitary disease and are similar to the changes of normal ageing. The benefits of GH replacement in the context of adults with multiple pituitary hormone deficiency, or in adults who have previously been treated for isolated GH deficiency as children, are very clear and indisputable. With ageing, there is a gradual decline in GH secretion, and consequent decline in IGF-1, although this is often associated with the presence of chronic disease and medications. The treatment of older patients with GH has not shown such indisputable results and there is ongoing controversy on the investigation and management of low serum IGF-1 in older people. Studies on GH treatment of older men and women with low IGF-1 showed some beneficial effects on the skin, bone density, muscle mass and muscle strength after 6 months or 1 year. Other studies have demonstrated that vigorous physical training can replicate most of these changes. A study that gave both GH and testosterone to older men also showed beneficial effects but had the significant side effects of glucose intolerance and gynaecomastia.

The oral GH secretagogues provide a more physiological GH secretion profile than injected GH and would be more convenient in older patients. Three GH secretagogues – tabimorelin, capromorelin and MK677 – have been studied and showed some beneficial effects in improving muscle strength and mobility in the short term. However, the pharmaceutical companies have been reluctant to conduct further studies on these compounds as the risk profile will remain very high in normal older people and the registration authorities have not accepted 'normal ageing' as a disease entity. A further complexity is the consistent finding that in many species (e.g. *C. elegans*, *Drosophila* spp. and various rodents and primates) within the laboratory setting, a GH/IGF deficiency state is associated with increased longevity and decreased incidence of cancer and atherosclerosis.

CONCLUSION

The endocrine system is unusual among the body systems in being age regulated and age timed in some of its 'normal' functions. The lessons from the early enthusiasm for oestrogen 'replacement' and subsequent restraint would urge caution as a wise principle in the evaluation of claims for rejuvenation by hormonal treatment. There will no doubt be more discussion and many further studies on endocrine treatment for ageing.

FURTHER READING

Chanson P, Epelbaum J, Lamberts S *et al.*, editors. *Endocrine Aspects of Successful Aging: genes, hormones and lifestyle*. Berlin and Heidelberg: Springer; 2010.

Sinclair AJ, editor. *Diabetes in Old Age*. 3rd ed. Chichester: Wiley-Blackwell; 2009.

Morley JE, van den Berg L, editors. *Endocrinology of Aging*. Totowa, NJ: Humana Press; 2000.

Vassiliadi DA, Tsagarakis S. Endocrine incidentalomas-challenges imposed by incidentally discovered lesions. *Nat Rev Endocrinol*. 2011; **7**(11): 668–80.

QUESTIONS: THE ENDOCRINE SYSTEM

1 There is an increase in the prevalence of autoantibodies with ageing. What is the most common associated consequence of this increase?
A amyloid accumulation within the endocrine glands
B decline in endocrine function
C increase in incidentalomas
D increase in 'toxicosis' in endocrine glands
E no consequence.

Answer: B

2 In normal healthy older men and women, there is a gradual increase in the body mass index (BMI). What is the most likely endocrine association of this increase in BMI?
A decline in circulating catecholamines
B decline in GH secretion
C decrease in insulin sensitivity
D increase in subclinical hypothyroidism
E increase in vitamin D absorption.

Answer: C

3 A 79-year-old man with a 20-year history of type 2 diabetes mellitus presents with prolonged hypoglycaemia caused by his oral glibenclamide. He had maintained good control of his diabetes in the last 8 years with metformin and glibenclamide, with an HbA1c of 7.6%. What is the most appropriate drug with which to replace his glibenclamide?
A gliclazide
B liraglutide
C pioglitazone
D pre-breakfast insulin
E sitagliptin.

Answer: E

4 A 72-year-old woman presents with a 3-month history of tiredness, poor memory and a weight gain of 3 pounds. Clinical examination is normal.

Investigations:
Serum fT4 = 19 pmol/L (9–22)
Serum TSH <0.01 mIU/L (0.4–4.5)

A diagnosis of subclinical hyperthyroidism is made. What is the most likely clinical development within the next 2 years if she is left untreated?

A   atrial fibrillation
B   goitre
C   proximal myopathy
D   thyroid eye disease
E   vertebral fracture.

Answer: A

5   A 78-year-old man is found to have mild hypercalcaemia in the course of inves-
tigations for polyuria. His polyuria resolved without treatment and investigations
showed hyperparathyroidism without any parathyroid adenoma localised with
ultrasound. He had no specific symptoms of hypercalcaemia. What is the most
appropriate treatment for his asymptomatic mild hypercalcaemia?
A   alendronate
B   metaiodobenzylguanidine (MIBG) scan and treatment
C   neck exploration and parathyroidectomy
D   no treatment
E   vitamin D antagonist.

Answer: A

Section 3

Frailty and quality of life

CHAPTER 18

Frailty and ageing

FINBARR C MARTIN

INTRODUCTION

Frailty has emerged again in the twenty-first century as an important concept for health and social care workers. It has been an almost pejorative term when applied to people generally, but in the context of old age medicine, it has become useful to distinguish the particular health-related vulnerability of some older people from the lazy and ageist assumption that the age of an individual was all you needed to know to guess what needed to be done or, more commonly, not done. By distinguishing frailty from chronological age, it becomes possible to be more specific about the challenges that older people may face and the solutions they need. By adding the measurement of frailty to the health assessment, it becomes possible to move on from the notion that a list of diagnoses is an adequate description of the patient.

Some history

Over half a century ago, Joseph Sheldon, the father of community geriatrics, coined the term 'frail ambulant', calling for a health policy on these individuals who were predominantly characterised as presenting a clinical challenge not soluble by established healthcare. His comments about defining illness still ring true:

> In general, the greater the age the greater the difficulty of such a simple classification, and the less likely it is to be continuously valid . . . and the greater the importance of flexibility and human understanding in the management of individual problems. (Sheldon JH. *BMJ.* 1960; **1**: 1223–6)

Bernard Isaacs introduced some classification by describing the common syndromes faced by older frail people in the last years of life as the four geriatric giants of immobility, instability (falls), incoherence (delirium and dementia) and incontinence. Of course, age-related changes are by definition universal, but the great variability among older people was highlighted by Rowe and Kahn, who distinguished 'usual' from 'successful' ageing, as the two ends of the spectrum of impairment seen in old age. There has been increasing focus in recent years on the lifelong sources of this variation in biomedical impairment, distinct from the focus on variation seen also in epidemiology of disease.

'Frailty' is the term that has emerged and become commonly used among clinicians and biogerontologists to describe an age-related vulnerability that is conceptually distinguishable from disease or disability. This was encapsulated in the definition of frailty as

> a condition or syndrome which results from a multi-system reduction in reserve capacity to the extent that a number of physiological systems are close to, or past, the threshold of symptomatic failure. As a result the frail person is at increased risk of disability or death from minor external stresses. (Campbell AJ, Buckner DM. *Age Ageing.* 1997; **26**(4): 315–18)

Noteworthy in this definition is that the causes of the 'reduction in reserve capacity' are not specified, thus might be combinations of distinct diseases with other age-related changes.

CAN FRAILTY BE SYSTEMATICALLY MEASURED?

So, the consensus understanding of 'frailty' is the heightened vulnerability to adverse health status change, in the face of illness, injury or psychosocial disruption. However, this understanding of the concept can lead to several views about how it can be identified. The common starting point is one or more specific measurable characteristics and the end point of an adverse outcome – for example, death, falls (or one of the other geriatric syndromes), disability in everyday functional activities or increased dependency such as admission to a care home. But different notions of frailty can be detected from the various approaches to its identification, which differ in how they secure their validity. For instance, the pragmatic operational approach is to identify which sets of measurable characteristics predict relevant outcomes, with statistical associations, without this necessarily signifying any proof of causal pathway. The pathophysiological approach, alternatively, situates frailty in the underlying biomedical driving forces that render the individual vulnerable.

Operational approaches

A number of studies have shown that it is feasible to achieve a definition of frailty derived from baseline measures with reasonable predictive accuracy and several operational tools have been developed to identify frailty as understood in this way, using two rather different approaches.

First, the 'phenotype' model of Fried *et al.*, which defines 'frailty' as the presence of impairment in three or more of five components:

- unintentional weight loss (self-reported or measured at follow-up)
- self-reported fatigue (self-assessed)
- diminished physical activity (estimate based on self-report)
- weakness (grip strength measurement)
- slowness (measured gait speed).

The final three in this list were defined as frailty indicators if the values were in the lowest quintile of relevant population age-standardised norms. Of course, the choice of what to measure to derive the key predictive components was not arbitrary, but based on previous empirical knowledge of their relationship to adverse outcomes. Notably, cognition, mood and social resources are not explicitly included, though all may actually affect the five measured domains. However, this does not matter, as the primary justification for this model is its empirically tested predictive power. The data were drawn from the Cardiovascular Health Study, a prospective observational study of 5201 men and women aged 65 years and older, with the later addition of 687 African American men.

Validity of this frailty definition is enhanced by the demonstration that greater degrees of frailty were associated with reduced life expectancy in this cohort. Also consistent with this notion of frailty as a distinct construct was the finding that even though frailty was more prevalent in those with the greatest burden of co-morbidity, chronic disease and frailty overlapped but did not map identically within the cohort.

Additionally, while frailty defined in this way is more prevalent in the oldest old, it is not universal. While some have found this tool useful, it may be that an even simpler approach would do the job, as suggested by the finding that the 'SOF' (Study of Osteoporotic Fractures index) approach based only on weight loss, chair rise performance and subjective low energy level was equally effective in predicting falls, disability and death of older men.

The second approach is to derive a global 'score' or category based on a full multidimensional clinical assessment, as refined in the 'accumulation of deficits' method in the Rockwood Frailty Index (*see* Box 18.1). It is a summation without weighting of the presence or absence of deficits and departs from the notion of frailty as a distinct set of impairments because the deficits can include specific components of disability or diseases.

BOX 18.1 **Estimation of the Rockwood Frailty Index**

- Tabulate the outcome of a comprehensive geriatric assessment in terms of either the presence or absence (dichotomise) of a specific disease, ADL (activities of daily living) capacity or impairment (e.g. visual) or trichotomise for a suitable impairment (e.g. normal, mild, moderate or severe cognitive impairment).
- Provide each item with a score:
  - dichotomised 0 or 1
  - trichotomised 0, 0.33, 0.66 or 1.0.
- Add all individual item scores.
- Divide by number of items.
- Sum the scores as the numerator.
- Sum the number of items as the denominator.
- Numerator/Denominator = Frailty Index and is between 0 and 1.

Adapted from Rockwood K, Mitnitski A, Song X *et al.* Long-term risks of death and institutionalization of elderly people in relation to deficit accumulation at age 70. *J Am Geriatr Soc.* 2006; **54**(6): 975–9.

The index is predictive of a full range of adverse outcomes including death. It has the potential for broad applicability because estimation of the index does not depend on standardisation of exactly what is assessed, as long as a sufficient number across a wide enough scope of domains is included. Validation is supported by the demonstration that the frailty index score was associated both with a higher incidence of delirium during acute illness and poorer survival among those who developed delirium.

The two approaches may identify similar people as frail. In three distinct populations of older people – independent community dwellers, those attending a day unit for treatment and rehabilitation and inpatients of a long-term care unit – the prevalence of frailty, as determined by Fried *et al.*'s definition, and the Rockwood Frailty Index were significantly different between the groups. The two methods were highly correlated, but the Rockwood Frailty Index was more discriminatory at the moderate/severe end of the frailty spectrum. In keeping with other longitudinal frailty studies, the cohort in the national population study of Canada, comprising 2740 participants aged 65–102 years, showed that frailty is age related and more prevalent in women than men, rising by age 85 to 39.1% of men and 45.1% of women.

One of the most convincing aspects of the frailty index approach to measuring frailty is the finding, from several populations, that there seems to be an upper limit in the index, at about 0.7, suggesting that accumulation of more deficits exhausts the redundancy required to sustain life.

A simpler approach to describing frailty has also been derived from the longitudinal dataset of the Canadian Study of Health and Aging. This is a seven-point Clinical Frailty Scale, based on the clinician's global judgement and supported by descriptions such as:

- moderately frail (level 6) = help is needed with both instrumental and non-instrumental activities of daily living
- severely frail (level 7) = completely dependent on others for the activities of daily living, or terminally ill.

Pathophysiological approach to defining frailty

Basic sciences, animal models, epidemiological and clinical studies can all contribute in suggesting potential parameters of interest to an understanding of the 'driving' forces in the process of becoming frail, and capturing these systematically might enable identification of an early stage of frailty, with consequent scientific and clinical utility. This reductive approach situates frailty within definable biomedical phenomena that have a credible putative role in downstream effects on bodily functioning. Subsequent work has generated a number of candidates to occupy this pathway, and these will be discussed in some detail further on in this chapter. Identifying frailty, perhaps at an early stage, through biomedical markers, could be clinically useful in the same way as the clinically based operational methods, to enable risk assessment and targeting of special measures in clinical settings. It is more difficult to picture it being useful at the public health level.

Can these approaches be combined?

A recent consensus process, which included most of the main authors of the operational work described above along with biogerontology researchers, attempted a sort of hybrid approach to capture frailty at several levels, bringing together clinicians and researchers from disparate fields. The aim of this endeavour was to reach a consensus definition of frailty that would be useful in daily practice. A number of statements about construct, diagnosis and prognostic factors achieved wide agreement among the members of the large expert group. No single biomarker alone or any combination of biomarkers was considered adequate for the assessment of frailty, but there was agreement that a comprehensive definition of frailty should include:

- assessment of physical performance
- assessment of gait speed
- assessment of mobility
- nutritional status
- mental health
- cognition.

However, agreement could not be reached on the specific variables to be measured to capture these domains or on the diagnostic criteria.

Clearly, more work remains to be done, though it is possible that within the umbrella of the frailty construct, there will be need of several methods of definition, depending upon the purpose.

Clinical utility of these approaches to defining frailty

All these tools could be helpful for clinical risk profiling. For example, frailty (Fried *et al.*'s definition) independently predicted post-operative complications, length of stay and discharge destination among 594 patients (aged 65 years and older) having elective surgery.

In a large prospective series of patients with a mean age of 82 years admitted to general medical and rehabilitation wards, baseline frailty on admission (Rockwood Frailty Index based on a comprehensive geriatric assessment) was associated with slower recovery of mobility function and poorer overall outcomes. This could be used prospectively to inform clinical decisions and, indeed, could be taken further by demonstrating that a clinical intervention that modifies the risk profile also affects outcomes – a step towards concluding a possible causal relationship.

At a public health level, a simple non-invasive tool that does not require clinician standard assessment, could be useful in several ways:

- as part of a population needs assessment, for resource allocation
- to identify at-risk groups, for example, those at increased risk of repeat hospitalisations or functional dependency, in order to target generic interventions such as exercise on prescription
- target interventions, such as community-based case management incorporating supervised programmes such as therapeutic exercise or nutritional interventions.

BIOLOGY OF FRAILTY

Life-course approach to development of frailty in old age

Disease and disability of older people is the result of the complex and cumulative interactions between genes, ageing-related molecular damage and environmental factors (*see* Chapter 2, 'The concept of ageing: theories and mechanisms'). Individuals 'carry their history on their back'; indeed, their parents' history as well, as shown by the growing evidence of intrauterine influences on health and disability in later life. Reduced foetal growth is strongly associated with chronic conditions in later life. The Barker hypothesis suggests that increased susceptibility results from adaptations made by the foetus in an environment limited in its supply of quality of nutrients, limited resources being adaptively invested in survival over maturation. It has been shown using birth weight records that chronic conditions in adulthood, including the metabolic syndrome, diabetes, hypertension and cardiovascular diseases, are impacted by these early life factors.

From birth onwards, there is an accumulating impact on the biomedical and psychosocial changes that result in frailty and its consequences. Socio-economic profile, including neighbourhood deprivation, income, life events, illness, diet, exercise and other health-related behaviours all play a part.

Ageing, frailty and disease

Making accurate diagnoses remains an important cornerstone of geriatric medical practice, but the simple view that we can strictly distinguish degenerative diseases from ageing at the pathophysiological level is no longer tenable. It is in this context of a spectrum of age-related change including degenerative diseases and cancer that frailty emerges. So, the question about the biology of frailty concerns what aspects of age-related changes seem to be key in driving the loss of physiological reserve that ultimately lead to the organism's decompensation and death. Current consensus about the key factors includes immune dysfunction, neuroendocrine decline and sarcopenia. Other chapters in this book explore some of these changes in more detail, so in this chapter their significance to frailty is considered. The scope of changes is large.

INFLAMMAGING

An inflammatory response to stressors is essential for health, and a muted response – during infection, for example – is generally a bad omen for the clinical outcome. Conversely, an exaggerated or prolonged response is counterproductive, as it contributes to the catabolic cost of the stress. A plethora of evidence has shown that ageing is associated with an altered inflammatory profile (*see* Chapter 4, 'The immune system'). The picture is one of a heightened pro-inflammatory steady state, with some evidence of exaggerated stress-induced responses. However, although this sounds like a potential advantage to respond to infection, the evidence does not support this. In addition, frailty (Fried *et al.* criteria) in a prospective clinical trial of community dwellers aged 70 years and older was associated with significant impairment in trivalent influenza vaccine-induced antibody titres and increased rates of clinical and laboratory-confirmed influenza infection.

Greater age-associated increases in interleukin IL-6, a pro-inflammatory cytokine, and C-reactive protein (CRP) levels are associated with disability and mortality. Elevated D-dimer levels add to this risk association.

In a further study from the Cardiovascular Health Study, greater long-term increases in CRP and IL-6 levels were associated with higher incidence of physical and cognitive impairments, cardiovascular disease and mortality. But is the disease burden the only factor? Perhaps not. Frailty (Fried *et al.* criteria) and the frailty index (Rockwood) were strongly associated with the inflammatory markers TNF-α, IL-6 and CRP after adjustment for age, sex, BMI category, smoking status, number of co-morbidities and number of prescribed medications among 110 patients aged over 75 years. High levels of these cytokines, IL-6, IL-1 and TNF-α, may induce skeletal muscle loss and aggravate neuroendocrine deregulation.

Among non-diabetic participants aged 80 years and older in the Women's Health and Aging Study II, frailty levels (Fried *et al.* criteria) were found to be associated with poorer glucose load clearance and higher insulin levels, despite similar baseline measures, suggesting an impaired responsiveness to the physiological stress.

Moreover, frailty, as judged by a nine-component scoring system mixing deficits and mobility-related impairments, was recently shown to be associated with lower vitamin D levels. Vitamin D insufficiency or deficiency is common in older people and already known to be associated with a number of adverse outcomes.

Oxidative stress and inflammation

There is accumulating genetic damage of mitochondria and nuclei, damage from mutation and oxidative stress from reactive oxygen species: mitochondrial DNA mutation and oxidative damage result in a progressive impairment to a cell's adenosine triphosphate production, which, if critical, may induce apoptosis. Oxidative damage accumulates with age and the net effects of genetic, muscle and lipid damage are sufficient to impair cellular and organ function (*see* Chapter 3, 'The ageing cell'). Oxidative stress triggers IL-6 production, and is a potential mechanism that leads to the age-associated pro-inflammatory state leading to frailty. Among older patients, frailty (Fried *et al.* criteria) was associated with circulating oxidative stress (relative excess of oxidised glutathione and higher levels of plasma protein adducts).

Antioxidant micronutrients play a critical role in decreasing this inflammatory response. In the longitudinal Baltimore Women's Health and Aging Study (WHAS), low baseline antioxidant levels were associated with both higher IL-6 levels and 5-year mortality rates. There is also damage to macromolecules associated with the damage caused by advanced glycation end products (AGEs). In view of the detrimental effects of both oxidative stress and AGEs, and the possible links between the two processes suggested by animal models, some researchers have suggested diabetes is an accelerated model of ageing; but the potential damage is not necessarily associated with hyperglycaemia. In long-term follow-up of adults aged 65 years and over without diabetes in the Cardiovascular Health Study, insulin resistance was associated with higher mortality, even after adjusting for renal function and other confounding characteristics.

Neuroendocrine decline

The well-established declines in the somatotrophic axis, the adrenal production of dehydroepiandrosterone (DHEA) and its sulphate, DHEAS, and reduced testosterone production have led to considerable research in the last two decades in the hope that replacement might offer a therapeutic approach to frailty. Growth hormone and circulating IGF-1 levels decrease with age and the similarity between the impairments and body composition seen in adults with growth hormone deficiency and ageing has attracted considerable interest and therapeutic investigation. However, no clear association has been established between IGF-1 levels and measurements of body composition, muscle strength and physical performance in older men, as large epidemiological studies have produced negative or conflicting findings. Even among cohorts with mild to moderate functional limitations, no association was recorded between IGF-1 and measures of physical function, body composition or strength. There may, however, be such a relationship for women, as shown for those aged between 70 and 79 years in the WHAS.

Despite this, IGF-1 levels may be important in combination with other factors. Interaction between IGF-1 and IL-6 in relation to disability has also been reported. Likewise, in a small study of community-dwelling older people, frail subjects had lower levels of both IGF-1 and DHEAS and higher levels of IL-6 and there was a trend towards an inverse correlation between IGF-1 and IL-6 in the frail, but not in the other participants, suggesting dysregulation in the interaction between the endocrine and inflammatory responses.

Furthermore, IGF-1 levels have not been consistently shown to be predictive of fragility fractures, although osteoporosis is more prevalent in growth hormone-deficient adults. In contrast, a positive association between cognitive performance and IGF-1 levels in older men has been conclusively demonstrated in a number of studies and a meta-analysis. Frail individuals certainly have lower average circulating IGF-1 levels but the pathophysiological significance of this is unclear. For example, delirium during acute illness is associated with lower IGF-1 levels. The suggestion is that low ambient IGF-1 levels may increase susceptibility of the brain damage induced by acute illness but research findings have been inconclusive so far.

Testosterone deficiency in younger men is associated with fatigue, reduced muscle mass and strength and mild anaemia, but the significance of the age-related decline is less clear-cut.

In the European male ageing study, higher levels of the frailty index (Rockwood) were significantly associated with lower levels of total and free testosterone and DHEAS but higher levels of gonadotrophins and binding globulins, which the authors interpreted as indicative of ageing-related disruptions of physiological regulation rather than an underlying pathophysiological mechanism for frailty.

In a large cross-sectional study of older people with varying levels of functional independence (n = 898), there was an association between frailty (Fried *et al.* criteria) and DHEAS levels. Gender did not impact on this association.

In a follow-up study of 254 independent men and women aged 65–70 years, lower baseline DHEAS levels along with higher differential white-cell counts (WCCs), and higher cortisol to DHEAS ratio were all significantly associated with increased odds of frailty (Fried *et al.* criteria) at 10 years. Baseline WCC and cortisol:DHEAS clearly discriminated between individuals who went on to be frail at follow-up, suggesting further evidence for a pro-inflammatory mechanism for frailty. Long-term therapeutic interventions with DHEA may clarify if the lower levels have significance for the development of frailty.

Sarcopenia

Sarcopenia is important both because muscle function is critical to functional performance and because muscle acts as a vital metabolic reserve during acute stress such as injury or illness. The pathogenesis of sarcopenia, therefore, has been a paradigm for the investigation of frailty. There is a need to unpick the specific features, clinically and pathogenically, of the range of muscle-wasting conditions.

The mechanisms underlying sarcopenia are not fully resolved, but all of the age-related changes mentioned so far have possible roles (*see* Chapter 14, 'The musculoskeletal system: muscle'). These include a catabolic inflammatory state, neuroendocrine decline and dysregulation, vitamin D deficiency, physical inactivity, and oxidative damage, and the interactions between these. For example, markers of oxidative muscle damage were associated with low grip strength in the Women's Health and Aging Study, but the oxidative damage and resultant cellular apoptosis induced via TNF-α may be responsible for the decline in muscle mass and strength.

THE ROLE OF CO-MORBIDITY IN THE GENERATION OF FRAILTY

Chronic disabling conditions such as cardiac failure and obstructive pulmonary disease are associated both with the metabolic features proposed as components of the pathophysiological frailty model and with the clinical features present in the operational model of frailty, such as fatigue and muscle weakness.

One mechanism is that the inflammatory component of these and other diseases contribute to the overall pro-inflammatory state characteristic of frailty. For example, cross-sectional analyses of 70–79-year-old community-dwelling participants from the Women's Health and Aging Study (WHAS) cohorts I and II demonstrated that a higher inflammatory disease burden increased the likelihood of frailty. A number of disease combinations contributed to this burden, suggesting that the pro-inflammatory state provides a common causal pathway between these diseases and frailty.

Using cross-sectional data from over 1000 participants in the two WHAS cohorts (covering the spectrum from high functioning to disabled), combined elevations in IL-6 and CRP were associated with the lowest pulmonary function levels. Without prospective study, the direction of causal relationship cannot be deduced.

Age-related conditions such as dementia, Parkinson's disease, atherosclerosis and non-insulin-dependent diabetes are all associated with elevated levels of inflammatory markers. The association of obesity and reduced physical activity levels with a pro-inflammatory profile provides a possible mechanism for their contribution to frailty.

Low vitamin D levels are now implicated in a host of adverse age-related phenomena, from susceptibilities to infection and cancer, fragility fractures and endothelial dysfunction. The mechanisms involved are the focus of extensive research. Data from the WHAS suggest that vitamin D deficiency is independently associated with poor pulmonary function in older disabled women. Clearly, relative pulmonary muscle weakness is a possible explanation, but the association of vitamin D with inflammatory processes and susceptibility to infection offer alternative pathophysiological pathways.

IMPACT ON CLINICAL PRACTICE

Disease-specific factors do not fully explain well-being and quality of life for individuals with long-term conditions and, along with myriad psychosocial factors, differing degrees of age-associated frailty may also contribute independently of disease.

Distinguishing frailty from both ageing and co-morbidity has potential clinical utility. If the underlying metabolic processes could be identified, then might it become possible to intervene at a preclinical stage of frailty, before the operational phenotypic criteria are evident? Furthermore, would addressing the frailty aspects offer an additional clinical approach to the management of patients with chronic diseases? Comprehensive geriatric assessment encompasses this approach, combining disease-specific and non-specific aspects in the assessment and treatment of older people. Therapeutic exercise, nutritional optimisation and social engagement are already established generic interventions. Frailty recognition is a refinement of this approach, particularly if biological agents become available that might affect the negative effects of oxidative damage, inflammation and so on. So far, approaches based on this premise have been largely unsuccessful, but these are early days.

Recognition of frailty through better definition may also improve clinical decision-making by informing the prediction of benefit or the risk of the adverse effects of clinical interventions including medications, surgical interventions and physical displacement. For example, the ability to improve prediction of post-operative functional recovery would be invaluable, as disease-based predictive models are far from perfect. At the level of the individual patient, laboratory tests and clinical assessments might each contribute to a 'risk profile'. The challenge, then, for twenty-first-century geriatrics would be to design and test clinical approaches that both modify standard interventions and address the specific underlying frailty processes.

CONCLUSION

The emerging consensus is that, just as there is no biological master clock dictating lifespan, there is no single common pathway for frailty. Conversely, as would be predicted by the disposable soma theory (*see* Chapter 2, 'The concept of ageing: theories and mechanisms'), evolution has resulted in sufficient but not excessively wasteful redundancy across the many cellular and physiological processes vital to life. Accumulation of damage in the form of highly variable age-related changes and specific diseases comes together to form a critical mass, reducing the reserve across a complex system. Recognition, measurement and modification of this frailty are the business of the twenty-first century, just as the last century was the era of disease.

FURTHER READING

Bortz WM 2nd. A conceptual framework of frailty: a review. *J Gerontol A Biol Sci Med Sci.* 2002; **57**(5): M283–88.

Campbell AJ, Buckner DM. Unstable disability and the fluctuations of frailty. *Age Ageing.* 1997; **26**(4): 315–18.

Fried LP, Tangen CM, Walston J *et al.* Cardiovascular Health Study Collaborative Research Group. Frailty in older adults: evidence for a phenotype. *J Gerontol A Biol Sci Med Sci.* 2001; **56**(3): M146–56.

Jones DM, Song X, Rockwood K. Operationalizing a frailty index from a standardized comprehensive geriatric assessment. *J Am Geriatr Soc.* 2004; **52**(11): 1929–33.

Kuh D. New Dynamics of Ageing (NDA) Preparatory Network. A life course approach to healthy aging, frailty, and capability. *J Gerontol A Biol Sci Med Sci.* 2007; **62**(7): 717–21.

Leng SX, Xue QL, Tian J *et al.* Inflammation and frailty in older women. *J Am Geriatr Soc.* 2007; **55**(6): 864–71.

Rowe JW, Kahn RL. Human aging: usual and successful. *Science.* 1987; **237**(4811): 143–9.

QUESTIONS: FRAILTY

1 Frailty is best understood as:
   A   a multi-system vulnerability
   B   a weakness of personality
   C   immune senescence
   D   low blood pressure
   E   sarcopenia.

   Answer: A

2 Fried *et al.*'s criteria for frailty includes:
   A   breathlessness
   B   cognitive impairment
   C   depression
   D   polypharmacy
   E   weakness compared with age-corrected norms.

   Answer: E

3 The Rockwood Frailty Index:
   A   cannot be estimated without age-standardised norms
   B   depends on the completion of a comprehensive geriatric assessment
   C   needs only 20 items
   D   requires standardised assessments of strength
   E   scores from 0 to 100.

   Answer: B

4 Frailty is probably due to:
   A   abnormal biochemistry due to adverse life events
   B   age-related immune senescence
   C   low IGF-1 levels
   D   multi-system impairment
   E   sarcopenia with cognitive impairment.

   Answer: D

5 Ageing is associated with:
   A   exaggerated responses to influenza vaccines
   B   high growth hormone levels in both sexes
   C   increased muscle protein turnover
   D   low testosterone levels in men
   E   reduced circulating levels of glycated proteins.

   Answer: D

CHAPTER 19

Quality of life and ageing

GURCHARAN S RAI AND AZA ABDULLA

INTRODUCTION

'Quality of life' (QoL) is an amorphous complex concept that researchers have tried to define in macro-societal (objective – based on income, employment, education, housing and other living circumstances) and micro-individual (subjective – based on an individual's experiences and values and may include indicators such as happiness, life satisfaction and well-being) terms.

The World Health Organization (WHO) defines QoL as an individual's perception of their position in life in the context of the culture and value systems in which they live and in relation to their goals, expectations, standards and concerns. It is a broad-ranging concept affected in a complex way by the person's physical health, psychological state, personal beliefs, social relationships and their relationship with salient features of their environment. Although there is a plethora of research on QoL indicators, there is no universally accepted standard measure of QoL.

There is also little consensus on a standard measure of QoL in older people. In defining QoL, some have advocated the inclusion of physical functioning and symptoms, social functioning, life satisfaction, emotional and behavioural functioning, ability to pursue personal interests and recreation, sexual functioning, energy, economic status and income as surrogate markers determining life expectancy and QoL, while others have suggested using an instrument that assesses well-being by asking individuals to assess this in areas of health, psychological well-being, happiness and physical environment.

A recently developed measure of QoL, the Older People's Quality of Life (OPQOL), is based on data derived from views of a representative sample of older people to open-ended questions about 'good things' that give life quality – research leading to development of this questionnaire found that the main factors contributing to QoL in old age include:

- good health and mobility
- psychological factors such as sense of optimism and realistic expectations
- engaging in large number of social activities and feeling supported
- feeling safe in one's environment
- having control over one's life
- maintaining independence and an adequate income
- good community facilities and infrastructure such as transport.

Of course, QoL in the older person can reflect his/her expectations of life at particular time of life. During illness, an older person's preference for survival may influence their perception of QoL – research on patients with cancer show that they are willing to accept toxic chemotherapy for minimal benefit in relation to prolongation of life. This may also explain why a patient's perception of QoL often differs from that rated by doctors.

SUCCESSFUL AGEING AND QOL

Much of the work on enhancing QoL has focused on achieving successful ageing using approaches that centre on health, social engagement, social functioning and activities, and psychological and lay themes. In various studies, older respondents have emphasised the importance of having good health; independence; having enough money, social relations and participation; living in a friendly neighbourhood; having a positive outlook; and having access to good local facilities (e.g. shops, transport). A recent study[1] on successful ageing has demonstrated that approaches that maximise psychological resources – namely, resilience and self-efficacy – improve/predict QoL. Measures that improve medical management, use of preventive measures and changes in lifestyle may improve health and increase life expectancy but may not improve QoL.

COMMONLY RECOMMENDED QOL INSTRUMENTS

Older people's quality of life questionnaire (OPQOL)

The OPQOL (*see* Appendix) is a 32–35-item measure of QoL. It has five-point Likert scales from 'strongly agree' to 'strongly disagree'. The 35-item OPQOL includes: life overall (four items); health (four items); social relationships and participation (eight items); independence, control over life, freedom (five items); home and neighbourhood (four items); psychological and emotional well-being (four items); financial circumstances (four items); and religion/culture (two items). It has potential for use in population surveys that assess health and social interventions in older people's lives to promote well-being.

Control, Autonomy, Pleasure and Self-realization (CASP-19)

The CASP-19 consists of 19 items comprising four domains: (1) control – the ability to intervene actively in one's own environment (four items), (2) autonomy – the right of an individual to be free from unwanted interference by others (five items), (3) pleasure – the sense of fun derived from more active aspects of life (five items) and (4) self-realisation – the active process of human fulfilment (five items), assessed by a four-point Likert scale. It is based on a theory of human needs satisfaction and self-actualisation. Items are scored, with a higher total score equating to better QoL, on a range from 0 (absence of QoL) to 57 (total satisfaction in all four domains).

World Health Organization Quality of Life Assessment of Older People (WHOQOL-OLD)

The WHOQOL-OLD (*see* Appendix) was developed from the WHOQOL-100 and cross-cultural studies. It is a multidimensional generic measure of QoL with items including: sensory abilities (assesses sensory functioning and the impact of loss of sensory abilities on QoL); autonomy (independence in old age); past, present and future activities; social participation (participation in activities of daily living, especially in the community); death and dying (relates to concerns, worries, and fears about death and dying); and intimacy (assesses being able to have personal and intimate relationships). It consists of 24 questions asking individuals to circle a response. Response scales are five-point and the wording varies ('not at all' to an 'extreme amount'/'completely' to 'extremely'; 'very poor' to 'very good'; 'very dissatisfied' to 'very satisfied'; 'very unhappy' to 'very happy'). Items are scored, with higher scores equating to higher QoL. The range of scores vary from 24 (lowest possible QoL) to 120 (highest possible QoL).

Short-Form 36 Health Status Questionnaire (SF-36)

The SF-36 comprises 36 questions that survey health and is used as a proxy for QoL. It was developed from work done by RAND Health and the Medical Outcomes Study. It is based on eight components of health status: physical function, mental health, role physical (problems with work or other daily activities as a result of physical illness), bodily pain, general health, role emotions (problems with work or daily activities as a result of emotional problems), social function and vitality. Each question has five responses. It is a generic measure that can be used to look at the usefulness of specific treatment(s) and to study burden of disease, although some researchers have suggested that several items may not be applicable to older people.

REFERENCE

1 Bowling A, Illiffe S. Psychological approach to successful ageing predicts future quality of life in older adults. *Health Qual Life Outcomes.* 2011; **9**: 13.

FURTHER READING

Bowling A. *Ageing Well: quality of life in old age.* Maidenhead: Open University Press and McGraw-Hill Education; 2005.

Bowling A, Stenner P. Which measure of quality of life performs best in old age? A comparison of the OPQOL, CASP-19 and WHOQOL-OLD. *J Epidemiol Community Health.* 2011; **65**(3): 273–80.

Hyde M, Wiggins RD, Higgs P *et al.* A measure of quality of life in early old age: the theory, development and properties of a needs satisfaction model (CASP-19). *Aging Ment Health.* 2003; **7**(3): 186–94.

Power M, Quinn K, Schmidt S. WHOQOL-OLD Group. Development of WHOQOL-OLD module. *Qual Life Res.* 2005; **14**(10): 2197–214.

RAND Health. *Medical Outcomes Study: 36-item short form survey.* Available at: www.rand.org/health/surveys_tools/mos/mos_core_36item.html (accessed 11 August 2012).

Ware JE Jr, Snow KK, Kosinski M *et al. SF-36 Health Survey: manual and interpretation guide.* Boston: New England Medical Center; 1993.

For copy of questionnaire and manual, email: mjpower@staffmail.ed.ac.uk

APPENDIX: QOL INSTRUMENTS
OPQOL

CONFIDENTIAL   **SERIAL NO.** ☐ ☐ ☐ ☐

Older People's Quality of Life Questionnaire (OPQOL-35)

We would like to ask you about your quality of life:
Please tick one box in each row. There are no right or wrong answers. Please select the response that best describes you/your views.

1. Thinking about both the good and bad things that make up your quality of life, how would you rate the quality of your life as a whole?

Your quality of life
as a whole is:

Very good	Good	Alright	Bad	Very bad
(1)	(2)	(3)	(4)	(5)
☐	☐	☐	☐	☐

2. Please indicates the extent to which you agree or disagree with each of the following statements.

Tick one box in each row

Life overall

(1) **I enjoy my life overall**

Strongly agree	Agree	Neither agree or disagree	Disagree	Strongly disagree
(1)	(2)	(3)	(4)	(5)
☐	☐	☐	☐	☐

(2) **I am happy much of the time**

Strongly agree	Agree	Neither agree or disagree	Disagree	Strongly disagree
(1)	(2)	(3)	(4)	(5)
☐	☐	☐	☐	☐

(3) **I look forward to things**

Strongly agree	Agree	Neither agree or disagree	Disagree	Strongly disagree
(1)	(2)	(3)	(4)	(5)
☐	☐	☐	☐	☐

(4) **Life gets me down**

Strongly agree (1)	Agree (2)	Neither agree or disagree (3)	Disagree (4)	Strongly disagree (5)
☐	☐	☐	☐	☐

Health

(5) **I have a lot of physical energy**

Strongly agree (1)	Agree (2)	Neither agree or disagree (3)	Disagree (4)	Strongly disagree (5)
☐	☐	☐	☐	☐

(6) **Pain affects my well-being**

Strongly agree (1)	Agree (2)	Neither agree or disagree (3)	Disagree (4)	Strongly disagree (5)
☐	☐	☐	☐	☐

(7) **My health restricts me looking after myself or my home**

Strongly agree (1)	Agree (2)	Neither agree or disagree (3)	Disagree (4)	Strongly disagree (5)
☐	☐	☐	☐	☐

(8) **I am healthy enough to get out and about**

Strongly agree (1)	Agree (2)	Neither agree or disagree (3)	Disagree (4)	Strongly disagree (5)
☐	☐	☐	☐	☐

Social relationships

(9) **My family, friends or neighbours would help me if needed**

Strongly agree (1)	Agree (2)	Neither agree or disagree (3)	Disagree (4)	Strongly disagree (5)
☐	☐	☐	☐	☐

(10) **I would like more companionship or contact with other people**

Strongly agree (1)	Agree (2)	Neither agree or disagree (3)	Disagree (4)	Strongly disagree (5)
☐	☐	☐	☐	☐

(11) **I have someone who gives me love and affection**

Strongly agree (1)	Agree (2)	Neither agree or disagree (3)	Disagree (4)	Strongly disagree (5)
☐	☐	☐	☐	☐

(12) **I'd like more people to enjoy life with**

Strongly agree (1)	Agree (2)	Neither agree or disagree (3)	Disagree (4)	Strongly disagree (5)
☐	☐	☐	☐	☐

(13) **I have my children around which is important**

Strongly agree (1)	Agree (2)	Neither agree or disagree (3)	Disagree (4)	Strongly disagree (5)
☐	☐	☐	☐	☐

Independence, control over life, freedom

(14) **I am healthy enough to have my independence**

Strongly agree (1)	Agree (2)	Neither agree or disagree (3)	Disagree (4)	Strongly disagree (5)
☐	☐	☐	☐	☐

(15) **I can please myself what I do**

Strongly agree (1)	Agree (2)	Neither agree or disagree (3)	Disagree (4)	Strongly disagree (5)
☐	☐	☐	☐	☐

(16) **The cost of things compared to my pension/ income restricts my life**

Strongly agree (1)	Agree (2)	Neither agree or disagree (3)	Disagree (4)	Strongly disagree (5)
☐	☐	☐	☐	☐

(17) **I have a lot of control** over the important things in my life

Strongly agree (1)	Agree (2)	Neither agree or disagree (3)	Disagree (4)	Strongly disagree (5)
☐	☐	☐	☐	☐

Home and neighbourhood

(18) **I feel safe where I live**

Strongly agree (1)	Agree (2)	Neither agree or disagree (3)	Disagree (4)	Strongly disagree (5)
☐	☐	☐	☐	☐

(19) **The local shops, services and facilities are good overall**	Strongly agree (1)	Agree (2)	Neither agree or disagree (3)	Disagree (4)	Strongly disagree (5)
	☐	☐	☐	☐	☐

(20) **I get pleasure from my home**	Strongly agree (1)	Agree (2)	Neither agree or disagree (3)	Disagree (4)	Strongly disagree (5)
	☐	☐	☐	☐	☐

(21) **I find my neighbourhood friendly**	Strongly agree (1)	Agree (2)	Neither agree or disagree (3)	Disagree (4)	Strongly disagree (5)
	☐	☐	☐	☐	☐

Psychological and emotional well-being

(22) **I take life as it comes and make the best of things**	Strongly agree (1)	Agree (2)	Neither agree or disagree (3)	Disagree (4)	Strongly disagree (5)
	☐	☐	☐	☐	☐

(23) **I feel lucky compared to most people**	Strongly agree (1)	Agree (2)	Neither agree or disagree (3)	Disagree (4)	Strongly disagree (5)
	☐	☐	☐	☐	☐

(24) **I tend to look on the bright side**	Strongly agree (1)	Agree (2)	Neither agree or disagree (3)	Disagree (4)	Strongly disagree (5)
	☐	☐	☐	☐	☐

(25) **If my health limits social/ leisure activities, then I will compensate and find something else I can do**	Strongly agree (1)	Agree (2)	Neither agree or disagree (3)	Disagree (4)	Strongly disagree (5)
	☐	☐	☐	☐	☐

Financial circumstances

(26) **I have enough money to pay for household bills**

Strongly agree (1)	Agree (2)	Neither agree or disagree (3)	Disagree (4)	Strongly disagree (5)
☐	☐	☐	☐	☐

(27) **I have enough money to pay for household repairs or help needed in the house**

Strongly agree (1)	Agree (2)	Neither agree or disagree (3)	Disagree (4)	Strongly disagree (5)
☐	☐	☐	☐	☐

(28) **I can afford to buy what I want to**

Strongly agree (1)	Agree (2)	Neither agree or disagree (3)	Disagree (4)	Strongly disagree (5)
☐	☐	☐	☐	☐

(29) **I cannot afford to do things I would enjoy**

Strongly agree (1)	Agree (2)	Neither agree or disagree (3)	Disagree (4)	Strongly disagree (5)
☐	☐	☐	☐	☐

Leisure and activities

(30) **I have social or leisure activities/hobbies that I enjoy doing**

Strongly agree (1)	Agree (2)	Neither agree or disagree (3)	Disagree (4)	Strongly disagree (5)
☐	☐	☐	☐	☐

(31) **I try to stay involved with things**

Strongly agree (1)	Agree (2)	Neither agree or disagree (3)	Disagree (4)	Strongly disagree (5)
☐	☐	☐	☐	☐

(32) **I do paid or unpaid work or activities that give me a role in life**

Strongly agree (1)	Agree (2)	Neither agree or disagree (3)	Disagree (4)	Strongly disagree (5)
☐	☐	☐	☐	☐

(33) **I have responsibilities to others that restrict my social or leisure activities**

Strongly agree (1)	Agree (2)	Neither agree or disagree (3)	Disagree (4)	Strongly disagree (5)
☐	☐	☐	☐	☐

(34) **Religion, belief**
     or philosophy is important
     to my quality of life

Strongly agree (1)	Agree (2)	Neither agree or disagree (3)	Disagree (4)	Strongly disagree (5)
☐	☐	☐	☐	☐

(35) **Cultural/religious**
     events/festivals are
     important to my
     quality of life

Strongly agree (1)	Agree (2)	Neither agree or disagree (3)	Disagree (4)	Strongly disagree (5)
☐	☐	☐	☐	☐

Thank you for your help.

WHOQOL-OLD

Instructions

This questionnaire asks for your thoughts and feelings about certain aspects of your quality of life and addresses issues that may be important to you as an older member of society.

Please answer all the questions. If you are unsure about which response to give to a question, please choose the one that appears most appropriate. This can often be your first response.

Please keep in mind your standards, hopes, pleasures and concerns. We ask that you think about your life in the last two weeks.

For example, thinking about the last two weeks, a question might ask:

How much do you worry about what the future might hold?

Not at all	A little	A moderate amount	Very much	An extreme amount
1	2	3	4	5

You should circle the number that best fits how much you have worried about the future over the last two weeks. So, you would circle the number 4 if you worried about your future 'Very much', or circle number 1 if you have worried 'Not at all' about your future. Please read each question, assess your feelings, and circle the number on the scale for each question that gives the best answer for you.

The following questions ask about *how much* you have experienced certain things in the last two weeks.

		Not at all	A little	A moderate amount	Very much	An extreme amount
1	To what extent do impairments to your senses (e.g. hearing, vision, taste, smell, touch) affect your daily life?	1	2	3	4	5
2	To what extent does loss of, for example, hearing, vision, taste, smell or touch affect your ability to participate in activities?	1	2	3	4	5
3	How much freedom do you have to make your own decisions?	1	2	3	4	5

		Not at all	Slightly	Moderately	Very much	Extremely
4	To what extent do you feel in control of your future?	1	2	3	4	5
5	How much do you feel that the people around you are respectful of your freedom?	1	2	3	4	5

		Not at all	A little	A moderate amount	Very much	An extreme amount
6	How concerned are you about the way in which you will die?	1	2	3	4	5

		Not at all	Slightly	Moderately	Very much	Extremely
7	How much are you afraid of not being able to control your death?	1	2	3	4	5
8	How scared are you of dying?	1	2	3	4	5

		Not at all	A little	A moderate amount	Very much	An extreme amount
9	How much do you fear being in pain before you die?	1	2	3	4	5

The following questions ask about *how completely* you experience or were able to do certain things in the last two weeks.

		Not at all	A little	Moderately	Mostly	Completely
10	To what extent do problems with your sensory functioning (e.g. hearing, vision, taste, smell, touch) affect your ability to interact with others?	1	2	3	4	5
11	To what extent are you able to do the things you'd like to do?	1	2	3	4	5

		Not at all	A little	Moderately	Mostly	Completely
12	To what extent are you satisfied with your opportunities to continue achieving in life?	1	2	3	4	5
13	How much do you feel that you have received the recognition you deserve in life?	1	2	3	4	5
14	To what extent do you feel that you have enough to do each day?	1	2	3	4	5

The following questions ask you to say how *satisfied, happy* or *good* you have felt about various aspects of your life over the last two weeks.

		Very dissatisfied	Dissatisfied	Neither satisfied nor dissatisfied	Satisfied	Very satisfied
15	How satisfied are you with what you have achieved in life?	1	2	3	4	5
16	How satisfied are you with the way you use your time?	1	2	3	4	5
17	How satisfied are you with your level of activity?	1	2	3	4	5
18	How satisfied are you with your opportunity to participate in community activities?	1	2	3	4	5

		Very unhappy	Unhappy	Neither happy nor unhappy	Happy	Very happy
19	How happy are you with the things you are able to look forward to?	1	2	3	4	5

		Very poor	Poor	Neither poor nor good	Good	Very good
20	How would you rate your sensory functioning (e.g. hearing, vision, taste, smell, touch)?	1	2	3	4	5

The following questions refer to any *intimate relationships* that you may have. Please consider these questions with reference to a close partner or other close person with whom you can share intimacy more than with any other person in your life.

		Not at all	A little	A moderate amount	Very much	An extreme amount
21	To what extent do you feel a sense of companionship in your life?	1	2	3	4	5
22	To what extent do you experience love in your life?	1	2	3	4	5

		Not at all	A little	Moderately	Mostly	Completely
23	To what extent do you have opportunities to love?	1	2	3	4	5
24	To what extent do you have opportunities to be loved?	1	2	3	4	5

QUESTIONS: QOL

1 Which one of these statements on QoL is correct?
   A QoL is easy to measure in older people
   B QoL assesses happiness and well-being only
   C QoL equates to satisfaction in life
   D QoL is difficult to define
   E there is consensus on a standard measure of QoL.

Answer: D

2 The OPQOL instrument:
   A can be used to assess the impact of drug therapy
   B consists of 32–35 items
   C is based on good health and sense of optimism
   D uses a four-point scale
   E uses happy and sad faces as responses.

Answer: B

3 With regard to the WHOQOL-OLD instrument:
   A the highest score equates to low QoL
   B it has been developed from the WHOQOL-90
   C it does not take into account participation in daily activities
   D it is a unidimensional measure
   E it uses a five-point scale.

Answer: E

4 The SF-36 questionnaire:
   A assesses components of health
   B directly assesses QoL
   C does not take into account social function and vitality
   D has six responses for each question
   E was developed by the American Medical Association.

Answer: A

5 With regard to the CASP-19 instrument:
   A a score of '0' signifies poor QoL
   B a score of '50' signifies total satisfaction
   C 'CASP' stands for control, autonomy, social well-being and pleasure
   D it consists of 19 items and gives a single overall measure of QoL
   E it uses a five-point Likert scale.

Answer: A

Index